Current Topics in Colorectal Surgery

Edited by John Camilleri-Brennan

Published in London, United Kingdom

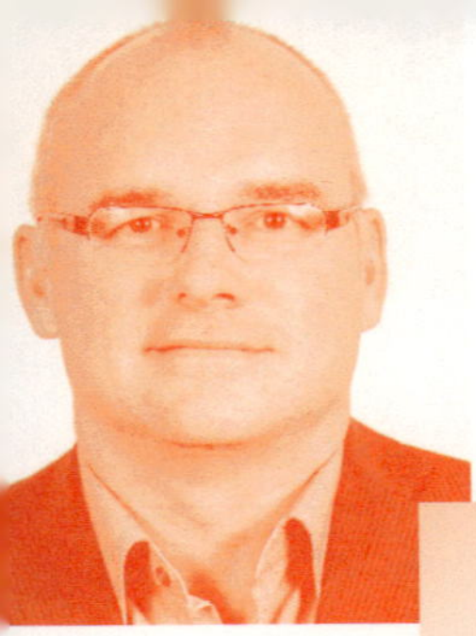
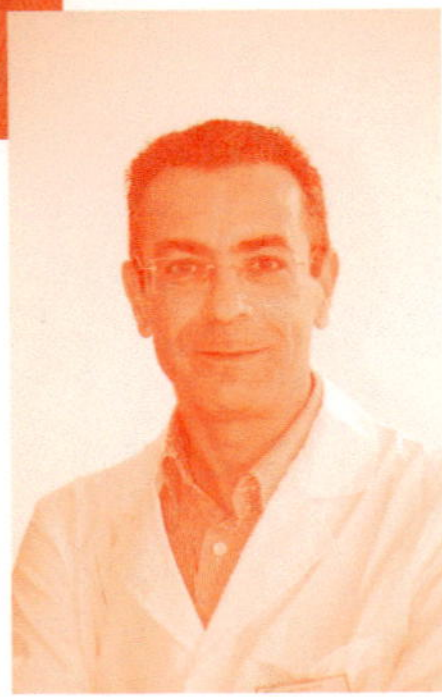
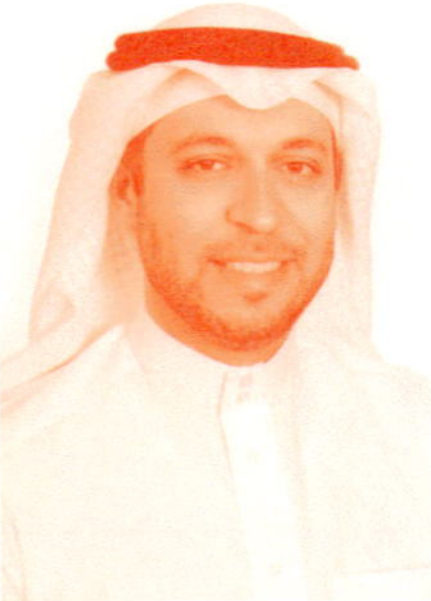
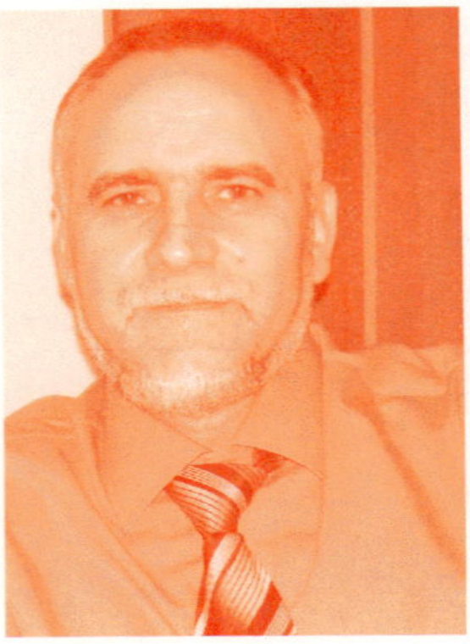
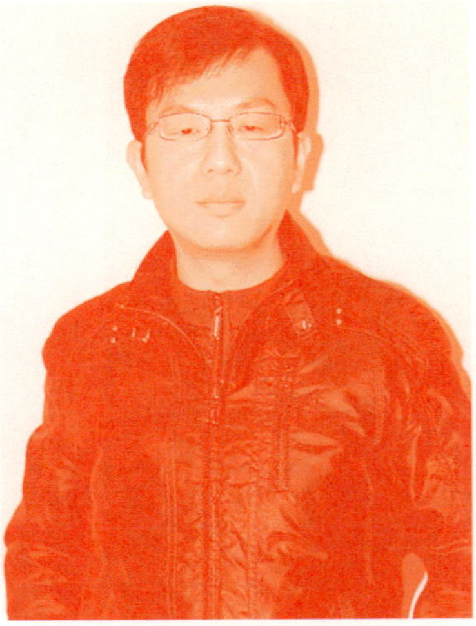
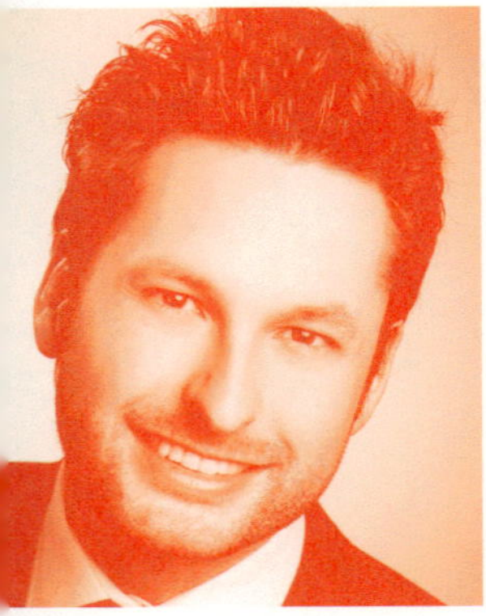
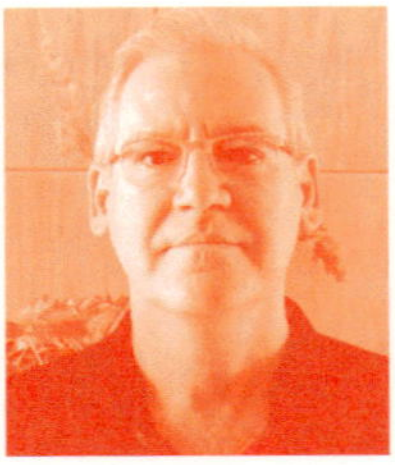

IntechOpen

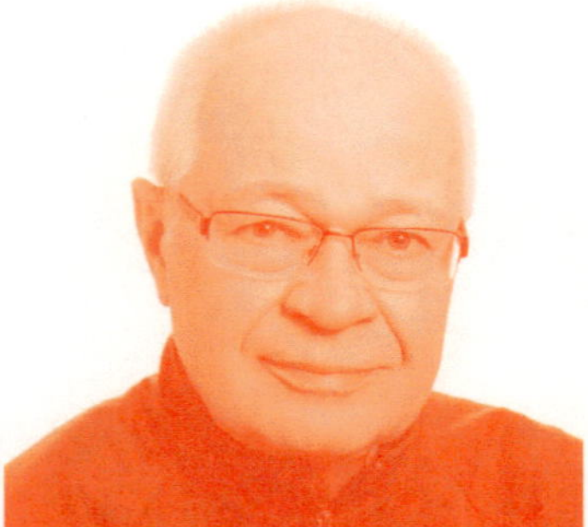
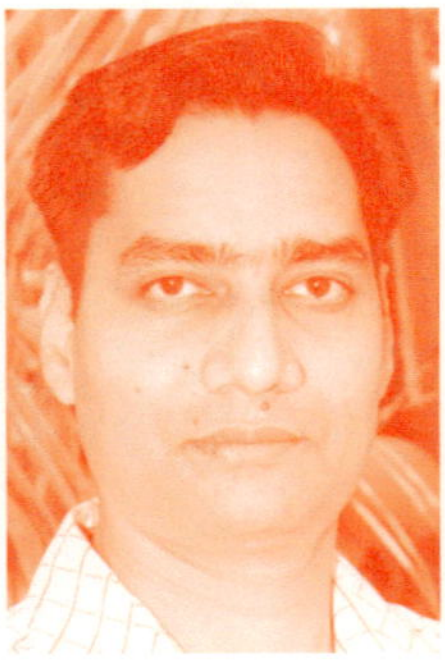
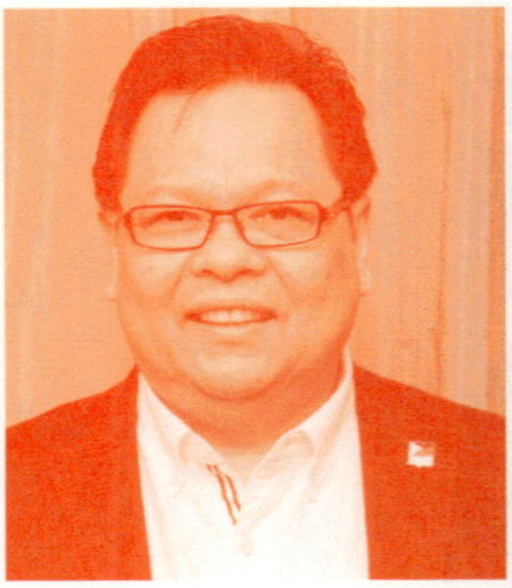
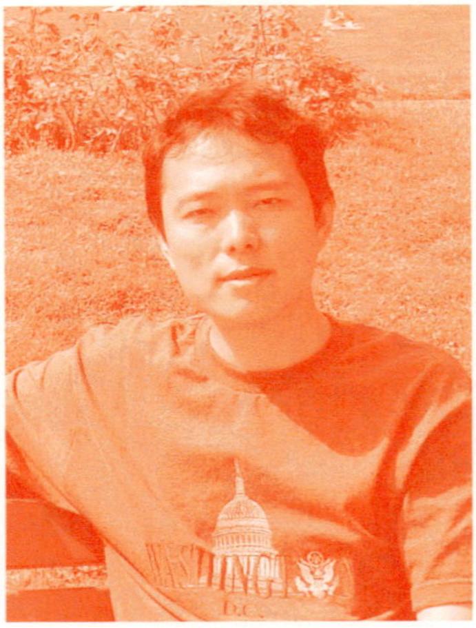
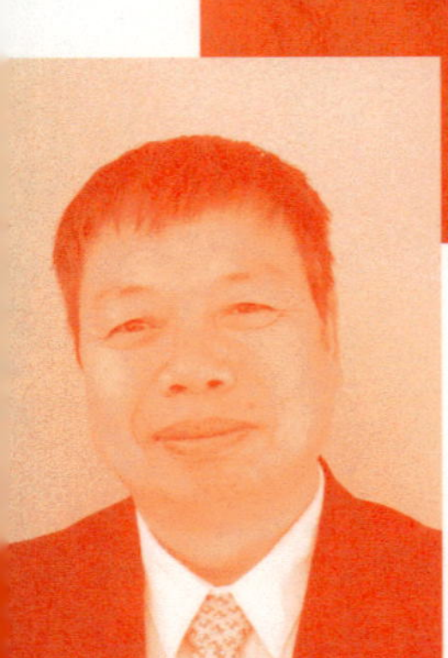
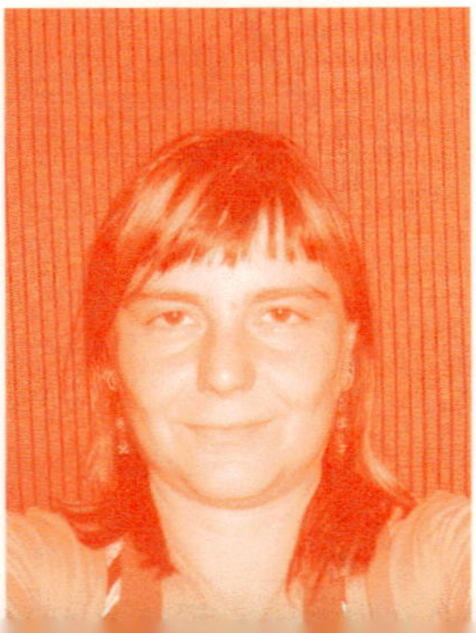

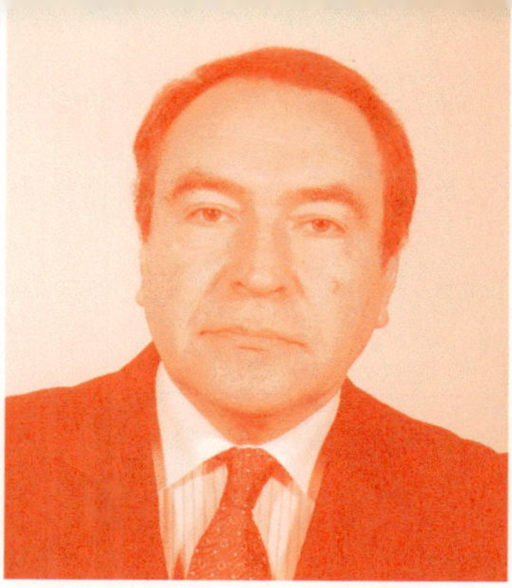
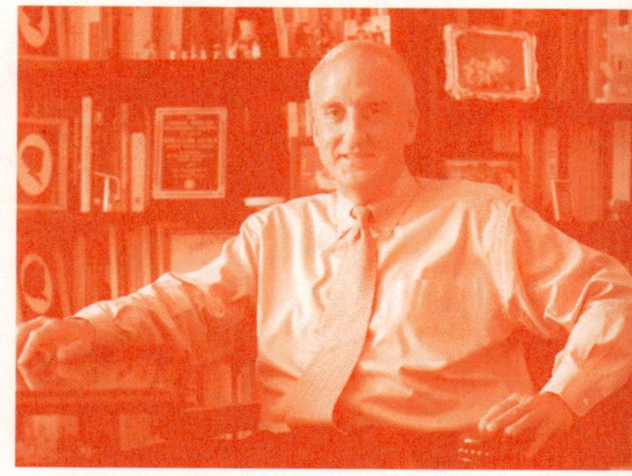
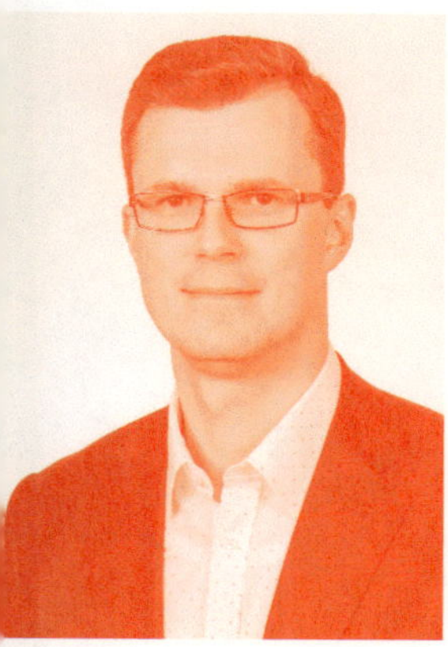
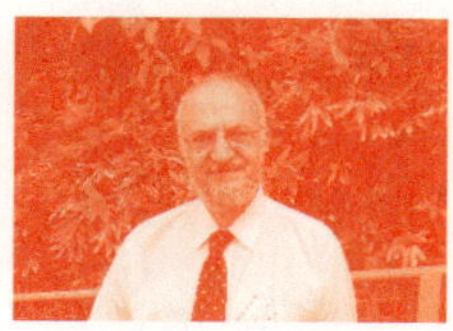
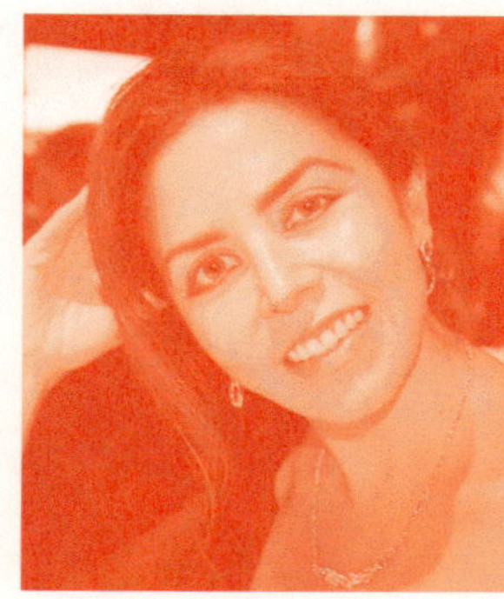

Supporting open minds since 2005

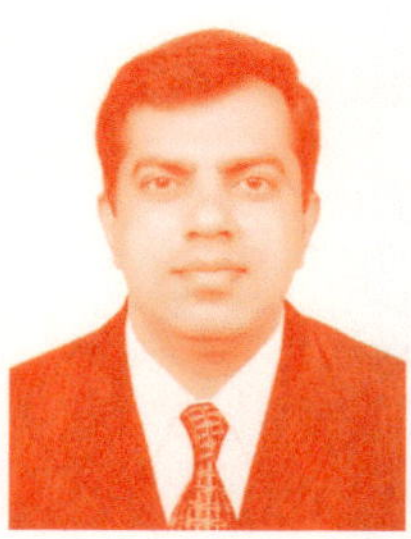
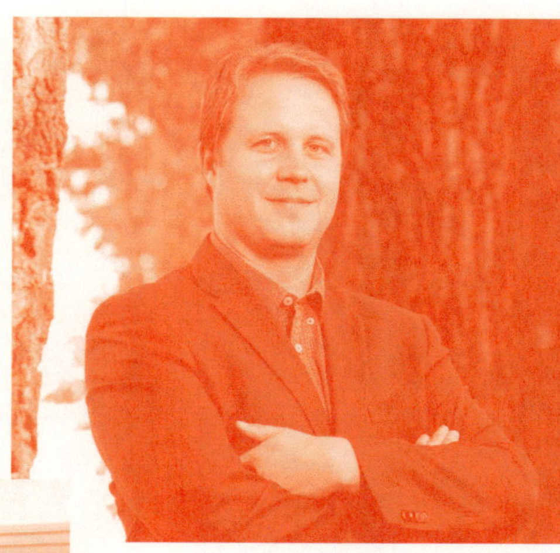
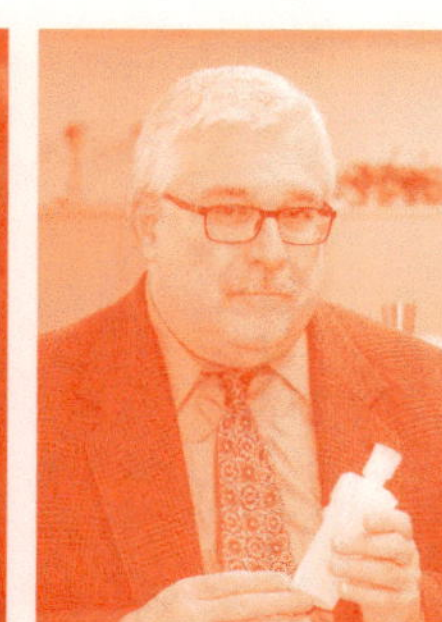
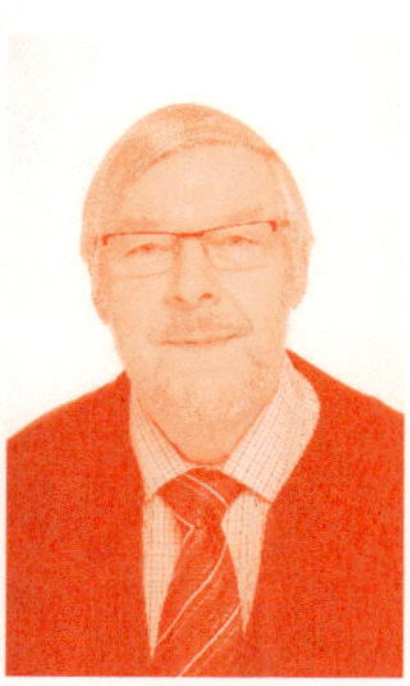
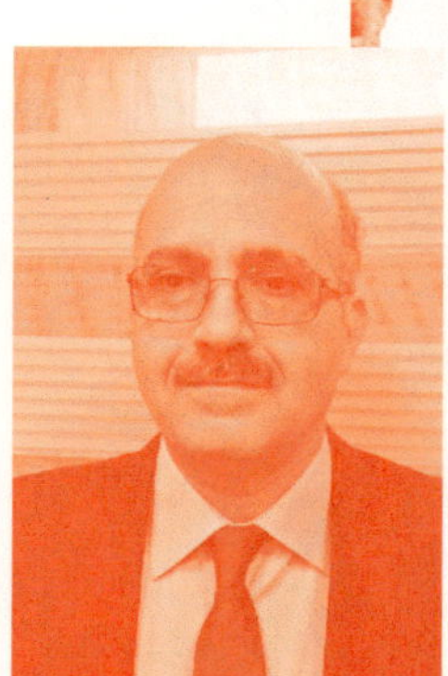
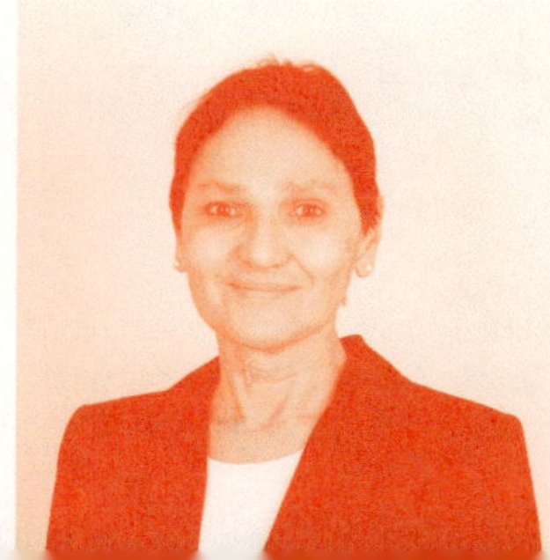
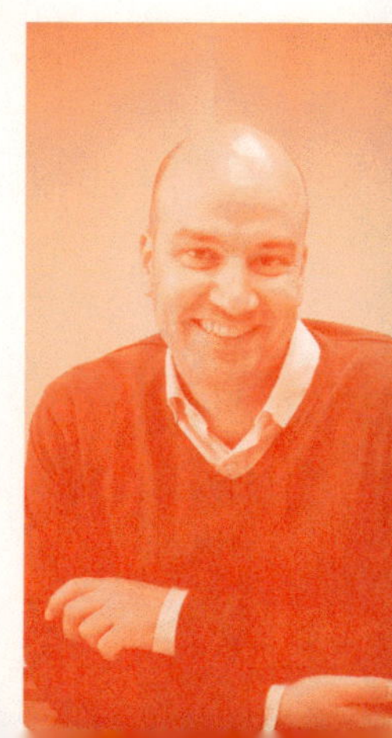

Current Topics in Colorectal Surgery
http://dx.doi.org/10.5772/intechopen.95173
Edited by John Camilleri-Brennan

Contributors
Dorian Kršul, Damir Karlović, Đordano Bačić, Marko Zelić, Muslim Abas Abed AlAdlee, Sahar Ghazi Imran, Ik Yong Kim, Sanghyun An, Marisa D. Santos, Eng (Eric) Kiat Yeoh, Kenneth Kher Ti K.T. Voon, Enio Chaves Chaves Oliveira, Mauro Bafutto, Salustiano Gabriel Neto, Alexandre Augusto Ferreira Bafutto, Jarbas Jabur Bittar Neto, Sinziana Ionescu, Călin Molnar, Nicolescu Cosmin, Andrei Suciu Bogdan, Adrian Tudor, Cristian Russu, Marian Botoncea, Mircea Gherghinescu, Vlad Olimpiu Butiurca, Catalin-Dumitru Cosma, Ciprian Duta, Stelu Pantea, Dan Brebu, Amadeus Dobrescu, Caius Lazar, Kitty Botoca, Cristi Tarta, Fulger Lazar, Ioana Hălmaciu, Nicolae Bacalbașa, Simu Patricia Maria Luminita, John Camilleri-Brennan, Alexia Farrugia

First published in London, United Kingdom, 2023 by IntechOpen
IntechOpen is the global imprint of INTECHOPEN LIMITED, registered in England and Wales, registration number: 11086078, 5 Princes Gate Court, London, SW7 2QJ, United Kingdom
Printed in Croatia

British Library Cataloguing-in-Publication Data
A catalogue record for this book is available from the British Library

Additional hard and PDF copies can be obtained from orders@intechopen.com

Current Topics in Colorectal Surgery
Edited by John Camilleri-Brennan
p. cm.
Print ISBN 978-1-83962-335-6
Online ISBN 978-1-83962-336-3
eBook (PDF) ISBN 978-1-83962-337-0

For EU product safety concerns:
IN TECH d.o.o., Prolaz Marije Krucifikse Kozulić 3, 51000 Rijeka, Croatia, info@intechopen.com or visit our website at intechopen.com.

Meet the editor

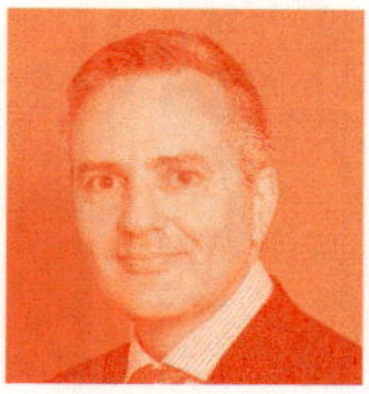

John Camilleri-Brennan MD (Melit), MD (Dundee), FRCS-Glas, FRCSGenSurg, MFSTEd, is a consultant in general and colorectal surgery and clinical lead in colorectal cancer with NHS Forth Valley, Scotland, and an honorary clinical associate professor with the University of Glasgow. He is also Associate Director of Surgical Examinations, Royal College of Physicians and Surgeons of Glasgow, and an elected member of the college's council. A graduate of the University of Malta, Dr. Camilleri-Brennan received his postgraduate surgical training primarily in Dundee and Aberdeen, Scotland. A travelling fellowship by the Royal College of Physicians and Surgeons of Glasgow enabled him to pursue further studies in colorectal surgery at the University of Minnesota, USA. His research on rectal cancer led to a doctorate from the University of Dundee, Scotland. He is the recipient of the William Cullen Prize from the Royal College of Physicians of Edinburgh for his innovative work in colorectal surgery.

Contents

Preface

Colorectal surgery continues to evolve at a fast pace. Minimal-access techniques, such as laparoscopic, endoanal, and robotic procedures, continue to gain ground. This book, *Current Topics in Colorectal Surgery*, reflects the evolving nature of colorectal disease and its treatment. The chapters cover a wide range of subjects and include original research as well as current and comprehensive reviews, especially in areas where recent developments have had a significant effect on clinical practice.

Written by international experts, the book is divided into six sections. Following the introductory chapter on surgical risk factors are sections on proctology and inflammatory bowel disease. Chapters on colorectal cancer predominate, with comprehensive reviews on surgical anatomy, preoperative and intraoperative investigative techniques, and treatment outcomes. Subsequent chapters discuss the latest advances in robotic technology.

This book is an invaluable resource for physicians, surgeons, nurses, and allied healthcare professionals who seek to refresh and expand their knowledge of coloproctology. It is also a source of excellent information for those preparing for professional examinations. I trust that the readers will find this book both enjoyable as well as educationally rewarding.

I hope this book contributes in some way to the understanding of the diverse aspects of colorectal disease and colorectal surgery. I am most grateful to the authors for their significant efforts and excellent contributions.

John Camilleri-Brennan MD (Melit), MD (Dundee), FRCSGlas, FRCSGenSurg, MFSTEd
Honorary Clinical Associate Professor,
University of Glasgow,
Glasgow, Scotland, UK

Section 1

Introducton

Chapter 1

Introductory Chapter: Challenges in Colorectal Surgery – Identifying Preoperative Risk Factors

John Camilleri-Brennan

1. Introduction

Many colorectal diseases, both benign and malignant, are managed surgically. The magnitude of surgical intervention varies from the minor incision to drain a perianal abscess to the complex exenteration for recurrent rectal cancer.

All operations are associated with a degree of risk of complications. The more complex the operation is, the higher the risk of complications. Postoperative complications have been noted in up to 35% of patients who undergo radical colorectal cancer surgery. Surgical complications contribute to increased mortality, length of hospital stay and an increased level of community care, as well as having a deleterious effect on quality of life.

Surgical complications may be classified in a number of ways. However, the classification by Clavien and Dindo [1] is the one that has gained most widespread acceptance. This classification, based on the type of intervention required to rectify the complication, is simple, reproducible, and reliable.

In general, complications can be divided into intra-operative and postoperative. Postoperative complications can be immediate, early, and late. Occurrence of intra-operative complications such as bleeding, bowel injury, ureteric and bladder injuries are affected by the presence of intra-abdominal adhesions, anatomic abnormalities, the experience of the surgeon, and many other factors. Major postoperative complications include anastomotic dehiscence, paralytic ileus, and bleeding [2].

2. Risk factors

Risk factors in emergency and in elective open, laparoscopic and robotic colorectal surgery should be recognised prior to surgery in order to reduce complications and to initialize individualised treatment as soon as possible. However, some risk factors such as age, gender, and prior abdominal surgery cannot be obviously modified before surgery [2, 3].

2.1 Non-modifiable risk factors

Increasing age itself remains an important risk factor for postoperative morbidity and mortality in patients having surgery for colorectal disease. Although morbidity and mortality rates in older patients could be similar to that of younger patients undergoing elective surgery, these rates could be up to nine times higher in cases of emergency surgery. With increasing age comes increasing frailty, and in general the risk of complications in frail patients is higher. The use of laparoscopic and other minimally invasive techniques results in less complications in the older patient when compared to emergency and open surgery.

Male patients have a higher risk of complications in open and laparoscopic colorectal surgery. Male gender is associated with increased anastomotic leakage rates after low rectal anastomoses, presumable due to the technical challenges associated with the male pelvis.

Prior abdominal surgery, especially open surgery, increases one's risk of developing postoperative adhesions. The presence of adhesions increases the rate of conversion from a laparoscopic to an open operation and increases the operating time. Adhesions are associated with increased risk of iatrogenic small bowel perforation leading to peritonitis and intra-abdominal abscess formation and postoperative ileus.

2.2 Modifiable risk factors

The presence of comorbid illnesses may adversely affect the outcome of colorectal surgery. Patients with higher levels of comorbidities, mainly cardiovascular and pulmonary disease, diabetes, and obesity, are expected to have significantly higher rates of complications, longer hospital stays and mortality. In many cases, a patient's general condition may be optimized if there is sufficient time prior to surgery. This applies to surgery for benign disease and early stage malignant disease. High risk assessment clinics and prehabilitation programs have been set up to identify modifiable risk factors and improve them. Such programs have certainly helped to improve cardiovascular and pulmonary function, improve nutritional status and muscle mass, optimize the haemoglobin levels, and achieve targeted weight loss and tighter control over blood sugar levels [3].

The use of mechanical bowel preparation (MBP) prior to elective colorectal surgery is controversial. Although it improves colonic handling especially during laparoscopic surgery, it is not without its risks. It may lead to severe fluid, electrolyte and acid-base abnormalities that may worsen cardiovascular and renal function. Some studies have shown an increased risk of anastomotic leaks and surgical site infection with MBP. Suboptimal MBP leads to liquid stool with a consequent increase in the rate of intra-operative spillage and therefore increasing the risk of postoperative intra-abdominal and wound infections. The author's view is that mechanical bowel preparation should only be used in elective surgery in patients undergoing restorative rectal resection such as when a defunctioning loop ileostomy is planned.

Several studies have shown an inverse relationship between the risk of complications and surgeons' experience. Greater surgeon experience performing colorectal surgery, especially in patients with complex conditions, is associated with reduced risk of surgical complications. Complications became significantly less frequent as the surgeons' learning and experience with the procedure increased. This is very relevant where certain skills are required, such as laparoscopic and robotic skills. In addition, hospital case load and surgical facilities are factors that are associated with complications. Therefore, more complex surgery demands the most experienced surgeon with the most experienced team to ensure the best outcome.

3. Risk scoring systems

In order to minimise and even avoid complications after colorectal surgery, it is vital to assess a patient thoroughly and identify the relevant risk factors. Rather than rely solely on the surgeon's "gut feeling," scoring systems have been developed to help clinicians assess risk and predict morbidity and mortality of various operations. These systems, using information gained during the preoperative assessment of the patient, evaluate the physiologic condition of the patient at the time of surgery, the severity of the surgery, and the age and general health of the patient to generate a score. Examples of commonly used scoring systems are the American Society of Anaesthesiologists (ASA) score, the Acute Physiology and Chronic Health Evaluation (APACHE) score, and the Physiological and Operative Severity Score for enUmeration of Mortality and Morbidity (POSSUM, and the more specific P-POSSUM and Cr-POSSUM). The National Emergency Laparotomy Audit (NELA) score is used to provide an estimate of the risk of death within 30 days of emergency abdominal surgery. These scoring systems however do not take into account the risks posed by surgical and anaesthetic inexperience and operative time [4].

Identifying pre-operative risk factors, assessing risk as accurately as possible, and optimizing a patient's clinical condition are crucially important to ensure the best outcome possible in colorectal surgery.

Author details

John Camilleri-Brennan[1,2]

1 Forth Valley Royal Hospital, Stirlingshire, Scotland, UK

2 The University of Glasgow, Glasgow, Scotland, UK

*Address all correspondence to: johncbrennan@doctors.org.uk

References

[1] Dindo D, Demartines N, Clavien PA. Classification of surgical complications: A new proposal with evaluation in a cohort of 6336 patients and results of a survey. Annals of Surgery. 2004;**240**(2): 205-213

[2] Kirchhoff P, Clavien PA, Hahnloser D. Complications in colorectal surgery: Risk factors and preventive strategies. Patient Safety in Surgery. 2010;**4**:5

[3] van Rooijen S, Carli F, Dalton SO, Johansen C, Dieleman J, Roumen R, et al. Preoperative modifiable risk factors in colorectal surgery: An observational cohort study identifying the possible value of prehabilitation. Acta Oncologica. 2017;**56**(2):329-334

[4] Chand M, Armstrong T, Britton G, Nash GF. How and why do we measure surgical risk? Journal of the Royal Society of Medicine. 2007;**100**(11): 508-512

Section 2

Proctology

Chapter 2

Understanding New Ideas in Cryptoglandular Fistula-in-Ano

Kenneth K.T. Voon

Abstract

Outcomes of surgical treatment for anorectal abscesses and chronic fistulas varies widely, as there is lack of unified classification and systematic surgical approach to address a wide range of disease pattern. Acute anorectal abscess and chronic fistula-in-ano should be considered the same disease at both end of a spectrum. This article describes in detail the pathogenesis and relevant anorectal anatomy to aid understanding of a new concept of classifying anorectal abscess and fistula based on natural patterns. A better understanding of patterns allows more accurate surgical treatment. Recent evidence shows that definitive surgical treatment for anal fistula during acute abscess stage is safe and feasible. An optimum surgical treatment should focus on eradication of intersphincteric infection, removal of secondary branches or abscesses, allow healing by secondary intention and preserve continence as best as possible. Common challenges faced by clinicians include confusion in classification, inaccurate delineation of fistula, challenging acute abscesses, unable to locate internal opening and facing complex features such as high fistula or multiple branches. Suggested solutions are discussed and a structured treatment strategy according to types and patterns is proposed. Surgical treatment should follow the principles above and combination of surgical techniques is beneficial compared to individual modality.

Keywords: anorectal abscess, fistula-in-ano, classification, natural patterns, combination surgical techniques

1. Introduction

Since the publications of Park and Eisenhammer in the 1960s to 1970s, we have gained better understanding on the pathogenesis of cryptoglandular infection leading to perianal abscesses and eventually fistula in ano. With this knowledge, we have moved in strides in producing numerous classifications and treatment options, ranging from minimally invasive techniques to surgical procedures that produces significant disruption to the anorectal anatomy.

Anorectal fistulous abscesses and chronic fistula-in-ano are the same disease. This view has been shared by both Parks and Eisenhammer [1, 2]. We tend to separate both topics and discuss the management separately. However, recent views suggest we should treat it as a same disease, both at different spectrum.

We have yet to achieve a gold standard as recurrence rates and success rates still varies widely across continent. I believe the reasons are:

- Lack of comprehensive classification of fistula-in-ano due to a lack of understanding of the natural pattern and progression of the disease.

- Lack of unified surgical approach to address different types of fistula-in-ano. Understanding and practices of surgical techniques varies according to institutions and regions.

Chapter Outline:

- Revisiting the pathogenesis of cryptoglandular infection.
- Relevant updates in anorectal anatomy.
- Understanding the natural patterns of cryptoglandular abscesses and fistulas.
- Review of practicality of classifications for fistula in ano.
- Using natural patterns to classify anorectal abscess and fistula.
- Definitive surgical treatment in acute abscess stage.
- Emerging concepts in managing cryptoglandular anal fistulas.

2. Revisiting the pathogenesis of cryptoglandular infection

In 1961, Park reported his study of 44 specimens of normal anorectal anatomy, and 30 resected specimens from fistula-in-ano surgery. Anal glands were racemose structure of widely ramifying ducts, opening internally via the anal crypts (at dentate line), and extended deep into internal sphincters or ends in the longitudinal layer. They never extend into external sphincter muscles. He concluded that, anal glands provided free channels for infection to pass from the anal lumen deep into the internal sphincter muscles [1]. This observation was echoed by Eisenhammer in 1966, who added that main concentration of large crypts was situated posteriorly, followed by the anterior commissure and last, laterally. Internal orifice of a fistula was always found at the crypt entrance in the pectinate line, at approximately the midlevel of the anal canal [2]. Another study in 1994 by Seow found that 1% of anal glands in fact do penetrate the external sphincter [3]. However, infection arising from external sphincter was never reported.

The term fistulous abscess was used by Eisenhammer; the acute stage represents the abscess, and the chronic stage represents the fistula [2]. Acute abscess progress to a recurrent acute abscess or a chronic infection within the anal glands [1]. Fistula is a granulation tissue tract, develops after abscesses spontaneously rupture or are surgically drainage, where it continues to discharge materials from infected anal gland/ducts. It is kept open by chronic granulomatous inflammation [1, 2].

Pyogenic infections constituting 90% of all cases [1, 2]. Parks noted that 73% of infections occurred at either anterior or posterior midline [1]. Eisenhammer postulated that this intermuscular infection is due to obstructive suppurative adenitis, where causative organism were intestinal bacilli, streptococcus or anaerobes [2].

The cryptoglandular infection pathogenesis remains relevant till present day. From the evidence of early studies, we can conclude that:

1. Anorectal abscess and fistula are essentially the same disease, both at different end of a spectrum, and therefore should always be treated as a single disease entity.

2. Origin of infection lies in deep to the internal anal sphincter and longitudinal layer, but not in the external sphincter based on clinical assessments. In the present-day practice, we understand this anatomical region as the intersphincteric space [4].

3. Majority of the origin of infection lies in either anterior or posterior aspect of anal canal.

4. Location of the internal opening should be predictable.

5. 90% are pyogenic infection, which can be dealt with appropriate surgery and antibiotics.

Why does complex fistula occur?

Of course, secondary causes of complex fistula-in-ano are not uncommon. It can be due to tuberculosis, Crohn's disease, perforated colonic diverticular disease or any form of pelvic sepsis [5, 6]. These are beyond the scope of this chapter.

Eisenhammer believes both spectrums of this disease have a pre-determined pattern and is predictable. He wrote: 'When faulty surgery is performed, natural anatomic barriers become disrupted, new planes of infections opened, leading to complex and complicated conditions' [6]. Recently, this concept is highlighted again. The pattern of spread should be predictable. Infection of the anorectal region should track in between the anogenital muscular and fascia layers rather than penetrating them, forming abscesses in various anorectal spaces. Anorectal musculature, fascias and spaces are constant. Therefore, the natural patterns of anal fistula should also follow a constant pattern [7].

To understand how cryptoglandular disease manifest as simple or complex disease, we should first discuss the natural patterns of cryptoglandular anorectal abscesses and fistulas.

3. Relevant updates in anorectal anatomy

Quoting Kurihara et al. in 2006, 'To be able to successfully treat cryptoglandular anorectal abscesses and fistulas, we need to understand the exact anatomy and extension course' [8]. Secondly, as mentioned before, we need to understand that infection will spread along the least resistant plane, along the planes of anorectal muscles and fascia to reach the respective anorectal spaces [7].

3.1 Review of relevant anorectal anatomy

Important anatomical structures are depicted in **Figure 1a** and **b**. The internal sphincter and the longitudinal muscle are continuation of the circular and longitudinal smooth muscles of rectum respectively in the anal canal. There are 3 components of external sphincters, subcutaneous, superficial and deep external sphincters, whereas puborectalis is a component of the levator ani [1, 2]. Recent publications suggest that puborectalis is also known to be the same entity as deep external sphincter [7, 9]. Perianal space and Ishio-rectal fossa were described by Parks as the 2 most common spaces for abscess formation [1]. However, his postulation that the source of infection was between internal sphincter and longitudinal muscle was later updated [1].

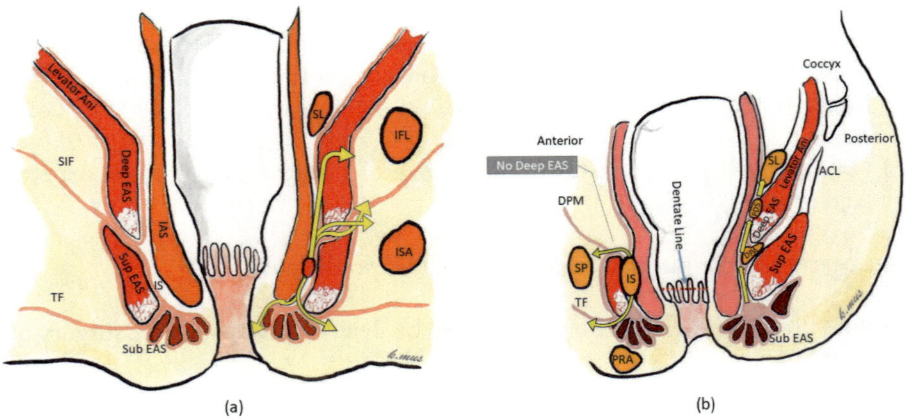

Figure 1.
Coronal view of the anorectal anatomy. Potential space for abscess to form; ISA: ischioanal space, IFL: Infralevator space, SL: Supralevator space, DPA: deep postanal space, PDS: posterior deep space (intersphincteric), IS: intersphincteric space, PRA: perianal space, SP: Superficial perineal space. SIF: septum of ischioanal fossa, TF: transversalis fascia, DPM: deep perineal membrane, ACL: anococcygeal ligament, IAS: internal anal sphincters. EAS: external anal sphincters, components: deep, sup (superficial) and sub (subcutaneous). Deep EAS is interchangeably termed puborectalis muscle. Sagittal view shows significant difference between anterior and posterior perineum. Deep perineal space lies above deep perineal membrane (DPM). Yellow lined arrows show postulated paths for intersphincteric sepsis to traverse the sphincter complex into respective anorectal spaces. Detailed explanation in segment 4.

3.2 Several updates in anorectal anatomy are summarized below

Internal sphincter circular muscles and longitudinal muscle layer are fused together, and the intersphincteric plane is a potential space between the longitudinal layer and the fascia of striated muscle external sphincters [4, 7] (see **Figure 1a** and **b**).

Deep external sphincter overlaps with puborectalis (part of levator ani), and superficial external sphincter overlaps with deep external sphincter, implicating that the external sphincter is not a continuous sheet of striated muscles. The author made a clear distinction between puborectalis and deep external anal sphincter as 2 separate entities, with weak connective tissue between each group [8].

However, other view states that the vertical portion of the levator ani's striated muscles around the anorectal ring is the puborectalis muscle, interchangeably known as the deep external sphincter [7]. This is supported by previous study by Shafik in 1975 confirming that puborectalis muscle and deep external sphincter are actually fused and functions as a single loop termed the top loop [9].

Both authors stipulate that there is a potential point of weakness between the vertical group and the horizontal group of striated muscles at the level of anorectal ring, allowing infection in the intersphincteric space to spread into the Infralevator space [7, 8].

The emerging terms of deep postanal space, posterior deep space and septum of ischiorectal fossa which will be explained next (refer to segments 4.2 & 4.5) [7, 8, 10, 11].

The anatomy of anterior perineum, especially superficial and deep perineal space are equally important to explain anterior patterns of abscesses and fistulas. Anterior perineum lacks puborectalis/deep external sphincter component. Posteriorly, there is a complex interconnection between intersphincteric space, supralevator space, posterior deep space and deep postanal space. (Shown in **Figure 1b**) Deep postanal space communicates with both ischioanal space and Infralevator space laterally and deep perineal space anteriorly (refer to segment 4.2) [7].

4. Understanding the natural patterns of cryptoglandular abscesses and fistulas

4.1 Simple and low abscesses and fistulas

The 2 most common fistulas described by Park in 1976 were intersphincteric fistula and transphincteric fistula, which accounts for 75% of his series. Eisenhammer in 1966 also reported that 80% in his series were low intermuscular type. Infection arising from anal gland forms suppuration in the intersphincteric space, forming an intersphincteric abscess. Alternatively, it can track along the potential intersphincteric space caudally to the intersphincteric groove or along the subcutaneous external sphincter fibers/septaes to form a perianal abscess. This forms an intersphincteric fistula once it ruptures outwards. However, if it spreads between subcutaneous and superficial external sphincter, it forms a low transphincteric fistula and results in a perianal or ischiorectal abscess. These 2 patterns are the most common findings reported and can occur anteriorly or posteriorly [1, 5–7, 12].

4.2 Depth of infection: depth of infections corresponds with the fascia layers

4.2.1 Posterior perineum

Posterior perineum divided into 2 compartments, infra-levator space and the clinical ischioanal space by a septum [8]. Abscess in the intra-levator space presents similarly as a clinical supralevator abscess and may not be apparent from external inspection. It can tract anteriorly to the deep perineal space. Infection/abscesses in the clinical ischioanal space is easily diagnosed by clinical examination externally due to inflamed, indurated or fluctuant ischioanal fossa.

4.2.2 Anterior perineum

There are 3 levels of soft tissue compartments [7].

- The lowest level consists of bulbus spongiosus and subcutaneous external sphincter, separated from the mid-level by transversalis fascia. Infection spreads radially in a linear fashion.

- The mid-level is termed superficial perineal space containing superficial transverse perineii muscles at the same level as the superficial external sphincter, separated from the deep level by perineal membrane. In males, infection in this space can extend to the scrotal area.

- The upper level is the deep perineal space, between the perineal membrane and the levator ani. It communicates posteriorly with the infra-levator space [7]. One should remember that in the deep perineal space, deep external sphincter or puborectalis is absent. Infection can spread between deep perineal space (anterior) and infra-levator space (laterally).

4.3 Transphincteric fistula

Low or high? This represents the level where infection extends through external sphincter into ischiorectal space. In clinical practice, we define low transphincteric fistula as those involving <1/3 of external sphincter, and high transphincteric fistula if >1/3 involved [12, 13]. Intersphincteric infection can pass through the external sphincter [1, 2, 8, 11], at junctions of each external sphincter portions [8]. If the infection passes through junction between levator ani and deep external sphincter, abscess may present as a Infralevator abscess, and the resulting fistula is a Suprasphincteric type as described by Park [5]. This typically occurs posteriorly and leads to horseshoe pattern (described in 2.2.5). On the other hand, if infection spread at the junction between superficial and deep external sphincter, it will cause ischioanal abscess and a high transphincteric fistula. A low transphincteric fistula results from infection spreading between the junction of superficial and subcutaneous external sphincter.

4.4 Anterior glands or posterior glands

Infection originating from anterior glands or posterior glands will results in typical patterns. Various authors reported internal openings found mainly at the anterior or posterior anal canal, which corresponds well with infected anal gland/crypt [1, 6].

Anterior gland infection that spreads via transphincteric route have predictable patterns. A low transphincteric pattern will tract along the subcutaneous tissue and below transversalis fascia in a linear fashion. A high transphincteric pattern will tract along the perineal space, in male, it extends into the scrotum. In female, it may result in ano-vaginal fistula or opens around the labia majora or causes perineal abscesses. Anterior horseshoe pattern has also been reported. It extends into the ischioanal space at 11 and 1 o'clock position [2, 6, 7].

Posterior gland infections are as described in 4.3 and 4.5.

4.5 Anatomy of the posterior perineum and deep posterior anal space

Hanley described the horseshoe pattern in detail; Infected anal glands originated from posterior midline of the anal canal, spreading along the longitudinal muscle cranially, passing superior or inferior to deep external sphincter (transphincteric extension) into the space known as deep postanal space. Deep postanal space communicates with both ischiorectal spaces above the surface of the superficial external sphincter. Pus will extend through the plane of least resistance into one or both ischiorectal spaces [10, 11].

In 2006, Kurihara made further anatomical discovery regarding posterior horseshoe pattern. Ischiorectal space is divided into 2 compartments by the septum of ischiorectal space, which starts at the Alcock's canal to border between puborectalis (part of levator ani) and deep external anal sphincter. This septum is important as the inferior rectal vessels and nerve runs along this fascia layer to penetrate the upper anal canal wall at the deep external sphincter level. At the point where inferior rectal vessels and nerve enters the external sphincter, tissue is loose. Infection spreads upwards along the intersphincteric plane, forms a nidus at the level of deep external sphincter within the intersphincteric space, which is termed as posterior deep space. It can extend via the weak points into either above or below the septum of ischiorectal space, spread either unilaterally or bilaterally to form horseshoe abscesses/fistulas [8]. Both authors however agreed that the internal opening is usually situated at the mid-anal canal posteriorly [8, 10]. Rojanasakul reports that the posterior high transphincteric fistula can occurs at 5 and 7 o'clock position of the anal canal [7].

4.6 Supralevator extension

In rare cases, intersphincteric sepsis tracks cranially, reaching the supralevator space via intersphincteric plane, limited only by the fascia of levator ani (extension of pelvic fascia) [2, 5]. It is unlikely that these collections spread across the levator ani. However, it is possible for the collection to enter the deep postanal space (posteriorly) or infra-levator space via a high transphincteric path or a suprasphincteric path as described above, forming an infra-levator abscess. These 2 are difficult to differentiate clinically, and erroneous drainage of these abscesses may lead to more complex iatrogenic fistulas such as extra-sphincteric fistula or a translevator fistula. Therefore, MRI imaging is advocated if such pattern is suspected [14, 15].

5. Review of practicality of various classifications for fistula in ano

There are numerous classifications of fistula in ano published over the last 4 decades. This chapter will focus on some of the most commonly used classifications to discuss the practicality in clinical scenario.

5.1 Park's classification

Park's classification of fistula-in ano remains popular as the standard terminology used by surgeons. It was published in 1976, based on operative findings of 400 patients over a span of 15 years [5]. The 4 main types are commonly used and reproduced in literatures. However, minimal attention was actually paid to the 14 sub-types in his original report (refer to **Figure 2**). Park's classification relied on intra-operative findings as it presented, and focused on the position or configuration of the fistula tract in relation to the external sphincter [5]. There were several disadvantages of this classification.

a. It does not stratify the complexity of each type of fistula, e.g. low or high fistula, single or multiple tracts.

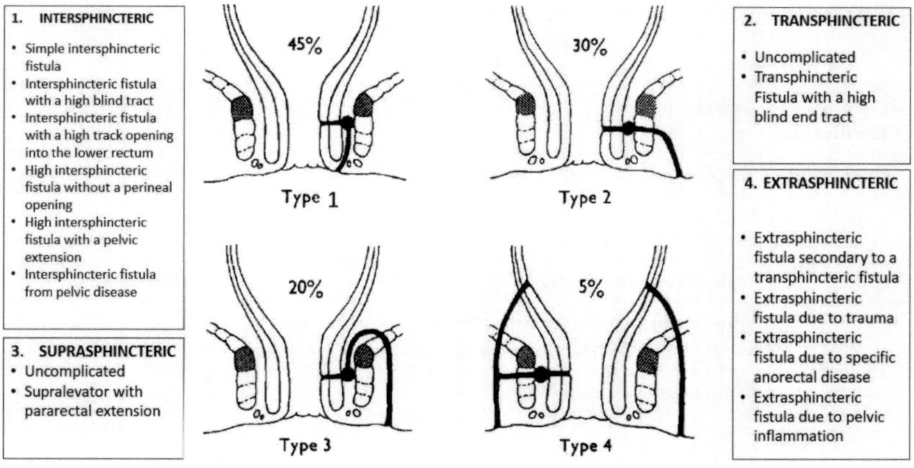

Figure 2.
Park's Classification in 1976. 4 main types with its sub-types (diagrams obtained from Park et al, 1976. A classification of fistula-in-ano. Br J Surg. 1976;63[1]:1–12). [5]

b. It does not guide clinicians in locating the source of intersphincteric sepsis and in selecting appropriate surgical treatment.

c. His clinical findings are recently disputed by several studies using modern imaging, especially the suprasphincteric and extrasphincteric type [8, 14, 16]. Even in 1976, Park described that some cases had difficult anatomy due to fibrosis (recurrence and previous surgery), thus exact anatomy was not entirely ascertained. There was no imaging to guide the findings back then.

5.2 Eisenhammer's classification

Eisenhammer published his final evaluation (refer to **Table 4**) based on low or high fistula, location of infection and pattern of spread. It was a useful guide for surgeons to predict the location of internal opening (intersphincteric infection) and course of fistula tract [6]. Eisenhammer stated that his series was mainly from private practice where all the patients presented to him were new cases, thus reporting the actual natural progression and patterns [6]. It is by far the most complete set of classification and focused on patterns of fistula, while stratifying each type by complexity. However, it did not gain popularity due to its' complex terminologies.

5.3 St James University Hospital classification

In year 2000, St James University Hospital improved Park's classification using Magnetic Resonant Imaging (MRI) studies. They analyzed 300 cases and classified fistula to five grades [16]. Essentially an anatomical classification, this classification refined the findings of Parks based on MRI (as shown in **Table 1**), splitting each of Park's type I (intersphincteric fistulas) & II (transphincteric fistulas) in two further grades (grade I into I & II and grade II into III & IV) and fused grade III & IV into one grade (grade V) [16]. This classification attempts to stratify fistula into simple or complex, allowing clinicians to judge the use of simple fistulotomy or more complex strategies/expert referrals. However, like Park's classification, it does not guide clinicians on the location of intersphincteric sepsis nor if the fistula is low or high. Furthermore, recent publications showed that not all intersphincteric fistulas are simple, and not all transphincteric fistulas are complex [7, 12].

St James's Classification	Description	Park's Classification
Grade 1	Simple Linear Intersphincteric Fistula	Type 1 – Intersphincteric
Grade 2	Intersphincteric Fistula with intersphincteric abscess and secondary fistulous tract	
Grade 3	Trans-sphincteric Fistula	Type 2 - Transphincteric
Grade 4	Trans-sphincteric Fistula with abscess or secondary track within the ischioanal or ischiorectal fossa	
Grade 5	Supralevator & Translevator Disease	Type 3 – Suprasphincteric
		Type 4 - Extrasphincteric

Table 1.
Comparison of St James Classification and Park's Classification. The former recognizes the need to stratify Park's Type 1 and 2 into simple and complex (information extracted from Morris et al, 2000. MR imaging classification of perianal fistulas and its implications for patient management, Radiographics 20 [2000] 623-635 discussion 635-7) [16].

5.4 Standard Practice Task Force

A practical and simple solution was created by Standard Practice Task Force in 2005, classified fistula-in-ano in just two categories-simple and complex [17]. The treatment of complex fistulas posed a high risk to anal continence and in simple fistulas, fistulotomy could be done safely without any risk of incontinence. The latter usually involved less than one-third of sphincter complex. Fistulotomy is not recommended in complex fistulas.

However, a study in 2017 showed that 32.1% (93/290) of complex fistulas were amenable to fistulotomy [12]. Simple and complex classification was shown to overestimate complexity of fistula. Furthermore, it was not particularly useful for clinicians in differentiating different types or patterns of complexity and determining the specific management.

5.5 Garg's classification

The most recent classification was introduced in 2017 and validated in 2020 with over 848 patients using combination of MRI study and intra-operative findings [12, 18]. This classification provided comprehensive and detailed grouping of anal fistula into 5 grades, from simple to complex grading (**Table 2**). In general, complexity was determined by low or high fistula, presence of multiple secondary tracts or collections. Intersphincteric and transphincteric fistulas were both recognized as simple if the fistula is low and safe for fistulotomy. This classification allows stratification of fistula-in-ano in a practical manner to guide their management strategies. Grade 1 and 2 fistulas were reported as safe to be treated with fistulotomy, whereas grade 3 to 5 requires more complex surgical strategy or expert referral (refer to **Table 2**) [12]. This method of stratification was validated to be safe. Following the Garg's new classification, patients underwent fistulotomy did not show significant changes in continence score post operatively [18]. However, this grading method relies heavily on MRI, which is not readily available in all

Grade 1	Low* Fistula with single branch	SIMPLE ¥
	Intersphincteric or Transphincteric	
Grade 2	Low* Fistula with multiple tracts, abscess or horseshoe.	
	Intersphincteric or Transphincteric	
Grade 3	High* Transphincteric with single branch	
	Anterior fistula in female	
	May have: Impaired continence, Crohn's disease or Previous radiation	
Grade 4	High* Transphincteric with	
	Multiple tracts, Abscess, Horseshoe.	
Grade 5	High* Transphincteric with Supralevator tract	
	Or Suprasphincteric	
	Or Extrasphincteric	

**Low transphincteric: <1/3 of external sphincter involved. High transphincteric: > 1/3 of external sphincter involved.*
¥Grade 1: Fistulotomy should be possible in almost all these fistulas (>95%). Grade 2: Fistulotomy should be possible in majority of these fistulas (>90%)

Table 2.
Garg's New Classification of Anal Fistulas (information extracted from Garg [18]).

institutions. Furthermore, there are many subclassifications to remember and challenging complex type such as suprasphincteric, supralevator and extrasphincteric types, were group into a single category even though each have unique patterns.

A useful classification allows clinicians:

- To categorize various subsets or presentations of a disease for better understanding.
- Stratification of a disease according to severity or complexity.
- To guide clinicians in treatment strategy and prognostication.

In general, most of the classifications above do not fulfill all 3 criteria above. Garg's classification was a significant improvement in categorizing, stratification and suggested treatment options for each grade. However, when faced with complex fistulas, there is still a general lack of understanding of its pathogenesis and optimal surgical treatment. This author believes, the step forward is to provide a more comprehensive treatment algorithm/guideline based on knowledge of natural patterns and progressions. To achieve this, the author believes classification based on natural patterns of cryptoglandular abscess and fistula will provide further insight.

6. Using natural patterns to classify anorectal abscess and fistula

6.1 Classifications that focuses on natural patterns

The new idea. Most classifications focus on anatomical configurations of fistula. It is possible to classify anorectal abscesses and fistula-in-ano based on natural patterns. This type of classification is beneficial as:

1. It helps clinician to understand the pathogenesis better, leading to a better understanding of different types and patterns of complex fistulas.
2. It helps clinician to predict the source of infected anal glands and intersphincteric sepsis, and the same time identify secondary extensions and external tracts.
3. This author postulate that it may reduce clinicians' reliance on imaging modalities.

Eisenhammer produced a classification method and later modified it in 1978 on his final evaluation of 800 patients over a span of 25 years. In general, the basis of his classification lied on low or high fistula/abscess, the position of the infected anal crypt (anterior or posterior), confined to intermuscular space (intersphincteric space) or spread to ischiorectal space [6]. However, it was not commonly utilized over the next few decades.

Rojanasakul proposed to classify the Natural Pattern of Anal Abscess and Fistula. It is effectively summarized into 5 main patterns and each pattern predicts the location of internal opening (refer to **Table 3**). This is paramount for surgeons to locate the offending anal gland/crypt for optimal treatment. Almost all patterns can be summarized by a simple classification of 5 patterns (refer to **Figure 3**) [7].

Type 4 and 5 can occur in combination. This is often complex and confusing to clinicians as it may present with a supralevator abscess concurrently with bilateral horseshoe or ischioanal abscesses (Shown in **Figure 3**). The key to managing this combination type is to address both the high intersphincteric tract and the high transphincteric tract with combination of surgical techniques (will be described in segment 8). When we compare both Eisenhammer's finding to this new classification of natural patterns, we find that all of the previously described types can be simplified into these 5 main patterns (refer to **Table 4**). Clinicians should be mindful that it is possible for 2 patterns to occur concurrently [7].

Pattern	Internal opening (& Intersphincteric tract)	Proportion
1. Intersphincteric pattern	Internal opening: any direction	3.8%
2. Low transphincteric pattern	Internal opening: any direction, most common anterior and posterior	26.9%
3. Anterior high transphincteric pattern	Internal opening: anterior. 11, 12 or 1 o'clock position	27.9%
4. Posterior high transphincteric pattern	Internal opening: posterior Common: posterior midline Less common: 5 and 7 o'clock position	31.7%
5. High intersphincteric pattern	Internal opening: posterior Common to occur concurrently with posterior high transphincteric fistula (horseshoe fistula)	9.6%

Table 3.
Summary of natural patterns of anorectal abscesses and fistulas with predicted internal opening, intersphincteric tract and proportion (information extracted with permission from Rojanasakul & Tsang, 2021. Emerging Concepts in Classification of Anal Fistulae. Pelvic Floor Disorders, Springer) [7].

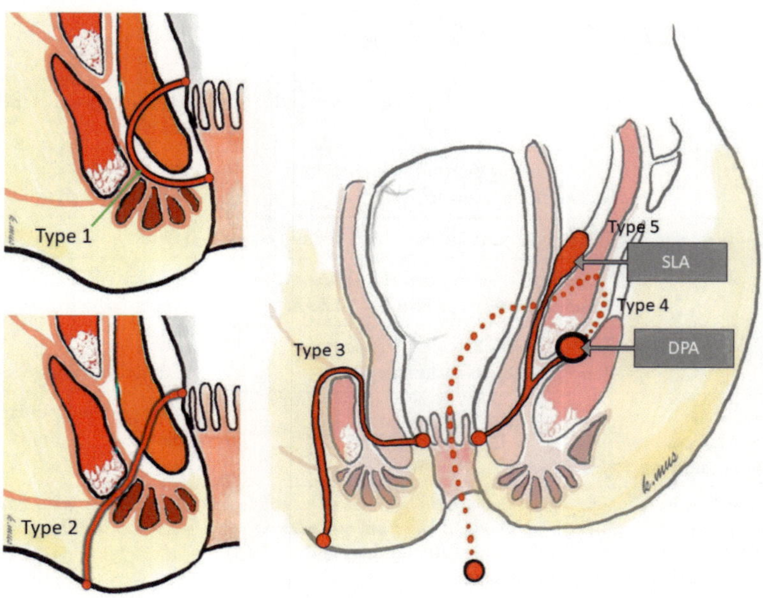

Figure 3.
Diagrammatic illustration of 5 types of natural patterns. SLA: Supralevator abscess. DPA: Deep post-anal abscess. Red dotted line represents the course of horseshoe pattern due to connection between deep post-anal space and ischioanal space/Infralevator space.

6.2 Controversies surrounding extra-sphincteric fistula

Park attributes extrasphincteric fistula to the following causes: secondary to a transphincteric fistula, trauma, specific anorectal disease and pelvic inflammation [5]. Eisenhammer's stated in both his initial series and final evaluation that extrasphincteric fistula was due to either iatrogenic probing or secondary causes such as pelvic sepsis, colonic diverticular diseases or inflammatory bowel disease [2, 6]. Garg's evaluation of more than 400 patients with anal fistula using MRI reported that there were no cases of extrasphincteric fistula in his series [12]. The most probable cause of extrasphincteric fistula: It is a combination of posterior high transphincteric fistula and high intersphincteric fistula situated posteriorly, resulting in both supra-levator collection and Infralevator collection. Incorrect drainage or probing of either can lead to a communication between the two collections across the levator ani [7]. Therefore, it is reasonable to conclude that extrasphincteric fistula does not fit into the natural pattern of cryptoglandular

	Eisenhammer's Classification	**Rojanasakul's Natural Patterns**
Group 1 – Intermuscular fistulous abscess and fistula		
Low:		
1	Posterior low intermuscular fistulous abscess and fistula	Intersphincteric and Low Transphincteric
2	Anterior low intermuscular fistulous abscess and fistula.	
3	Posterior low intermuscular superficial ischiorectal, unilateral horseshoe, fistulous abscess and fistula. [*]	Posterior High Transphincteric
4	Anterior low intermuscular superficial ischiorectal, bilateral horseshoe, fistulous abscess and fistula. [Ω]	Anterior High Transphincteric
High:		
1	High intermuscular fistulous abscess and fistula – mostly posterior	High Intersphincteric
2	High anovulvar intermuscular fistulous abscess and fistula – anterior. [π]	Anterior High Transphincteric
Group 2 – Intermuscular Transphincteric Ischiorectal fistulous abscess and fistula		
1	The Posterior Ischiorectal Horseshoe Fistulous Abscess and Fistula – bilateral [Σ]	Posterior High Transphincteric
2	The Anterior Ischiorectal Fistulous Abscess and Fistula – unilateral [μ]	Anterior High Transphincteric
Group 3 – Acute, non-cryptoglandular, non-fistulous abscess		Non-cryptoglandular diseases

[Ω π μ] *Anterior high transphincteric pattern can present as bilateral horseshoe, anovulvar tract or unilateral horseshoe. Bilateral anterior horseshoe pattern tends to have a lower internal opening compared to unilateral anterior horseshoe pattern [2, 6]. However, no other studies reported similar findings.*
[*] *Infection occurs in the clinical ischiorectal space.*
[Σ] *Infection occurs in the infra-levator space.*

Table 4.
Comparing current classification of natural patterns with Eisenhammer's updated description and classification in 1978 [6, 7].

infection. Its finding should alert surgeons of possibility of previous erroneous surgery or secondary sepsis originating from pelvis/abdomen [6].

6.3 Clinical application of the natural pattern and the role of adjunct imaging modalities

Understanding the pathogenesis and natural pattern helps in management of fistula-in-ano. Lessons from early publications showed that successful treatment of fistula-in-ano lies on the ability of surgeons to eradicate the source of infection, which is the infected anal crypt/gland and the intersphincteric abscess/tract [1, 2, 10, 19]. Recent publications further emphasized on eradicating secondary tracts or abscesses to prevent recurrences [15, 20, 21]. Therefore, objective clinical assessment should assist clinicians to:

a. Identify the internal opening & intersphincteric tract/abscess.

b. Identify the location of anorectal space involved.

c. Identify the external tract and secondary branches.

d. Ascertain the level of sphincter involved.

In the author's view, using the knowledge and classification of the Natural Patterns of Anal Abscess and Fistula [7], the above information can be actively sought after using a combination of clinical assessment and imaging modalities.

6.3.1 Clinical examination or examination under anesthesia

In cases of acute abscess, clinical examination generally elicits tenderness and fluctuation around perianal or ischioanal fossa. However, detailed assessment is usually informative with sedation, local or regional anesthesia. In high intersphincteric abscesses or Infralevator abscesses, tenderness is elicited on digital rectal examination at the anorectal ring. Examination under anesthesia may reveal pus discharge from internal opening upon insertion of anoscope. Perianal abscess is typical of type 1 (Intersphincteric) and type 2 (Low Transphincteric) patterns, and internal opening usually corresponds with the location of abscess. Ischioanal fossa abscess is the usual presentation of type 3 and 4 (high transphincteric) patterns. However, it should also be remembered that type 4 pattern produces Infralevator abscess, where internal opening is almost always posterior. Type 5 pattern produces high intersphincteric abscess and internal opening is usually posterior [6, 7].

In cases of chronic fistula, location of external opening and course of fistula tract should direct clinicians to the possible patterns. Low fistulas are clinically palpable as thickened fibrous cord extending from the external opening towards the infected anal crypt (internal opening). In high fistulas, tracts are usually not palpable subcutaneously. Digital examination may reveal chronic induration over the anorectal ring adjacent to lateral wall of rectum. External tracts usually runs deep and parallel with the anal canal on probing [6].

In cases where internal opening is not apparent, there are several techniques described to facilitate the identification of internal openings [6, 15].

a. Hard, board like changes to the deep surface of the internal sphincter usually represents the location of infected anal crypt.

b. Offending anal crypt retracts into a funnel on pulling the external tract.

c. Palpation of cord-like fibrous tract.

d. Internal opening probing: using hook or right-angled blunt tip forceps.

e. Gentle probing from external sinus: using small sized urethral catheter. Lacrimal probe is not advisable as it may cause false tracts.

f. Injection of dye (methylene blue solution) or water via external sinus.

g. Sensitivity of clinical examination in detecting the primary fistula tract is 68.7%, followed by 62.1% for secondary extension, and 59.7% for localizing internal opening [22]. Therefore, imaging is required as adjunct.

6.3.2 Imaging modalities as adjunct to classify the abscess/fistula pattern

Magnetic resonant imaging (MRI) and Endoanal ultrasound (EAUS) are the 2 most reliable imaging modality to delineate anorectal abscess and fistula. Conventionally, both modalities are equally sensitive in detecting anal fistula, but MRI has slightly superior specificity compared to EAUS [23]. MRI is not readily available in all institutions, whereas EAUS is operator dependant and requires significant learning curve.

Kim et al. in 2009 reported that 3 dimensional endoanal ultrasound is the preferred method, and use of hydrogen peroxide contrast may increase the detection rate of anal fistula. Sensitivity in detecting primary fistula tract is 84.4%, 81.8% for secondary extension and 84.2% for localizing the internal opening [22].

Recently, the interest in MRI has surged, in line with renewed efforts from various institutions to produce new classifications [16, 18]. With the availability of MRI scan, the fistula could be assessed in all three dimensions (axial, coronal and sagittal) [14]. The sensitivity and specificity of MRI in diagnosing fistula tracts were 98.8 and 99.7%, and in identifying internal opening were 97.7 and 98.6% respectively [14]. In addition, MRI is able to reclassify simple fistula based on clinical assessment to complex fistula, as it has the extra benefit of detecting additional secondary tracts, horseshoe tracts and supralevator extensions [18].

Clinical assessment and imaging adjunct helps clinicians to identify internal opening and intersphincteric tract/abscess, location of abscess, external tracts and secondary tracts. It also helps to define low and high fistula. This information will assist clinicians to recognize the type of anal fistula/abscess, thus allowing stratification and planning for appropriate surgical treatment. Surgical treatment will be discussed in the next segments.

7. Definitive surgical treatment in acute abscess stage

Eisenhammer wrote: '*single stage definitive surgery during the acute abscess phase is the correct timing to provide definite treatment and is associated with remarkably high healing rate, as long as the offending anal crypt is correctly identified and dealt with.*' [6] The idea of definitive surgery for fistulous anorectal abscess is not a recent concept, but one which never took off for the past few decades due to concerns of incontinence [24].

7.1 Benefits and disadvantages

Major guidelines recommend that immediate fistulotomy should be undertaken only by experienced surgeons, and a more conservative practice of simple abscess drainage in most circumstances is safest. Fistulotomy should only be done in low or simple fistulas [13, 25, 26]. This approach is known to be beneficial for 2 reasons: 1) Simple incision and drainage procedure, especially as an office procedure, allows quick return of function and daily living, thus avoiding prolong wound healing and hospital stay [2, 27]. 2) Less experienced surgeons may be confused with the exact anatomy of the fistula, or may cause iatrogenic injury and incorrect fistulotomy [6].

However, in the author's view, definitive surgery during the acute abscess stage has its advantage. Sharing Eisenhammer's view, the ideal management should be during the acute abscess stage [6]. Treating the fistula during acute abscess stage will reduce the number of chronic fistula formation [19]. A meta-analysis showed that definitive treatment leads to a risk reduction of 83% in recurrent fistula [24]. Furthermore, this is cost effective for health care facilities in general as the burden of treating chronic fistula is greatly reduced by reducing the need for re-operations.

7.2 Challenges

7.2.1 No standardized approach

Conventionally, several techniques were described in treating fistula during acute abscess stage. For perianal and ischioanal abscesses with identifiable fistula tract, fistulotomy, fistulectomy and cutting seton were used [19, 24–26]. Internal sphincterotomy was reported for intersphincteric abscess [6, 13]. Oliver reports performing immediate fistulotomy only for low transphincteric, intersphincteric and subcutaneous type, with recurrence rate of 5% [28].

7.2.2 Difficulty in localizing internal opening

A meta-analysis in 2006 analyzed 5 studies with a total of 405 patients showed that internal opening is not found in 10–17% of cases [24]. Inability to locate internal opening leads to higher recurrence rate as the source of infected anal crypt is not dealt with. Recurrence rate increased from 5–29% when internal opening was not found [28]. Imaging modalities are not readily available in cases of acute abscess.

7.2.3 Risk of incontinence

The same meta-analysis reported that sphincter-cutting procedures like fistulotomy and cutting seton during acute abscess is associated with 2-fold increase of risk of fecal incontinence to flatus and soiling. Severe incontinence rate was reported up ranging from 0 to 40%, although sample sizes for most studies were small [24].

7.3 Feasibility

The principles of treating acute fistulous abscess were laid down by McElwain:

1. Identification and excision of offending anal crypt [19] – position of infected gland and internal opening

2. Laying open the intermuscular abscess cavity [19] – drainage of intersphincteric space

3. Create a superficial external drainage for abscess beyond the external sphincter [19] – drainage of extrasphincteric abscesses

This author adds another 2 important principles:

1. Keeping wound open for drainage and to allow secondary healing.

2. Preservation of continence as best as possible.

In line with sphincter preservation as an important principle, a recent prospective study showed promising results utilizing sphincter preserving techniques for drainage and definitive treatment of fistulous anorectal abscess [29]. 86 patients with anorectal abscesses were operated by a single surgeon with intention of definitive single stage surgery and preservation of sphincter muscles. Using Rojanasakul's Natural Patterns of Anorectal Abscess and Fistula classification as guide, this study proposes 2 important steps: 1) Drainage of the perianal abscess at its most bulging point, 2) Exploration of the intersphincteric space to locate internal opening and intersphincteric tract/abscess. Internal opening was found in 95% of cases and intersphincteric tract was found in 77% of cases. Intersphincteric tract is treated with ligation as per LIFT procedure [4], whereas intersphincteric abscess were drained with suture closure of internal opening. Intersphincteric exploration wound is loosely closed with tube drains to promote drainage and secondary healing. This method reported overall healing rate of 83%, where the best results is obtained if intersphincteric tract is well formed. There were no cases of post-op incontinence. The remaining 17% non-healing group went on to elective surgery for definitive surgery of chronic fistula [29].

It is well known that in patients with anorectal abscesses undergoing simple drainage, 2/3 will progress to chronic fistula [27]. Definitive treatment of fistula may reduce the incidence of chronic fistula to an estimated below 30% based on recent evidence [28, 29]. With emerging sphincter preserving approaches, guided by our understanding of patterns of infection spread and imaging modalities, we are better equipped to approach acute fistulous abscesses with intention of single stage surgery.

8. Emerging concepts in managing cryptoglandular anal fistulas

Principle of surgical treatment of chronic fistula-in-ano should include the following:

1. Identification and removal of the source of sepsis in the intersphincteric space [1, 4, 6, 30].

2. Eradication of external and secondary tracts or abscesses [15, 20].

3. Maintaining the intersphincteric space open to heal by secondary intention [15].

4. Preservation of continence as best as possible [13, 25, 26].

5. An ideal surgical procedure should fulfill all 4 criteria above. Various surgical techniques have been described in literatures, ranging from sphincter cutting procedures to minimally disruptive biomaterials or novel techniques. In this segment, the author attempts to classify various surgical procedures into

categories, thereby assessing its suitability for specific fistula types and adherence to the above principles.

8.1 Sphincter cutting procedures for low fistula

Fistulotomy is the oldest, simplest, and most widely used procedure for anal fistulae. Most major guidelines recommend fistulotomy as a suitable and safe procedure for simple or low fistula [13, 25, 26]. This procedure involves laying open the entire fistula tract, together with the sphincter muscles it traverses, with adequate curettage to remove all granulation tissue tract [13, 31]. Marsupialization of the edges appears to speed up wound healing and reduces post-op pain and bleeding, but reported benefits were not significant [13]. Success rate is more than 90%, but incontinence rate is reported as high as 28% in elective setting [31]. According to Garg et al. in 2020, fistulotomy performed on low intersphincteric and low transphincteric fistulas (Garg's Classification grade 1 & 2) is safe. Post-operative mean continence score increased from 0.044 to 0.135, without reaching statistical significance. Low fistula is defined as involvement of less than 1/3 of external sphincter [18]. Failure of treatment or recurrence is associated with inappropriate selection of patients with high fistula or multiple tracts [31].

Internal sphincterotomy was first reported by Eisenhammer in 1966 to treat low intermuscular fistula (low intersphincteric type) which accounted for majority of cases in his series [2]. The principle is similar to fistulotomy, where the only difference is only lower half of internal sphincter muscles were laid open to eradicate intersphincteric sepsis. This technique gradually became synonymous with fistulotomy in various literatures as later studies showed that low intersphincteric type is far less common than low transphincteric type [7, 12]. In recent decade, ASCRS Practice Parameters introduced it as a treatment for intersphincteric fistulous abscess [13]. This technique is suitable for low intersphincteric type and does not cause incontinence [6].

8.2 Sphincter preservation or sphincter reconstruction procedures for both low and high fistula

Surgeons generally try to avoid sphincter cutting techniques. Ligation of Intersphincteric Tract (LIFT) procedure avoids sphincter cutting, using a small incision to explore the intersphincteric space to ligate and excise the intersphincteric tract [4] or to drain intersphincteric abscess [29]. Additional procedure in combination with LIFT such as closure of internal opening, excision of external tract and bioprosthetic mesh have been reported to improve outcomes [32]. A recent report from the original birthplace of LIFT procedure reported 10 year overall primary healing rate of 87.65%, and overall healing rate after re-operation was 99.2%. True recurrences were due to recanalization as a result of incorrect identification of intersphincteric tract. However, majority of recurrences were due to infection in the intersphincteric wound, leading to intersphincteric fistula which was easily treated by fistulotomy [20]. Other reports cited Crohn's disease, complex multiple fistulas and horseshoe pattern as a common cause of recurrences [33], stressing the importance of identification of secondary tracts and abscesses. In the author's view, LIFT procedure is best combined with additional curettage, drainage or excision of external fistula tracts/abscess. Recently, the original author reported slight modification where LIFT incision was loosely approximated and tube drain inserted to reduce intersphincteric space infection and promote secondary healing [29]. A recent meta-analysis and systematic review reported overall pooled success rate of 76.5% and incontinence rate of 1.4% [21].

Excision of fistula with immediate sphincter reconstruction is an alternative to reduce the risk of incontinence, at the same time completely eradicate intersphincteric and secondary tracts. It is suitable for both low and high transphincteric fistula. Procedure is similar as described in 8.1, with additional sphincter repair to restore continuity. Term as Fistulotomy or fistulectomy with primary sphincteroplasty (FIPS), Ratto reports 93.2% overall success rate, with a low morbidity rate [33]. Overall postoperative worsening continence rate was 12.4% mainly post-defecation soiling, without significant changes in anorectal manometry parameters [33]. In general, this technique produces higher success rate compared to LIFT procedure, albeit variations of techniques and terms used across institutions [34]. Incontinence is still a major concern, despite being much lower than fistulotomy alone. It is recommended in the German's S3 guideline but not in other major guidelines [26]. In the author's recent experience, this procedure produces excellent outcome in both low and high transphincteric chronic fistula, and extrasphincteric secondary (branching) tracts can be excised or curetted concurrently. However, in acute abscess stage, initial seton drainage is preferred prior to FIPS to reduce the risk of breakdown of sphincter repair [34].

8.3 Role of seton in complex fistula

Loose draining seton allows initial control of sepsis prior to definitive surgery to improves success rate. German S3 guideline used the term fibrosing seton [26]. It allows drainage of abscess and forms a thick fibrous fistula tract, which can be dealt with easily on the next elective surgery. Draining seton before LIFT shows no added benefits [32]. However, seton before fistulotomy and sphincter reconstruction showed benefits in downstaging high transphincteric to low transphincteric type [34]. From personal experiences, seton drainage can also be utilized to drain ischioanal/Infralevator collections with multiple external openings after debridement or curettage to prevent extensive wounds in the perineum.

8.4 Sphincter saving biomaterials and novel techniques

Many sphincter saving biomaterials and novel techniques surfaced in the last 4 decades to deal with complex fistula with wide variation of success rates across continents. Among those are anal fistula plug [35, 36], fibrin glue [26], laser procedures [37], Video Assisted Anal Fistula Tract Treatment (VAAFT) [38] and endoscopic clips (OTSC) [39]. Across the board, none of these procedures have reported very high success rate. This is likely due to the fact that most procedures, in their attempt to avoid cutting sphincters, only focus on the closure of internal opening and/or the fistula tract, but do not eradicate the intersphincteric sepsis and its secondary tracts. The author's opinion is that these procedures are highly specialized and are often based on selected specialized institutions. Therefore, usage of these techniques should be reserved to experts of the respective fields.

8.5 Approach for high intersphincteric fistula and extensions

Garg described an improved procedure in 2017 for high fistulas termed Transanal Opening of the Intersphincteric Space (TROPIS) [30]. High intersphincteric tracts and abscesses are typically difficult to reach via intersphincteric approach or conventional probing from external opening, and usually branching. TROPIS procedure allows lay open and drainage of these tracts into the anal canal, thus eradicating septic nidus at the high intersphincteric plane, which is usually posterior and was termed as the posterior deep space in the previous segment 4.5. This is done through the internal opening and external sphincter is not cut. The external branching tracts in the ischiorectal fossa were curetted. The space is left open for secondary healing. In the initial prospective cohort of 61 patients, success rate was 84.6% with no significant changes in continence score. The series consist of a mixture of high transphincteric type (anterior and posterior) and high intersphincteric type [30]. Incision on the internal

Type of pattern	Suitable procedure	Intersphincteric sepsis eradication	Eradication of external and secondary tracts/ abscesses	Healing by secondary intention	Preservation of continence
1. Low Intersphincteric	Fistulotomy or Internal Sphincterotomy	Yes	NA	Yes	Yes
	FIPS	Yes	NA	NA	Yes
2. Low Transphincteric	Fistulotomy	Yes	Yes	Yes	Unpredictable
	FIPS	Yes	Yes	NA	Yes
	LIFT	Yes	Yes	**Mod**	Yes
3. Anterior High Transphincteric	FIPS*	Yes	Yes	NA	Yes
	LIFT	Yes	**Add**	**Mod**	Yes
4. Posterior High Transphincteric	FIPS	Yes	Yes	NA	Yes
	LIFT	Yes	**Add**	**Mod**	Yes
	TROPIS	Yes	**Add**	Yes	Yes
5. High Intersphincteric	TROPIS	Yes	Yes	Yes	Yes
6. Combination type 4 & 5	Combination: TROPIS + **CED**	Yes	**Add**	Yes	Yes
	Staged approach. TROPIS, draining seton and delayed LIFT or FIPS	Yes	Yes	Yes	Yes

CED: Short for closure of external sphincter defect. After lay open of intersphincteric tracts and abscesses, an attempt is made to close the defect where transphincteric tract traverses the external sphincter. This can be done transanally or via external opening wound.
Mod: Modification by loosely approximate incision with tube drains to allow drainage and secondary healing of intersphincteric wound [29].
Add: Additional procedures includes drainage of ischioanal/Infralevator abscess, curettage or excision of external tracts, insertion of drains to the ischiorectal space [15, 29, 30].
Seton: Use of loose draining seton for drainage, induce fibrosis to form thickened tract and allows downgrading of high to low transphincteric fistula [34].
NA: Not applicable.
**Caution in performing FIPS in anterior transphincteric fistula, especially in female patients where external sphincter is thin, lack of support anteriorly and risk injuring perineal body.*

Table 5.
Summary of appropriate surgical treatment for different types of fistula pattern based on the principles of surgical treatment. No single procedure is 100% successful, therefore our clinical judgment is important in deciding on additional procedures, combination, staged approaches or modification to achieve our goal.

sphincter is shown to be safe without worsening incontinence [2, 30, 40]. In author's personal experience, TROPIS procedure is an excellent approach for high intersphincteric type and posterior high transphincteric type, especially if transphincteric fistula is located at the puborectalis level. However, like LIFT procedure, combination with drainage, curettage or excision of external tracts is necessary to reduce recurrences.

8.6 Deciding on the best surgical approach

To achieve good outcomes for anal fistula surgery, the author concludes that; 1) Understanding of type and natural patterns of fistula is extremely important, 2) The 4 principles of surgical treatment should be adhered to as closely as possible, and 3) No one surgical technique is suitable for all types of fistula. Therefore, selecting the appropriate procedure is important and to our best knowledge, no guidelines or classifications so far outlines a complete treatment algorithm especially on complex fistulas. Based on this review of evidence and best clinical judgment of the author, **Table 5** below attempts to summarize reasonable treatment options available for different fistula types to guide surgeons, where combination of procedures, additional procedures or modification of procedures is preferred over single modality (refer to **Table 5**).

9. Conclusions

Revisiting the anatomy and pathogenesis facilitates us to understand the natural patterns of anorectal abscess and fistula. With this new idea, we are able to classify and stratify this disease according to level of complexity and sphincter involvement, thus selecting the appropriate tool to manage it. Definitive treatment in acute abscess stage is feasible if the principles are followed. Surgical options and strategies should be carefully selected to suite each pattern, while adhering to the principles of surgical treatment. Challenges in managing cryptoglandular fistula-in-ano are summarized in Appendix (**Table 6**). The proposed solution is carefully selected from the current review of evidence and the experience of a high-volume tertiary centre.

Acknowledgements

The author would like to acknowledge Dr. Khairul Mustaqim Mazlan, Hospital Universiti Sains Malaysia (Kota Bharu) for contributing the graphics and figures in this paper, and Dr. Ng Hui Been, Hospital Raja Pemaisuri Bainun (Ipoh) for her contribution in prove reading and language editing.

Conflict of interest

The author declares no conflict of interest.

Notes/thanks

Special gratitude to my beloved wife, Dr. Ingrid Ting for her unwavering support in the process of completing this writing.

Appendix

Challenges	Complications	Proposed solution
i. Confusion in classification	• Wrong diagnosis	Adapting classifications that allows clear delineation of patterns, stratification of severity and guides management [7, 12]
	• Wrong stratification into simple or complex	
ii. Incorrect delineation of pattern	• Wrong procedure	Combination of clinical assessment and imaging modalities: MRI, EAUS
	• Risk of recurrence and incontinence	
iii. Acute abscess	• Develop chronic fistula	McElwain's principle [19]
		Consider intersphincteric exploration [29]
iv. High fistula	• Difficult to delineate	Role of MRI [15]
	• High risk of incontinence if treated with sphincter cutting surgery	TROPIS procedure [30]
v. Multiple secondary tracts and abscesses	• Risk of recurrence if not completely treated	Role of MRI and natural patterns classification [7, 14]
	• Technically more demanding	Additional procedures: drainage, curettage, excision.
vi. Internal opening not found	• Risk of recurrence	Combination of clinical assessment and imaging modalities: MRI, EAUS
		Attempt closure of internal opening at its predicted site [29].

Table 6.
Challenges in managing fistula-in-ano, with summary of its complications and proposed solutions.

Author details

Kenneth K.T. Voon
Selayang Hospital, Selangor, Malaysia

*Address all correspondence to: kenneth.voon@ummc.edu.my

References

[1] Parks AG. Pathogenesis and treatment of fistula-in-ano. Br Med J. 1961;1(5224):463–469.

[2] Eisenhammer, S. (1966). The anorectal fistulous abscess and fistula. Diseases of the Colon & Rectum, 9(2), 91–106.

[3] Seow-Choen F, Ho JM. Histoanatomy of anal glands. Diseases of the colon and rectum. 1994;37(12):1215–1218

[4] Rojanasakul A, Pattanaarun J, Sahakitrungruang C, Tantiphlachiva K. Total anal sphincter saving technique for fistula-in-ano; the ligation of intersphincteric fistula tract. J Med Assoc Thai. 2007;90(3):581–586.

[5] Parks AG, Gordon PH, Hardcastle JD. A classification of fistula-in-ano. Br J Surg. 1976;63(1):1–12.

[6] Eisenhammer S. The final evaluation and classification of the surgical treatment of the primary anorectal cryptoglandular intermuscular (intersphincteric) fistulous abscess and fistula. Dis Colon Rectum. 1978;21(4): 237–254.

[7] Rojanasakul A., Tsang C.B. (2021) Emerging Concepts in Classification of Anal Fistulae. In: Santoro G.A., Wieczorek A.P., Sultan A.H. (eds) Pelvic Floor Disorders. Springer, Cham. https://doi.org/10.1007/978-3-030-40862-6_80

[8] Kurihara H, Kanai T, Ishikawa T, Ozawa K, Kanatake Y, Kanai S, Hashiguchi Y. A new concept for the surgical anatomy of posterior deep complex fistulas: the posterior deep space and the septum of the ischiorectal fossa. Dis Colon Rectum. 2006 Oct;49 (10 Suppl):S37–S44. doi:10.1007/s10350-006-0736-6.

[9] Shafik A. New concept of the anatomy of the anal sphincter mechanism and the physiology of defecation. II. Anatomy of the levator ani muscle with special reference to puborectalis. Invest Urol. 1975 Nov;13 (3):175–182.

[10] Hanley PH. Conservative surgical correction of horseshoe abscess and fistula. Dis Colon Rectum 1965;8:364–368.

[11] Hanley PH, Ray JE, Pennington EE, Grablowsky OM. Fistula-in-ano: a ten-year follow-up study of horseshoe abscess fistula-in-ano. Dis Colon Rectum 1976;19:507–515.

[12] Garg P. Comparing existing classifications of fistula-in-ano in 440 operated patients: Is it time for a new classification? A Retrospective Cohort Study. Int J Surg. 2017 Jun;42:34–40. doi: 10.1016/j.ijsu.2017.04.019.

[13] Vogel JD, Johnson EK, Morris AM, Paquette IM, Saclarides TJ, Feingold DL, Steele SR. Clinical Practice Guideline for the Management of Anorectal Abscess, Fistula-in-Ano, and Rectovaginal Fistula. Dis Colon Rectum. 2016 Dec;59 (12):1117–1133. doi: 10.1097/DCR.0000000000000733.

[14] Garg P, Singh P, Kaur B. Magnetic Resonance Imaging (MRI): Operative Findings Correlation in 229 Fistula-in-Ano Patients. World J Surg. 2017 Jun;41 (6):1618–1624. doi: 10.1007/s00268-017-3886-x.

[15] Garg P, Sodhi SS, Garg N. Management of Complex Cryptoglandular Anal Fistula: Challenges and Solutions. Clin Exp Gastroenterol. 2020;13:555–567. https://doi.org/10.2147/CEG.S198796M.H.

[16] J. Morris, J.A. Spencer, N.S. Ambrose, MR imaging classification of perianal fistulas and its implications for patient management, Radiographics 20 (2000) 623–635 discussion 635–7.

[17] Whiteford, J. Kilkenny 3rd, N. Hyman, W.D. Buie, J. Cohen, C. Orsay, G. Dunn, W.B. Perry, C.N. Ellis, J. Rakinic, S. Gregorcyk, P. Shellito, R. Nelson, J.J. Tjandra, G. Newstead, Practice parameters for the treatment of perianal abscess and fistula-in-ano (revised), Dis. Colon Rectum 48 (2005) 1337–1342.

[18] Garg P. Assessing validity of existing fistula-in-ano classifications in a cohort of 848 operated and MRI-assessed anal fistula patients - Cohort study. Ann Med Surg (Lond). 2020 Sep 19;59:122–126. doi: 10.1016/j.amsu.2020.09.022.

[19] McElwain JW, MacLean MD, Alexander RM, Hoexter B, Guthrie JF. Anorectal prlblems: experience with primary fistulectomy for anorectal abscess, a report of 1,000 cases. Dis Colon Rectum. 1975 Nov-Dec;18(8): 646–649. doi: 10.1007/BF02604266.

[20] Malakorn S, Sammour T, Khomvilai S, et al. Ligation of intersphincteric fistula tract for fistula in ano: lessons learned from a decade of experience. Dis Colon Rectum. 2017;60: 1065–1070.

[21] Emile SH, Khan SM, Adejumo A, Koroye O. Ligation of intersphincteric fistula tract (LIFT) in treatment of anal fistula: An updated systematic review, meta-analysis, and meta-regression of the predictors of failure. Surgery. 2020 Feb;167(2):484–492. doi: 10.1016/j. surg.2019.09.012.

[22] Kim Y, Park YJ. Three-dimensional endoanal ultrasonographic assessment of an anal fistula with and without H2O2 enhancement. World J Gastroenterol 2009;15:4810–4815.

[23] Siddiqui MR, Ashrafian H, Tozer P, Daulatzai N, Burling D, Hart A, Athanasiou T, Phillips RK. A diagnostic accuracy meta-analysis of endoanal ultrasound and MRI for perianal fistula assessment. Dis Colon Rectum. 2012 May;55(5):576–585. doi: 10.1097/ DCR.0b013e318249d26c.

[24] Quah HM, Tang CL, Eu KW, Chan SY, Samuel M. Meta-analysis of randomized clinical trials comparing drainage alone vs. primary sphincter-cutting procedures for anorectal abscess-fistula. Int J Colorectal Dis. 2006 Sep;21(6):602–609. doi: 10.1007/ s00384-005-0060-y.

[25] Williams, G. & Williams, Andrew & Tozer, Philip & Phillips, Robin & Ahmad, A. & Jayne, D. & Maxwell-Armstrong, C.. (2018). The treatment of anal fistula: second ACPGBI Position Statement – 2018. Colorectal Disease. 20. 5–31. doi: 10.1111/codi.14054.

[26] Ommer A, Herold A, Berg E, Fürst A, Post S, Ruppert R, Schiedeck T, Schwandner O, Strittmatter B. German S3 guidelines: anal abscess and fistula (second revised version). Langenbecks Arch Surg. 2017 Mar;402(2):191–201. doi: 10.1007/s00423-017-1563-z.

[27] Scoma JA, Salvati EP, Rubin RJ. Incidence of fistulas subsequent to anal abscesses. Dis Colon Rectum.1974;17: 357–359.

[28] Oliver I, Lacueva FJ, Pérez Vicente F, Arroyo A, Ferrer R, Cansado P, Candela F, Calpena R. Randomized clinical trial comparing simple drainage of anorectal abscess with and without fistula track treatment. Int J Colorectal Dis. 2003 Mar;18(2):107–110. doi: 10.1007/ s00384-002-0429-0.

[29] Rojanasakul A, Booning N, Huimin L, Pongpirul K, Sahakitrungruang C. Intersphincteric Exploration With Ligation of Intersphincteric Fistula Tract or Attempted Closure of Internal Opening for Acute Anorectal Abscesses. Dis Colon Rectum. 2021 Apr 1;64(4): 438–445. doi: 10.1097/DCR. 0000000000001867.

[30] Garg P. Transanal opening of intersphincteric space (TROPIS) - A new procedure to treat high complex anal fistula. Int J Surg. 2017 Apr;40:130–134. doi: 10.1016/j.ijsu.2017.02.095.

[31] Göttgens KW, Janssen PT, Heemskerk J, et al. Long-term outcome of low perianal fistulas treated by fistulotomy: a multicenter study. Int J Colorectal Dis. 2015;30:213–219.

[32] Hong KD, Kang S, Kalaskar S, Wexner SD. Ligation of intersphincteric fistula tract (LIFT) to treat anal fistula: systematic review and meta-analysis. Tech Coloproctol. 2014 Aug;18(8):685–691. doi: 10.1007/s10151-014-1183-3.

[33] Ratto C, Litta F, Donisi L, Parello A. Fistulotomy or fistulectomy and primary sphincteroplasty for anal fistula (FIPS): a systematic review. Tech Coloproctol. 2015 Jul;19(7):391–400. doi: 10.1007/s10151-015-1323-4.

[34] Voon KKT, A Shanwani, KM Mazlan, Z Zakaria. Modified-2-staged fistulectomy with sphincter repair (m2fisr) procedure for transphincteric fistula-in-ano: a modified surgical approach. Brunei Int Med J. 2020;16: 117–123.

[35] Ommer A, Herold A, Joos AK, Schmidt C, et al. (2012b) Gore BioA Fistula Plug in the treatment of high anal fistulas—initial results from a German multicenter-study. GMS German Medical Science 10

[36] McGee MF, Champagne BJ, Stulberg JJ, Reynolds H et al. (2010) Tract length predicts successful closure with anal fistula plug in cryptoglandular fistulas. Dis Colon rectum 53:1116–1120: Doc13

[37] Giamundo P, Esercizio L, Geraci M, Tibaldi L et al. (2015) Fistula tract Laser Closure (FiLaC): long-term results and new operative strategies. Tech Coloproctol 19:449–453

[38] VAAFT - Meinero P, Mori L (2012) Video-assisted anal fistula treatment (VAAFT): a novel sphincter-saving procedure to repair complex anal fistulas. Tech Coloproctol 16:469–470

[39] Prosst RL, Joos AK. Short-term outcomes of a novel endoscopic clipping device for closure of the internal opening in 100 anorectal fistulas. Tech Coloproctol. 2016 Nov;20(11):753–758. doi: 10.1007/s10151-016-1537-0.

[40] Parks AG, Stitz RW. The treatment of high fistula-in-ano. Dis Colon Rectum. 1976;19(6):487–499

Chapter 3

Sphincter Preserving Techniques in Anal Fistula Treatment

Dorian Kršul, Damir Karlović, Đordano Bačić and Marko Zelić

Abstract

Complex anal fistulas present a challenge to even a seasoned colorectal surgeon due to high rate of recurrence and a real possibility of fecal incontinence if treated with conventional methods (e.g., fistulotomy, fistulectomy, seton placement). Although the illness is benign in nature, it can significantly decrease patient's quality of life because of symptoms like pain and soiling. Given those facts, minimally invasive or sphincter preserving methods of treatment were introduced. Some of these include: Video-assisted anal fistula treatment (VAAFT), ligation of intersphincteric fistula tract (LIFT), Fistula-tract laser closure (FILAC), rectal advancement flap (RAF), treatment with platelet cells and combinations of techniques. This chapter would be an overview of these novel techniques with reference to latest clinical trials and meta-analyses.

Keywords: VAAFT, LIFT, RAF, FiLaC, anal fistula, sphincter preserving, proctology

1. Introduction

Anal fistula is a chronic abnormal connection between the anal canal and the perianal skin. It is a tract lined with granulation tissue which supports chronic inflammation. Incidence of the disease is about 10 cases per 100 000 individuals with male to female ratio of 2:1. It mostly develops after an abscess of cryptoglandular origin although it can be associated with inflammatory bowel disease (IBD), trauma and carcinomas [1, 2].

Various classifications are proposed, but most widely used is the Parks classification. It relates to the course of fistula in relation to the sphincter mechanism [3]. Nowadays, fistulas can also be classified as simple and complex according to the relation of the proportion of the anal sphincter mechanism they pass through. Simple anal fistulas have one tract that crosses less than 30% of the external anal sphincter. They are treated best by fistulotomy or fistulectomy with very low incidence of continence disturbance. Other fistulas are classified as complex. These tracts cross external anal sphincter at a point that involves more than 30% of the external anal sphincter and can be associated with multiple tracts. Complex fistulas also include those anteriorly positioned in a female, recurrent fistulas and those related to IBD. In case they are treated by lay-open techniques, there is a high risk of postoperative continence disturbance [4].

The average rate of continence disturbance following treatment with a cutting seton is up to 12% which increased when the internal opening of fistula tract was positioned more proximally [5]. Following lay open techniques, the incidence of flatus incontinence or liquid stool leakage was observed in 20–25% of the patients [6]. This effect on continence has resulted in these techniques being less favorable for complex anal fistulas and the appetite for the use of minimally invasive techniques is increasing.

Various sphincter preserving techniques were introduced in clinical practice in the last 10–15 years with different success rates. This chapter serves as an overview of these techniques. This chapter covers treatment of cryptoglandular anal fistula. Anal fistula associated with Crohn's disease present a somewhat different problem and are not the scope of this chapter.

It is important to note that, given the novelty of some of these techniques, exact indications and contraindications do not exist as such. There are, however, some recommendations made in publications concerning various respective techniques, and these are referred to in the reference section. Authors of this chapter, given our experience in using these novel techniques, will fill in the gaps that may exist, extrapolated from our clinical practice.

2. Sphincter preserving techniques

2.1 Video-assisted anal fistula treatment (VAAFT)

Video-assisted anal fistula treatment is a sphincter preserving procedure that was developed by Italian surgeon Piercarlo Meinero in 2011 where he and others have described long and short-term results.

The operation is performed under spinal or general anesthesia using fistuloscope and specially designed equipment developed by Karl Storz (GmbH, Tuttlingen, Germany).

VAAFT procedure has two phases: diagnostic and therapeutic. The aim of the diagnostic phase is to visualize the entire fistula tract as well as the internal opening and to identify any possible secondary tracts and abscess cavities (**Figure 1**). In the therapeutic phase, complete destruction of the main and any secondary fistula tracts are preformed using monopolar electrode introduced to the fistula tract through working canal of the fistuloscope (**Figure 2**). This is followed by removal of necrotic detritus and closure of internal opening [7].

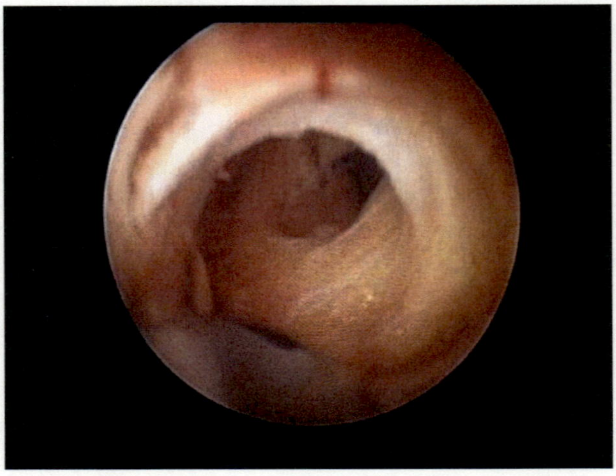

Figure 1.
Exploration of anal fistula tract using fistuloscope.

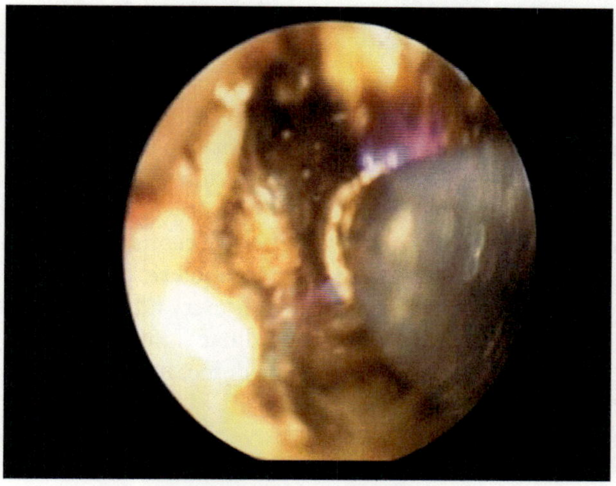

Figure 2.
Electrofulguration of anal fistula tract using monopolar electrode.

The main indication for VAAFT is operative treatment of complex anal fistulas, where there is a high possibility of continence disturbance if the sphincter were to be divided, and complex anal fistulas with multiple tracts [5, 8]. The VAAFT technique is comparable with other sphincter preserving techniques in relation to healing and patient satisfaction [9]. Diminished postoperative pain, earlier recovery after surgery and smaller postoperative perianal wounds allows for earlier return to normal activities. Although simple fistulas were treated with this technique, it is our opinion that VAAFT technique offers no benefit in this setting and should be reserved for complex anal fistulas.

The VAAFT technique allows multiple attempts in case the procedure is not successful in the first instance. The proposed mechanism whereby repeated procedures have an incremental effect is converting a complex fistula with multiple tracts into a more manageable, low, or simple fistula, which can be called conversion of the fistula [10].

To date, the VAAFT has been shown to be safe and associated with good functional outcomes and very low incidence of complications [7, 8, 11], which was shown in a published meta-analysis (Emile et. al). It showed recurrence rate ranging from 7,5 to 33.3% with a weighted mean recurrence rate of 17,7%. Recurrence rates varied significantly depending on the method of internal fistula opening closure (mattress suture, stapler, rectal advancement flap). No affection of anal continence was documented [12].

Compared with other minimally invasive techniques, VAAFT is the only procedure which allows intraoperative visualization of entire fistula tract, possible secondary tracts and the internal fistula opening from within the tract. Limitations of the technique are that it uses rigid instrument to examine curved tracts. Although this is not an issue in most operations due to elasticity of tissue, some fistulas, such as suprasphincteric, may prevent complete examination of the tract due to sharp angle tract makes when it passes above external anal sphincter. This could also lead to creation of false tracts if diathermy is applied unselectively or too much force is used to push fistuloscope when advancing through the tract. When operating on suprasphincteric fistulas, modification of the approach can be used so that the fistuloscope is inserted through internal opening as well as external opening. That way surgeon can explore complete length of the fistula from openings to the curve of suprasphincteric fistula.

2.2 Ligation of intersphincteric fistula tract (LIFT)

LIFT is a sphincter sparing technique introduced by dr. Arun Rojanasakul in 2007. It is based on the concept of secure closure of the internal opening and concomitant removal of infected cryptoglandular tissue in the intersphincteric plane.

The procedure is performed by identifying fistula tract and internal opening using jet irrigation through external opening or by using metal probe. Next step is making a curvilinear incision on the anocutaneous border and identifying Intersphincteric plane with fistula tract. Intersphincteric portion of fistula tract is then ligated on the side of the internal anal sphincter and cut (**Figure 3**). Rest of the tract is excised along with affected cryptoglandular tissue followed by curettage of the rest of tract through external opening. The defect in the external anal sphincter is sutured and the incision closed [13].

Two available meta-analyses showed that overall rate of success was 76.4 and 78% respectively. The weighted mean complication rate was 5,5–13.9%. The most common complication was wound dehiscence, others being infection, bleeding, anal discharge, anal fissure, and hematoma. Fecal incontinence was recorded in 1.4% of patients, but only of minor grade [14, 15].

LIFT has an advantage over other methods in that it is easily reproducible without investment in potentially costly equipment. Due to specific surgical technique and access in the intersphincteric plane, it is logical to conclude that its role lies mostly in treatment of transsphincteric anal fistula. In case of procedure failure or persistence of fistula, repeated LIFT on the same place might be a problem because of the tissue scaring. Therefore in such cases it would be best to consider some other sphincter preserving technique like VAAFT that has the added value of visualizing branching tracts that might have been the cause of failure in the first place.

While it is always best for transsphincteric fistula to heal primarily, an important observation when dealing with wound dehiscence after LIFT on the anocutaneous border is that loose seton can be inserted through the wound, which converts

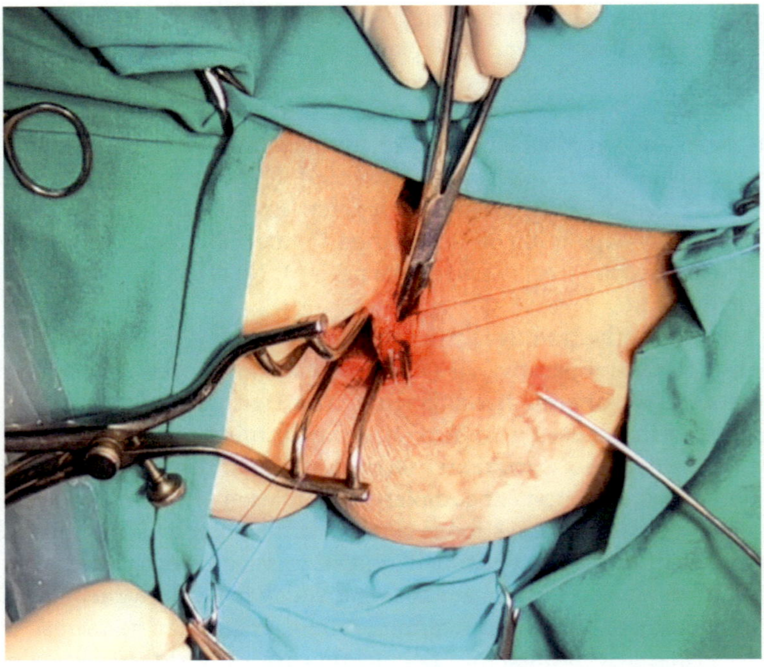

Figure 3.
Anal fistula tract dissected and ligated in the intersphincteric plane.

transsphincteric into simple intersphincteric fistula that can be dealt with later by lay open technique without fear of continence disturbances.

2.3 Anal fistula laser closure (FiLaC™)

Fistula laser closure was first introduced in 2011 by Wilhelm. The procedure involves destruction of fistula tract using radial emitting laser probe by applying energy while retracting laser probe that was inserted through perianal opening [16]. It was proposed initially to close the site of internal opening with anorectal flap, but procedure was later modified by Giamundo to exclude any form of internal opening closure by using the shrinking effect of laser energy to obliterate the opening, as well as remaining fistula tract [17]. It is postulated that this approach has an advantage over simple diathermy because diathermy cannot elicit shrinking effect on surrounding tissues, and it is more difficult to regulate thermal damage on anal sphincter complex [18].

Since the technique introduction, multiple observational studies were reported and published but only one systematic review and meta-analysis currently exists (Elfeki et al). Overall, mean rate of primary healing among the analyzed studies was 67,3% which was increased to 69.7% with a repeated procedure. Only 5,5% of patients had complications, but those were all minor, scoring I or II on Clavien-Dindo scale. Weighted mean rate of fecal incontinence was 1% but was not statistically significant [19].

Drawback of this procedure is argued to be lack of visualization of fistula tract. Even though energy of the probe can be adjusted to different power settings, and therefore different depth of tissue penetration, there is still an issue of branching tracts that cannot be adequately accessed by blind insertion. On the other hand, increasing power of the laser diode in order to widely affect perianal tissue, could result in inadvertent damage of anal sphincter complex.

As the probe itself is a flexible instrument, it could potentially reach parts of fistula tract that are otherwise inaccessible behind the sharp angle such is often the case in suprasphincteric fistulas.

2.4 Rectal advancement flap (RAF)

This is the oldest sphincter preserving technique, primarily reserved for treatment of complex anal fistulas. It was first described by Elting in the beginning of the 20th century but was implemented in everyday practice during the last few decades [20]. Many publications about the technique can be found under different names, such as endorectal, endoanal, transanal advancement flap etc.

First step in this procedure is to identify and excise internal fistula opening. Then the U-shaped or rhomboid flap with wider base side should be performed by dissecting anorectal mucosa and adjacent internal anal sphincter muscle. Curettage and irrigation of the whole of fistula tract should be performed followed by suture of defect in sphincter complex left by earlier fistula tract. Site is then covered by previously prepared flap and sutured (**Figure 4**).

Much research has been made about optimal flap thickness, whether be it only mucosal flap or full thickness flap which involves full transection of the rectal wall. Researchers found that there was statistically higher rate of primary healing in group with thicker flaps, but also noticed that there was higher rate of postoperative mild continence disturbance which was more severe the thicker flap was [21–23]. Another frequently discussed issue was necessity to use loose seton prior flap operation to rase the rate of primary healing. Even though there have not been clear statistical findings, many surgeons advocate seton placement as an important step

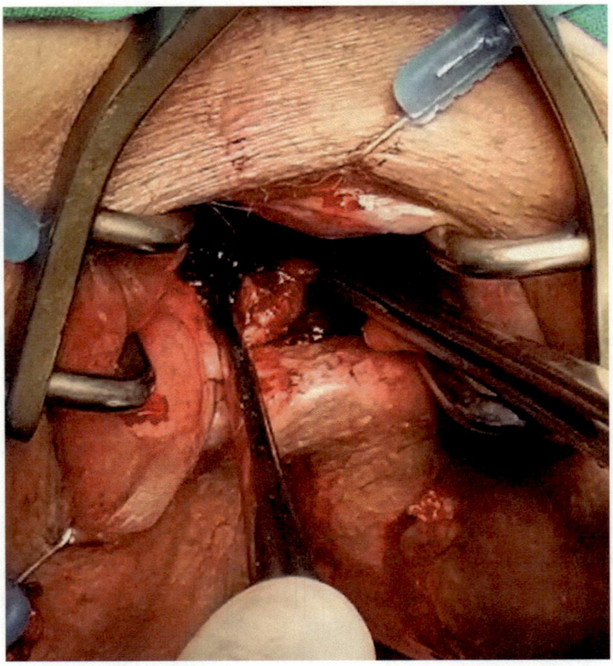

Figure 4.
Mobilized full-thickness rectal advancement flap.

before flap operation [24]. Factors that could affect healing after flap procedure are obesity and smoking, so patients should be advised to quit smoking and to try to reduce their weight prior flap operation [25–27].

There have been many publications and several systematic reviews and meta-analyses on this technique where the effectiveness was shown to be 60–80%, but same cases also reported some degree of postoperative fecal disturbance [23, 28, 29]. That is why we cannot talk about pure sphincter preserving technique, even though this technique was developed primarily for treatment of complex high anal fistulas that would otherwise have high postoperative risk of fecal disturbance if treated by lay open techniques.

It is important to note that although RAF is a treatment technique, it is used by itself as a method of internal fistula opening closure when preforming other sphincter preserving procedures. This type of internal opening closure can be made in all cases, but is most appropriate when large openings are present, and when tension on the suture line is presumed to be increased by simple mattress suturing. RAF is also technically most demanding to preform, because it involves dissection and suturing in a confined space, often deeply in anal canal. Flap itself has to be rhomboid in shape or U-shaped with wider base, so that circulation is adequate to avoid dehiscence or flap ischemia. Excessive grasping should also be avoided as well as too big a strain on the suture line.

2.5 Autologous platelet rich plasma (APRP)

Although autologous platelet rich plasma (APRP) is used as treatment in other fields of medicine, such as plastic surgery, orthopedics, and dental medicine, treatment of anal fistula using this technique has emerged in the last decade.

Autologous platelet-rich plasma (APRP) is platelet concentration derived from centrifuged full blood after removal of red blood cells. Such plasma is a rich source of growth factors implicated in tissue healing and regeneration [30, 31].

Treatment itself consists of removal of granulation tissue lining the fistula tract followed by irrigation and closure of the internal opening. APRP injection, which was previously prepared using gravitational platelet separation procedure from autologous blood sample, is then injected into the fistula tract [32]. Specifics of the separation procedure are beyond the scope of this chapter. Majority of publications combined mucosal advancement flap with APRP injection [33–36].

There have been several publications with the reported average healing rate from 60 to 90% [34–36]. All of publications had relatively small number of patients enrolled and still no meta-analyses exist on the subject. No continence disturbances were reported.

This is still somewhat experimental procedure and not widely used. Platelet separation procedures require specialized equipment that is often only available in larger institutions. Cost per patient also exceeds that of the other techniques, which is why this technique needs more solid evidence for patient benefit before it can be considered to become one of the mainstream sphincter preserving treatments.

2.6 Hybrid sphincter preserving techniques

Hybrid sphincter preserving techniques combine two techniques into a single procedure. Some of the reported combinations are as follows.

LIFT-VAAFT is used with intention of combining internal fistula opening closure in the intersphincteric plane with VAAFT to destroy remaining fistula tract and to check for any branching tracts [37]. A new and yet unpublished report combines VAAFT and FiLaC procedures with the same fundamental philosophy [38]. VAAFT was also combined with RAF in order to close especially large internal openings that would not be suitable for closure with mattress suture [10].

BioLIFT combines LIFT with insertion of bioprosthetic graft in the intersphincteric plane. On a study of 31 patients, success rate was reported to be 94% in a one-year follow-up period [39]. Another study combined LIFT and human acellular dermal matrix as a bioprosthetic plug with reported success rate of 95% on 21-patient sample [40].

Advancement flap was combined with injection of porcine dermal collagen implant through external opening in a study of 24 patients with success rate of 82,5% in a 14-month follow-up period [41].

It was to be expected that surgeons, encouraged by initial promising results, started combining sphincter preserving techniques in order to achieve even better healing rates. Some of these procedures were more successful than others, but majority of reports are on a single institution basis or case reports and relatively few patients. Idea of combining two (or more) techniques in order to recruit the individual one's advantage is sound. For example LIFT combined with VAAFT has potential to resolve pathology in intersphincteric plane as well as find additional tract branches. VAAFT in conjunction with FiLaC can visualize branching tracts while managing to reach fistula behind sharp angle etc.

For now, as there is no evidence to the contrary, we can use hybrid techniques in order to take advantage of one's strong suits, overcome the shortages of another and vice versa. Until evidence is found that one technique, or combination of techniques, has significantly better results over the others, they should be tailored individually depending on patient's case.

3. Discussion and conclusions

Complex anal fistulas present a complex problem, although they are often not perceived as such. Operation of anal fistula is usually one of the first operations that a surgical resident will do in the course of their residency as it is thought as simple and straightforward procedure. The actuality is that unless patient requires only seton placement, no treatment of complex fistulas should be made if surgeon is not acquainted with sphincter preserving procedures or knows how to repair anal sphincter if treatment using traditional techniques results in fecal incontinence. The most difficult cases should be treated in high-volume institutions only, as successfully treated fistula resulting in any degree of fecal incontinence is not a good outcome.

Important point in every operation is to try to identify internal opening even when one is not evident. This is especially important in very complex cases, such as horseshoe fistulas, when multiple internal openings might be present but not all of them immediately visible. Goodsall's rule is a good waypoint as to where the opening might be. Failure of dealing with internal opening is almost certain to result in procedure failure. Surgeon should take care not to use excessive force when identifying the opening to avoid creation of false openings or false tracts. Easy way to find the opening is to inject hydrogen peroxide through external opening and look for the spurt of foam in the anal canal.

Several things can be considered to increase the chance of healing, especially when preforming RAF. It might be a good idea to try to reduce intraoperative fecal matter and postoperative stool passage through the anal canal by applying enema. Postoperatively stool regulation by avoiding hard stool and excessive straining should be advised. Although not specific to this pathology, flavonoid use after hemorrhoidectomy has been observed to reduce inflammatory reaction and pain by reducing leukocyte adherence, so the same can be considered after these types of procedures [42].

There is also the issue of direct repair of fistula or seton placement in the first act. It is observed that seton placed and held for several weeks or months helps draining perianal sepsis and promotes fibrosis of the tract, making the subsequent sphincter preserving procedure easier. Therefore, an effort should be made to decrease perianal inflammation before attempting definite procedure, if possible. This opinion is not uniform between surgeons however. Other opinion is that the incidence of false tracts creation with metal probes while placing setons is unacceptably high, so that in this case, the wrong tract ends up being treated and reccurence is certain. This kind of belief is mostly anecdotal and there is no evidence in scientific literature.

Many new methods of sphincter preserving techniques for treating anal fistula emerged in the last 10–15 years. The shear fact that so many different procedures are proposed, shows that there is no best technique, and those that initially showed exceptional results usually could not be replicated in another institution. This speaks volumes about the complexity of anal fistula problem for the colorectal surgeon and hints that there is much that we still do not understand.

Nevertheless, several techniques gained somewhat wider acceptance, such as LIFT, VAAFT and RAF. Problem in choosing the best procedure lies in heterogeneity of fistulas and still no algorithm exists to rely on, so it is actually no surprise that a wide variety of procedures exist in the first place. We have tried to summarize characteristics of aforementioned techniques along with proposed indications and their pros and cons, but ultimately decision on what technique to choose should still be made on individual basis, surgeon's preference and on equipment availability.

Still, more randomized studies are needed. It is to be expected that success rate of these procedures will increase somewhat as the time passes given that a lot of publications reported initial results that are burdened by surgeon's learning curve. With increasing amount of sphincter preserving procedures being underwent, we will probably have more results to rely on in the future and to extrapolate better conclusions.

Conflict of interest

The authors declare no conflict of interest.

Author details

Dorian Kršul*, Damir Karlović, Đordano Bačić and Marko Zelić
Clinical Hospital Center Rijeka, Rijeka, Croatia

*Address all correspondence to: dorian.krsul@hotmail.com

References

[1] Mappes HJ, Farthmann EH. Anal abscess and fistula. Munich: Zuckschwardt; 2001.

[2] Hamalainen KP, Sainio AP. Incidence of fistulas after drainage of acute anorectal abscesses. Dis *Colon Rectum*. 1998; 41:1357-1361.

[3] Parks AG, Gordon PH, Hardcastle JD. A classification of fistula-in-ano. Br J Surg. 1976; 63:1-12.

[4] Whiteford MH, Kilkenny J III, Hyman N, Buie WD, Cohen J, Orsay C et al. Practice parameters for the treatment of perianal abscess and fistula-in-ano (revised). Dis *Colon Rectum*. 2005; 48:1337-1342.

[5] Ritchie RD, Sackier JM, Hodde JP. Incontinence rates after cutting seton treatment for anal fistula. Colorectal Dis. 2009;11(6):564-571.

[6] Atkin GK, Martins J, Tozer P, Ranchod P, Phillips RKS. For many high anal fistulas, lay open is still a good option. Tech Coloproctol. 2011;15(2):143-150.

[7] Meinero P, Mori L. Video-assisted anal fistula treatment (VAAFT): A novel sphincter-saving procedure for treating complex anal fistulas. Tech Coloproctol. 2011;15(4):417-422

[8] Schwandner O. Video-assisted anal fistula treatment (VAAFT) combined with advancement flap repair in Crohn's disease. Tech Coloproctology. 2013;17(2):221-225.

[9] García-Aguilar J, Davey CS, Le CT, Lowry AC, Rothenberger DA. Patient satisfaction after surgical treatment for fistula-in-ano. Dis *Colon Rectum*. 2000;43(9):1206-1212.

[10] Zelić M, Karlović D, Kršul D, Bačić Đ, Warusavitarne J. Video-assisted anal fistula treatment (VAAFT) for treatment of complex cryptoglandular anal fistulas with 2 years follow up period – our experience. J Laparoendosc Adv Surg Tech A. 2020 Dec;30(12):1329-1333.

[11] Walega P, Romaniszyn M, Nowak W. VAAFT: A new minimally invasive method in the diagnostics and treatment of anal fistulas – initial results. Pol Przegl Chir. 2014;86(1):7-10.

[12] Emile SH, Elfeki H, Shalaby M, Sakr A. A Systematic review and meta-analysis of the efficacy and safety of video-assisted anal fistula treatment (VAAFT). Surg Endosc. 2018 Apr;32(4):2084-2093.

[13] Rojanasakul A. LIFT procedure: a simplified technique for fistula-in-ano. Tech Coloproctol. 2009 Sep;13(3):237-240.

[14] Hong KD, Kang S, Kalaskar S, Wexner SD. Ligation of intersphincteric fistula tract (LIFT) to treat anal fistula: systematic review and meta-analysis. Tech Coloproctol. 2014 Aug;18(8):685-691.

[15] Emile SH, Khan SM, Adejumo A, Koroye O. Ligation of intersphincteric fistula tract (LIFT) in treatment of anal fistula: An updated systematic review, meta-analysis, and meta-regression of the predictors of failure. Surgery. 2020 Feb;167(2):484-492.

[16] Wilhelm A. A new technique for sphincter-preserving anal fistula repair using a novel radial emitting laser probe. Tech Coloproctol. 2011 Dec;15(4):445-449.

[17] Giamundo P, Geraci M, Tibaldi L, Valente M. Closure of fistula-in-ano with laser-FiLaC™: an effective novel sphincter-saving procedure for complex disease. Colorectal Dis. 2014 Feb;16(2):110-115

[18] Limura E, Giordano P. Modern management of anal fistula. World J Gastroenterol. 2015 Jan 7; 21(1): 12-20.

[19] Elfeki H, Shalaby M, Emile SH, Sakr A et al. A systematic review and meta-analysis of the safety and efficacy of fistula laser closure. Tech Coloproctol. 2020 Apr;24(4):265-274.

[20] Elting AW. X. The Treatment of Fistula in Ano: With Especial Reference to the Whitehead Operation. Ann Surg 1912; 56:744-752.

[21] Balciscueta Z, Uribe N, Balciscueta I, Andreu-Ballester JC, Garcia-Granero E. Rectal advancement flap for the treatment of complex cryptoglandular anal fistulas: a systematic review and meta-analysis. Int J Colorectal Dis 2017; 32:599-609.

[22] Dubsky PC, Stift A, Friedl J, Teleky B, Herbst F. Endorectal advancement flaps in the treatment of high anal fistula of cryptoglandular origin: fullthickness vs. mucosal-rectum flaps. Dis Colon Rectum 2008; 51:852-857.

[23] Khafagy W, Omar W, El Nakeeb A, Fouda E, Yousef M, Farid M. Treatment of anal fistulas by partial rectal wall advancement flap or mucosal advancement flap: a prospective randomized study. Int J Surg 2010; 8:321- 325

[24] Mitalas LE, van Wijk JJ, Gosselink MP, Doornebosch P, Zimmerman DD, Schouten WR. Seton drainage prior to transanal advancement flap repair: useful or not? Int J Colorectal Dis 2010; 25:1499-1502.

[25] Zimmerman DD, Delemarre JB, Gosselink MP, Hop WC, Briel JW, Schouten WR. Smoking affects the outcome of transanal mucosal advancement flap repair of trans-sphincteric fistulas. Br J Surg 2003; 90:351-354.

[26] Ellis CN, Clark S. Effect of tobacco smoking on advancement flap repair of complex anal fistulas. Dis Colon Rectum 2007; 50:459-463

[27] Schwandner O. Obesity is a negative predictor of success after surgery for complex anal fistula. BMC Gastroenterol 2011; 11:61

[28] Schouten WR, Zimmerman DD, Briel JW. Transanal advancement flap repair of transsphincteric fistulas. Dis Colon Rectum 1999; 42:1419-1422.

[29] Ozuner G, Hull TL, Cartmill J, Fazio VW. Long-term analysis of the use of transanal rectal advancement flaps for complicated anorectal/vaginal fistulas. Dis *Colon Rectum* 1996; 39:10-14. 7.

[30] Eppley BL, Woodell GE, Higgins J. Platelet quantification and growth factor analysis from platelet-rich plasma: implications for wound healing. Plast Reconstr Surg. 2004; 114:1502-1508

[31] Bai MY, Wang CW, Wang JY, Lin MF, Chan WP. Threedimensional structure and cytokine distribution of platelet-rich fibrin. Clinics (Sao Paulo). 2017; 72:116-124

[32] Van der Hagen SJ, Baeten CG, Soeters PB, van Gemert WG. Autologous platelet-derived growth factors (platelet-rich plasma) as an adjunct to mucosal advancement flap in high cryptoglandular perianal fistulae: a pilot study. Color Dis. 2011; 13:215-218

[33] Pérez-Lara FJ, Moreno Serrano A, Ulecia Moreno J, HernándezCarmona J, Ferrer-Márquez M, Romero-Pérez L, del Rey Moreno A, Oliva-Muñoz H (2015) Platelet-rich fibrin sealant as a treatment for complex perianal fistulas: a multicentre study. J Gastrointest Surg 19:360-368

[34] Moreno-Serrano A, García-Díaz JJ, Ferrer-Márquez M, AlarcónRodríguez R,

Álvarez-García A, Reina-Duarte Á (2016) Using autologous platelet-rich plasma for the treatment of complex fistulas. Rev Esp Enferm Dig (Madrid) 108:123-128

[35] Göttgens KW, Vening W, van der Hagen SJ, van Gemert WG, Smeets RR, Stassen LP, Baeten CG, Breukink SO (2014) Longterm results of mucosal advancement flap combined with plateletrich plasma for high cryptoglandular perianal fistulas. Dis *Colon Rectum* 57:223-227

[36] Göttgens KWA, Smeets RR, Stassen LPS, Beets GL, Pierik M, Breukink SO (2015) Treatment of Crohn's disease-related high perianal fistulas combining the mucosa advancement flap with platelet-rich plasma: a pilot study. Tech Coloproctol 19:455-459

[37] Karlović D, Kršul D, Bačić Đ, Zelić M. Video-assisted anal fistula treatment in combination with ligation of the intersphincteric fistula tract in the treatment of complex transsphincteric fistulas - a video vignette. Colorectal Dis. 2020 Sep;22(9):1204-1205. doi: 10.1111/codi.15050.

[38] Yao Y-B, Xiao C-F, Wang Q-T, Zhou H, Dong Q-J, Cao Y-Q, Wang C. AAFT plus FiLaC™: a combined procedure for complex anal fistula. Tech Coloproctol. 2021 Jan 21. doi: 10.1007/s10151-021-02411-0. Online ahead of print.

[39] Ellis CN. Outcomes with the use of bioprosthetic grafts to reinforce the ligation of the intersphincteric fistula tract (BioLIFT procedure) for the management of complex anal fistulas. Dis Colon Rectum 2010 Oct;53(10):1361e4

[40] Han JG, Yi BQ, Wang ZJ, Zheng Y, Cui JJ, Yu XQ, et al. Ligation of the intersphincteric fistula tract plus a bioprosthetic anal fistula plug (LIFT-Plug): a new technique for fistula-in-ano. Colorectal Dis 2013 May;15(5):582e6.

[41] Sileri P, Boehm G, Franceschilli L, Giorgi F, Perrone F, Stolfi C,et al. Collagen matrix injection combined with flap repair for complex anal fistula. Colorectal Dis. 2012 Dec;14(Suppl. 3): 24e8.

[42] La Torre F, Nicolai AP. Clinical use of micronized purified flavonoid fraction for treatment of symptoms after hemorrhoidectomy: results of a randomized, controlled, clinical trial. Dis *Colon Rectum*. 2004 May;47(5):704-710.

Chapter 4

Pathophysiology, Natural History and Approaches to Treatment and Prevention of Radiation Proctitis

Eng (Eric) Kiat Yeoh

Abstract

Chronic radiation proctitis (CRP), characterized by increased frequency and urgency of defecation, fecal incontinence and rectal bleeding, is an under-estimated cause of morbidity after pelvic irradiation for urological and gynecological malignant diseases. Despite improvements in radiotherapy technology, 90% of patients have persistent long term symptoms and 50% of all patients report impairment of quality of life after pelvic radiotherapy. Research by an Australian group of clinician scientists, including prospective, longitudinal and retrospective studies as well as a randomized trial of two current approaches used for the treatment of haemorrhagic radiation proctitis over a time span exceeding two decades, have provided important insights into the prevalence, pathophysiology natural history and treatment of CRP. The findings have important implications for the management and amelioration if not prevention of CRP. Data from 4 selected studies conducted by the Australian group, each characterizing changes in anorectal function and anal sphincteric morphology, are first presented. This is followed by discussion of how the findings have led to the development of more rational therapeutic interventions for CRP and how novel approaches designed to reduce the prevalence of CRP when combined could lead to its elimination in the foreseeable future.

Keywords: Pelvic cancer, radiotherapy, anorectal physiology, haemorrhagic proctitis, quality of life

1. Introduction

Among the estimated 300,000 patients per year worldwide undergoing radiotherapy for pelvic malignant diseases such as carcinoma of the uterine cervix and corpus, bladder and prostate, nine out of 10 will develop a permanent change in their bowel habit [1]. Furthermore, this UK group and an Australian group of clinician scientists have independently reported that 50% of all patients report an adverse impact on activities of daily living (ADL) after pelvic radiotherapy [1, 2].

The radiation induced bowel symptoms which have the greatest adverse effect on ADL are anorectal symptoms such as increased frequency and urgency of defecation, fecal incontinence and rectal bleeding collectively referred to as Chronic Radiation Proctitis (CRP) [1–3].

IntechOpen

The prevalence of CRP is uncertain. Studies using physician based questionnaires such as the Radiation Therapy Oncology Group (RTOG) scales report a prevalence of only 5–10% [4]. However, because these scales do not evaluate common anorectal symptoms such as urgency of defecation and fecal incontinence, physician based scales probably under-estimate the prevalence of CRP. In support of this, studies that have included patient-based questionnaires such as the Late Effect Normal Tissue – Subjective Objective Management Analytic (LENT – SOMA) scales have reported that up to 78% of patients have persistent anorectal symptoms after radiotherapy for prostate carcinoma [5–9]. Although persistent anorectal symptoms impair the daily activities of 50% of all patients 5 years after pelvic radiotherapy, the pathophysiology of anorectal dysfunction has not been fully characterized and its treatment is unsatisfactory. Previous physiological studies in patients with anorectal dysfunction after radiotherapy have been limited either by methodological inadequacies [10] or lack of follow-up studies beyond 2 years [11, 12].

The rationale for the selection of each of the 4 listed studies for discussion in this chapter are provided under the sub-headings below:

1. Pathophysiology and natural history of anorectal sequelae following radiation therapy for carcinoma of the prostate [2]

   In view of the limitations of previous physiological studies of anorectal function after radiotherapy for prostate carcinoma, 5 year data from an Australian prospective, longitudinal study of a subset of patients who participated in a Phase III randomized trial comparing a 4 week course of (hypofractionated) radiotherapy with the then conventional 6.5 week schedule of radiotherapy for carcinoma of the prostate [13] will first be presented.

2. A retrospective study of the effects of pelvic irradiation for gynecological cancer on anorectal function [14]

   As at least a third of patients, who have had pelvic radiotherapy for gynecological cancer are reported to suffer significant radiation bowel sequelae [1], anorectal function data from the above retrospective study will be presented next.

3. Argon Plasma Coagulation Therapy versus Topical Formalin for intractable rectal bleeding and anorectal dysfunction after radiation therapy for prostate carcinoma [15]

   As rectal bleeding is the second most common reason for referral to a gastroenterologist after pelvic radiotherapy even though it impairs the ADL's of only 6% of patients [1], data from the only randomized trial of two current approaches used in the treatment of haemorrhagic radiation proctitis above will follow.

4. Pudendal nerve injury impairs anorectal function and health related quality of life measures ≥2 years after 3D conformal radiotherapy for prostate cancer [16]

   Previous studies of the pathophysiology of anorectal dysfunction after radiotherapy for carcinoma of the prostate including our own have implicated weakness of the external anal sphincter (EAS) and internal anal sphincter (IAS), decreased rectal compliance, increased rectal sensitivity and faster distal colonic transit [2, 17, 18]. The underlying pathogenesis proposed for the observed changes in anorectal dysmotility is either myogenic or neurogenic. However, as muscle tissue particularly striated muscle constituting the EAS is more resistant to radiation damage than neural tissue [2], evidence of pudendal nerve injury after radiotherapy for prostate cancer is presented in the above study [16]. In addition, the editorial accompanying the publication states that the findings show the way forward for the restoration of bowel health of patients who have been adversely affected following pelvic radiotherapy for urological and gynecological malignant diseases [19].

2. Eligibility criteria, experimental protocol, data presentation and interpretation of the studies selected for presentation in this chapter

2.1 Pathophysiology and natural history of anorectal sequelae following radiation therapy for carcinoma of the prostate

2.1.1 Subject selection criteria

The 34 patients, median age = 68 (range 54–79) years, selected for the above study met the following eligibility criteria:

i. Were part of the 217 total patient population participating in a previous Phase III randomized trial of two radiation dose schedules [13]

ii. Have completed (7) serial evaluations (before radiotherapy, at 1 month and at 1 yearly intervals to 5 years after completion of radiotherapy) of anorectal function using the same manometric assembly

iii. Have not needed treatment intervention likely to influence anorectal function such as a constant requirement for antidiarrhoeal medication and argon plasma coagulation therapy (APC) for rectal bleeding

iv. Have provided signed informed consent

Of the total patient population of 217 patients, 86 patients (57 completed two serial evaluations of anorectal function using an earlier manometric assembly which meant that later serial measurements were no longer comparable, 5 started radiotherapy before baseline evaluation and 24 patients died before 5 years), failed to meet eligibility criterion (ii), 12 patients, who required APC for rectal bleeding after radiotherapy, failed eligibility criterion (iii) and 85 patients, who withdrew consent for anorectal manometry after radiotherapy because of distant domicile from the laboratory, failed eligibility criterion (iv).

2.1.2 Experimental protocol

Each of the 34 patients meeting all eligibility criteria for the study underwent evaluations of (i) gastrointestinal symptoms (modified LENT-SOMA scales including effect on activities of daily living (ADL), (ii) anorectal motor and sensory function (manometry with a perfused sleeve and multiport assembly incorporating a highly compliant polyethylene bag in the rectum) and (iii) anal sphincteric morphology (endoanal ultrasound) before radiotherapy and at 1 month, then yearly for 5 years after completion of radiotherapy.

2.1.3 Data presentation and interpretation

Total GI symptom scores increased after radiotherapy and remained above baseline levels at 5 years (**Table 1**). At this time, 48% of patients reported impairment of ADL [2].

The prevalence of persistent urgency of defaecation (44%) was doubled that of rectal bleeding (21%) at 5 years. The % of patients free from the risk of urgency of defecation was significantly less than that of rectal bleeding (**Figure 1**).

All measures of anorectal motor function remained below baseline levels at 5 years (**Table 2**). Furthermore, anal pressures in response to voluntary squeeze and increased intra-abdominal pressure progressively decreased after radiotherapy.

The volume for first perception of rectal distension and that associated with the desire to defaecate both decreased after radiotherapy although only threshold

	Baseline	1 mo	1 y	2 y	3 y	4 y	5 y	ANOVA P value
Stool frequency	0(0–2)	1(0–2)	1(0–2)	1(0–2)	1(0–1)	1(0–2)	1(0–1)	0.05
Stool Consistency	0(0–1)	0(0–2)	0(0–2)	0(0–2)	0(0–2)	0(0–1)	0(0–2)	ns
Rectal Pain	0(0–1)	0(0–3)	0(0–1)	0(0–1)	0(0–1)	0(0–1)	0(0–2)	<.01
Rectal mucous discharge	0(0–2)	0(0–4)	0(0–3)	0(0–3)	0(0–3)	0(0–3)	0(0–3)	<.01
Urgency of defecation	0(0–3)	0(0–4)	1(0–3)	1(0–3)	1(0–4)	1(0–3)	1(0–3)	ns
Rectal bleeding	0(0–2)	0(0–2)	0(0–2)	0(0–3)	0(0–3)	0(0–2)	0(0–4)	ns
Total GI symptom	2(0–4)	3(0–10)	3(0–9)*	3(0-9)*	3(0-7)†	3(0–9)*	3(0-9)*	<.01

Abbreviations: *ANOVA, analysis of variance; GI, gastrointestinal; ns, not significant.*

**P < .05 Compared with baseline.*

†P < .01 Compared with baseline.

From Yeoh et al. [2], with permission.

Table 1.
Median (range) anorectal symptoms at baseline and 1 month, annually to 5 years after radiation therapy for prostate carcinoma.

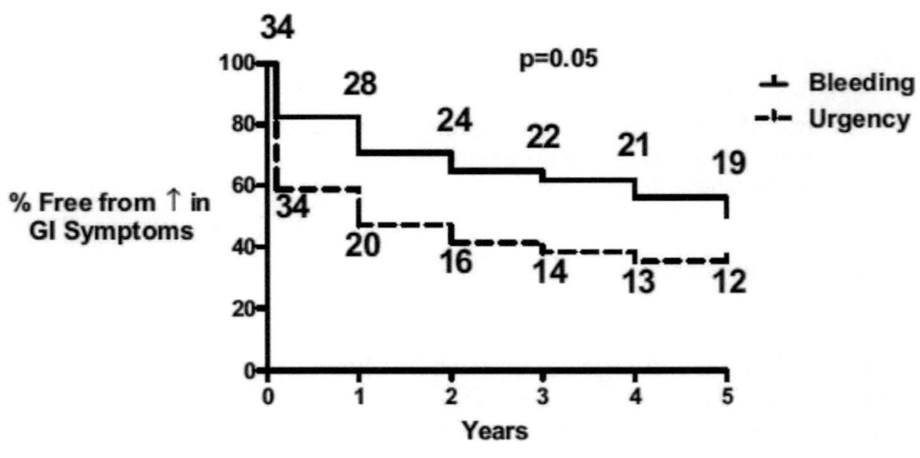

Figure 1.
Percent of patients free from urgency of defaecation vs. rectal bleeding 5 years after radiation therapy. GI = gastrointestinal. (From Yeoh et al. [2], with permission).

DOI: http://dx.doi.org/10.5772/intechopen.99269

	Baseline	1 mo	1 y	2y	3y	4y	5y	ANOVA *P* Value
Basal pressure (mm Hg)	65 ± 3	63 ± 3	59 ± 3	60 ± 3	$54 \pm 3^{\dagger}$	57 ± 3	$56 \pm 3^{*}$	<.001
Squeeze Pressure (mm Hg)	128 ± 10	126 ± 9	$106 \pm 6^{*}$	$105 \pm 6^{\dagger}$	$104 \pm 5^{\dagger}$	$103 \pm 6^{\dagger}$	$99 \pm 6^{\ddagger}$	<.0001
Increased intra-abdominal Pressure (mm Hg)	104 ± 5	99 ± 4	96 ± 5	99 ± 5	94 ± 4	92 ± 5	$90 \pm 5^{*}$	<.05
First Perception (mL)	24 ± 2	$17 \pm 1^{\dagger}$	$17 \pm 1^{\dagger}$	$15 \pm 1^{\ddagger}$	$14 \pm 1^{\ddagger}$	$14 \pm 1^{\ddagger}$	$15 \pm 1^{\ddagger}$	<.0001
Desire to defecate (mL)	63 ± 7	44 ± 5	58 ± 6	$40 \pm 4^{*}$	42 ± 3	51 ± 6	60 ± 8	<.0001
Rectal compliance(mL)	8.2 ± 0.6	7.4 ± 0.5	6.8 ± 0.7	$6.2 \pm 0.8^{*}$	6.4 ± 0.7	$5.7 \pm 0.5^{\dagger}$	$5.5 \pm 0.6^{\dagger}$	<0.001
IAS thickness(mm)	2.4 ± 0.1	2.2 ± 0.1	2.2 ± 0.2	2.1 ± 0.1	2.1 ± 0.1	2.2 ± 01	2.3 ± 0.1	ns
EAS thickness (mm)	10.7 ± 0.5	11.2 ± 0.5	11.2 ± 0.5	10.5 ± 0.5	10.3 ± 0.7	9.6 ± 0.4	9.7 ± 0.7	Ns

Abbreviations: *ANOVA, analysis of variance; EAS, external and sphincter; IAS, internal anal sphincter; ns, not significant; SE, Standard error.*

$^{*}P < .05$ compared with baseline.

$^{\dagger}P < .01$ compared with baseline.

$^{\ddagger}P < .0001$ compared with baseline.
From Yeoh et al. [2], with permission.

Table 2.
Mean (± SE) anal pressurres (sleeve), rectal sensory volumes, rectal compliance, and anal sphincter thickness at baseline and I month, annually to 5 years after radiation therapy for prostate carcinoma.

volumes for sensory perception at 5 years remained below those recorded at baseline (**Table 2**). Rectal compliance progressively reduced with time after radiotherapy and remained persistently lower at 5 years compared with that recorded at baseline **Table 2**).

Radiotherapy had no effect on the thicknesses of the IAS and EAS (**Table 2**).

There were no differences in any of the GI symptoms nor in any anorectal functional and anal sphincteric morphological measurements between patients randomized to the 2 radiation dose schedules.

5 years after radiotherapy for carcinoma of the prostate, persistent GI symptoms continue to have a significant impact on ADL of almost 50% of all patients. At this time, the prevalence of urgency of defecation (44%) was doubled that of rectal bleeding (21%). Increased GI symptoms after radiotherapy were associated with progressive or persistent reductions of basal anal pressures and pressures in response to voluntary squeeze and increased intra-abdominal pressures, rectal compliance and volumes of sensory perception and desire to defaecate. These physiological changes, which suggest weakness of the IAS and EAS as well as stiffness of the rectal wall and consequent increased rectal sensitivity, are the pathogenetic basis for anorectal dysfunction after radiotherapy for carcinoma of the prostate. The etiology of the motility changes is likely to be neurogenic in the intrinsic neural network in the bowel wall and/or extrinsic nerve supply such as the pudendal nerves since muscle tissue, particularly striated muscle is more resistant to radiation damage.

2.2 A retrospective study of the effects of pelvic irradiation for gynecological cancer on anorectal function

2.2.1 Subject selection criteria

The 15 patients, median age = 67 (range 47–84) years, selected for the study met the following eligibility criteria:

i. Were part of the 33 total patient population who completed pelvic and abdominal irradiation 5–10 years earlier for carcinoma of the cervix (n = 30) and endometrium (n = 3) who participated in a previous prospective longitudinal study of changes in gastrointestinal function after pelvic radiotherapy [20]

ii. Had not needed treatment intervention likely to influence anorectal function such as a constant requirement for antidiarrhoeal medication

iii. Had provided signed informed consent

Of the original total patient population of 33 patients, 6 had died and 2 had been lost to follow-up since completing the previous study [20]. The 25 remaining patients were invited to participate in this study, 10 refused including two patients who had intermittent episodes of rectal bleeding.

9 healthy females, median age = 63 (range 41–70) years served as control subjects.

2.2.2 Experimental protocol

The following parameters were assessed in each subject: (i) anorectal symptoms (questionnaire), (ii) anorectal motor and sensory function (manometry with a perfused sleeve and multiport assembly incorporating a highly compliant latex balloon in the rectum and concurrent electromyography of the anal sphincters) and (iii) anal sphincteric morphology (endoanal ultrasound).

2.2.3 Data presentation and interpretation

Total anorectal symptom scores was significantly greater in the patients compared with the control subjects (**Table 3**). Urgency of defaecation was the most frequent symptom, occurring in 10 of the 15 patients (67%). Four of these patients also had fecal incontinence [14]. Urgency of defecation in eight of the 10 patients resulted in changes in lifestyle such that the patients were either housebound or could only go out if there was a toilet nearby [14].

Basal minimum pressures just proximal to the anal canal (4 cm from the anal verge) were lower in the patients than the control subjects ($p = 0.05$) and there was a trend for lower basal maximum pressures at the same site ($p = 0.07$, **Table 4**).

Squeeze pressures measured at the sleeve sensor and at 4 cm from the anal verge were lower in the patients ($p < 0.05$, **Table 4**) and were below the control range in five patients [14].

In the patients, residual anorectal pressures measured at 0.5 cm from the anal verge in response to rectal distension were less ($p \leq 0.05$) at volumes of 10 ml, 20 ml and 40 ml (**Table 5**). There was also a trend for lower pressures in the patients at the highest (100 ml) volume ($p = 0.09$).

A higher proportion of patients perceived the desire to defecate at lower rectal volumes than the controls ($p < 0.05$, **Figure 2**). The slope of the pressure/volume relationship associated with rectal distension volumes of 20 ml, 40 ml, 60 ml, 100 ml and overall slope was greater in the patients ($p < 0.05$, $p < 0.01$, $p < 0.001$, $p < 0.001$ and $p < 0.05$ respectively than the controls, suggesting that rectal compliance was reduced in the patients (**Figure 3**).

There were no differences in external anal sphincteric electrical activity between the patients and control subjects in response to voluntary squeeze and blowing up a party balloon (**Table 4**). Either basal pressures, pressures generated in response to rectal distension, voluntary squeeze and blowing up a party balloon were below the control range in 14 of the 15 patients, including all 10 patients with anorectal symptoms [14].

There was no difference in mean EAS and IAS thickness between the two groups (**Table 4**) nor difference in thicknesses of the EAS and IAS in patients with and without urgency of defaecation [14].

The data indicate that (i) urgency of defaecation, occurring in 10 out 15 (67%) of patients 10–15 years after pelvic irradiation for gynecological cancer resulted in eight of the 10 patients being either housebound or only able to go out if there was a toilet nearby, (ii) anorectal symptoms were associated with multiple parameters of anorectal dysfunction including weakness of the external anal sphincter, stiffness of the rectal wall and consequent increase in rectal sensitivity.

2.3 Argon plasma coagulation therapy versus topical formalin for intractable rectal bleeding and anorectal dysfunction after radiation therapy for prostate carcinoma

2.3.1 Subject selection criteria

The 30 patients, median age = 72 (range 49–87) years selected for the study met the following eligibility criteria:

i. Had completed radiotherapy for prostate carcinoma ≥6 months previously

Parameters/ subjects	Fecal incontinence			Urgency of defecation	Symptom score*	No. of bowel actions/ week*	No. of babies*	No. with large babies	No. who had forceps
	Diurnal	Nocturnal	Both						
Patients	3/15	1/15	10/15	10/15†	3‡(0-8)	13(13-28)	3(0–12)	4/15	3/15
Normal	0/9	0/9	1/9	1/9	0(0)	7(7–14)	3(0–4)	2/9	2/9

Median (range).

†$P < 0.01$.

‡$P < 0.001$ *Compared to normals.*
From Yeoh et al. [14], with permission.

Table 3.
Anorectal symptoms including bowel habits and obstetric parameters in patients and normal subjects.

	Normal	Patients	p-Value
EAS (mm)	8.8 ± 0.5	9 ± 0.4	0.78
IAS (mm)	2.8 ± 0.2	2.3 ± 0.2	0.65
B_{max} (mmHg)			
Anal 0.5 cm†	64 ± 12.5	45.1 ± 5.5	0.13
Sleeve	58.7 ± 6.3	53.3 ± 6.2	0.58
Anorectal 4 cm†	22 ± 5.8	12.1 ± 1.9	0.07
B_{min} (mmHg)			
Anal 0.5 cm†	32.2 ± 8.2	33.1 ± 5.0	0.93
Sleeve	44.3 ± 5.6	41.5 ± 5.9	0.75
Anorectal 4 cm†	14.1 ± 3.3	8.1 ± 1.0	0.05
Voluntary squeeze (mmHg)			
Anal 0.5 cm†	108.2 ± 21.6	70 ± 10.0	0.08
Sleeve	103 ± 10.2	68.1 ± 7.2	0.01
Anorectal 4 cm†	26.4 ± 4.6	16.3 ± 1.8	0.03
Change EMG activity (mm)	6.7 ± 1.8	6.2 ± 0.8	0.75
Blowing up a party balloon			
Anal 0.5 cm†	61.8 ± 11.6	49.4 ± 0.8	0.35
Sleeve	70.1 ± 7.5	65.6 ± 7.8	0.7
Anorectal 4 cm†	35.8 ± 3.7	30.5 ± 2.2	0.21
Change EMG activity (mm)	3.8 ± 1.0	3.4 ± 0.5	0.75

**Data are mean values ±SEM.*
†Manometric port distances from anal verge.
From Yeoh et al. [14], with permission.

Table 4.
Maximum thickness of IAS and EAS and anorectal pressures (basal, in response to voluntary squeeze and blowing up a party balloon).

ii. had intractable rectal bleeding (defined as ≥1x per week and/or requiring blood transfusions) attributed to CRP at colonoscopy

iii. had no constant requirement for medications likely to influence anorectal motility such as opioid analgesics and anti-diarrhoeal agents

iv. Had provided signed informed consent

2.3.2 Experimental protocol

The 30 eligible patients were randomized to treatment with APC (n = 17) or topical formalin (n = 13).

Each patient underwent evaluations of (i) anorectal symptoms (validated questionnaires including modified LENT-SOMA scales for GI symptoms and visual analogue scales for rectal bleeding), (ii) anorectal motor and sensory function (manometry with a perfused sleeve and multiport assembly incorporating a highly compliant polyethylene bag in the rectum) and (iii) anal sphincteric morphology (endoanal ultrasound) before and after the treatment endpoint (defined as reduction

	Normal	Patients	*p*-Value
RD 10			
Anal 0.5 cm†	47.3 ± 10.8	27.7 ± 4.1	0.05
Sleeve	41.6 ± 7.9	30.8 ± 4.3	0.2
Anorectal 4 cm†	8.6 ± 1.5	8.1 ± 0.6	0.77
RD 20			
Anal 0.5 cm*	40.2 ± 5.9	24.6 ± 3.0	0.02
Sleeve	34.2 ± 7.5	26.7 ± 3.4	0.31
Anorectal 4 cm†	10.4 ± 1.9	9.1 ± 0.7	0.44
RD 40			
Anal 0.5 cm†	35.6 ± 4.8	23.1 ± 3.2	0.04
Sleeve	30.2 ± 4.7	30.3 ± 3.7	0.99
Anorectal 4 cm†	12 ± 1.7	10.2 ± 0.8	0.3
RD 60			
Anal 0.5 cm†	43.5 ± 12.0	29.9 ± 7.6	0.33
Sleeve	31.1 ± 6.0	30.9 ± 4.0	0.98
Anorectal 4 cm†	17 ± 2.5	12.8 ± 1.3	0.12
RD 100			
Anal 0.5 cm†	43.8 ± 11.8	20.1 ± 6.3	0.09
Sleeve	30.5 ± 6.9	35.5 ± 5.7	0.59
Anorectal 4 cm†	13.7 ± 2.5	19 ± 6.6	0.49

**Data are mean values ± SEM.*

†Manometric port distances from anal verge.
From Yeoh et al. [14], with permission.

Table 5.
*Residual anorectal pressures in response to rectal distension (RD), with 10 ml, 20 ml, 40 ml, 60 ml and 100 ml**

of rectal bleeding to 1x per month or better, reduction of visual analogue scales to ≤25 mm, no longer needing blood transfusions). Cross-over to the other therapy was allowed if the treatment endpoint was not reached after 4 treatment sessions.

2.3.3 Data presentation and interpretation

Rectal bleeding was controlled in twenty nine of the 30 patients after a median of 2 treatment sessions of APC or topical formalin. One patient, initially treated with APC, failed after 4 treatment sessions but achieved control after 3 sessions of cross-over topical formalin, Control of rectal bleeding was evidenced by reductions of its frequency to ≤1x per month, VAS ≤ 25 mm (**Figures 4** and **5**, **Table 6**) and no further requirement for blood transfusion in the 2 patients (1 each in APC and topical formalin groups) needing this before randomization to therapy.

The durability of control of rectal bleeding by APC and topical formalin was evidenced by only 1 patient in each group needing further therapy after a median (range) follow-up of 111 (29–170) months [15].

No effect on other anorectal symptoms, such as increased frequency and urgency of defecation and fecal incontinence, was observed (**Table 6**).

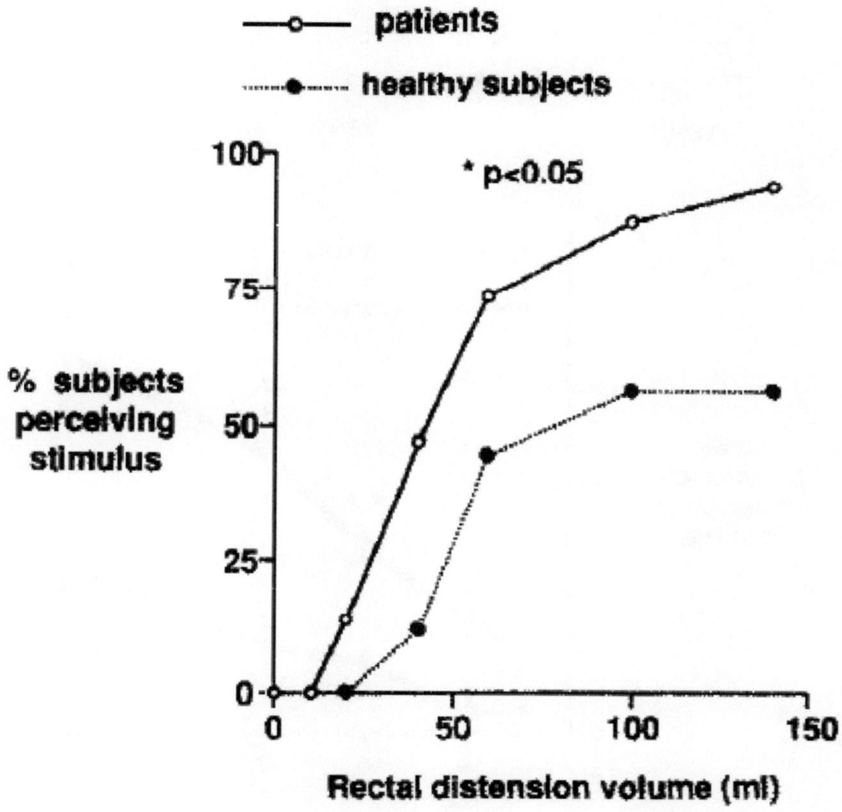

Figure 2.
Rectal volumes at which patients and normal subjects felt desire to defaecate. (From Yeoh et al. [14], with permission).

Other than a reduction in rectal compliance and volumes of sensory perception after APC, no effects on parameters of anorectal function and anal sphincteric morphology were observed (**Table 7**).

APC and topical formalin had comparable efficacy in the durable control of rectal bleeding associated with chronic radiation proctitis but no beneficial effect on anorectal dysfunction.

2.4 Pudendal nerve injury impairs anorectal function and health related quality of life measures ≥2 years after 3D conformal radiotherapy for prostate cancer

2.4.1 Subject selection criteria

The 25 patients, median age = 76 (range 64–83) years, selected for the above study met the following eligibility criteria:

i. Were part of 80 patients still attending follow up ≥2 years after 3D conformal radiotherapy ± high dose rate brachytherapy (HDR) for localized prostate carcinoma under the supervision of the same tertiary institution based Radiation Oncologist

ii. Had no clinical or radiological signs of relapse

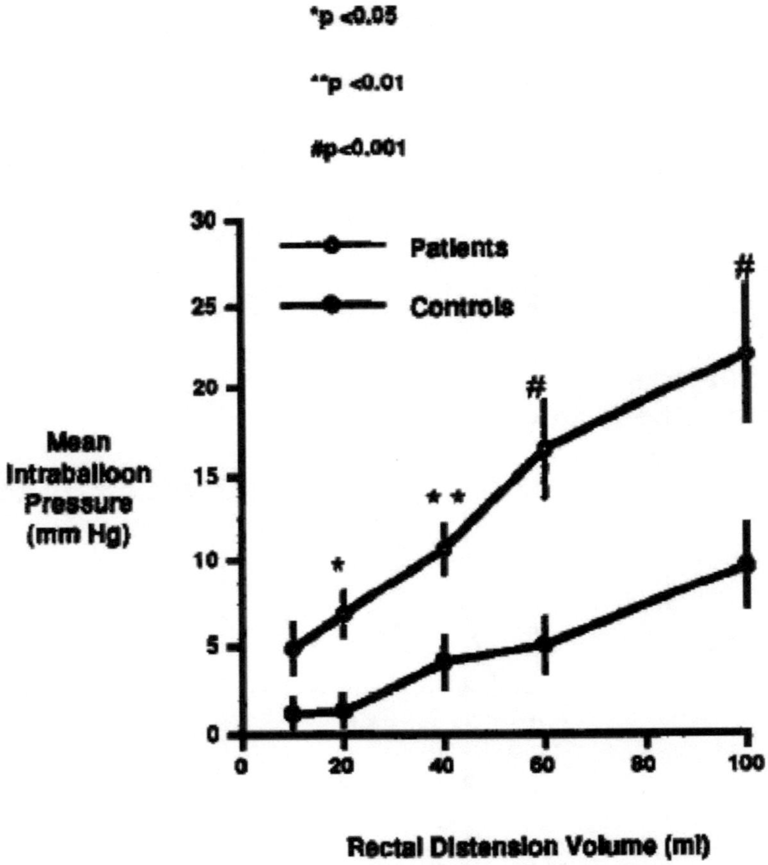

Figure 3.
Pressure/volume relationship in patients and controls associated with rectal distension (from Yeoh et al. [14], with permission).

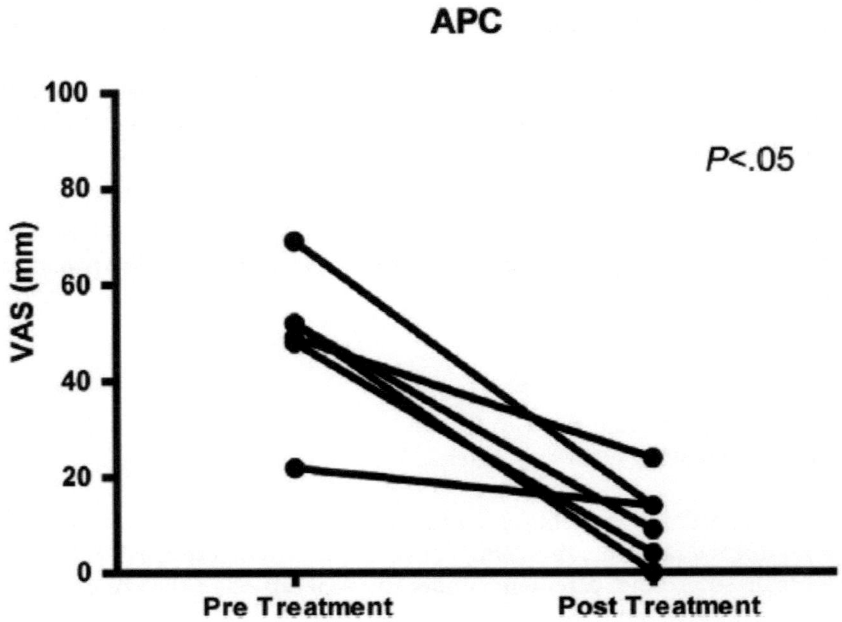

Figure 4.
Visual analogue scale (VAS) before (pre) and after (post) APC treatment. (From Yeoh et al. [15], with permission).

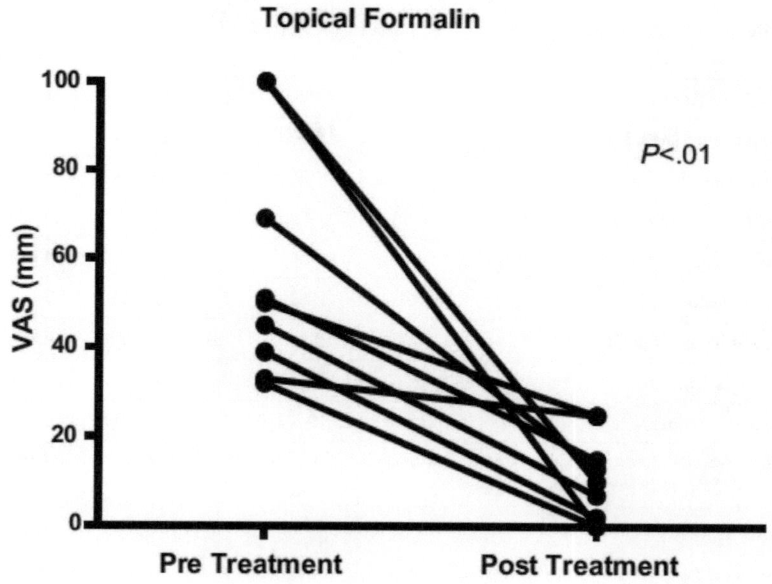

Figure 5.
Visual analogue scale (VAS) before (pre) and after (post) topical formalin treatment. (From Yeoh et al. [15], with permission).

Wilcoxon rank sum test for listed parameters	Before APC	After APC	*P*	Before formalin	After formalin	*P*
No. of bowel actions per week	14(4–39)	16(7–46)	NS	16(3–32)	14(4–42)	NS
Fecal incontinence scores	0(0–10)	0(0–4)	NS	0(0–3)	0(0–2)	NS
Urgency of defecation scores	3(0–6)	4(0–6)	NS	4(0–6)	4(0–6)	NS
Rectal bleeding scores	3(1–4)	1(0–2)	.0001	3(2–4)	1(0–2)	.001
VAS for rectal bleeding (mm)	52(22–75)	14(0–34)	.05	50(32–100)	13(0–25)	.01

Abbreviations: NS, not significant; VAS, visual analogue scale; Values are median (range).
From Yeoh et al. [15], with permission.

Table 6.
Effect on anorectal symptom parameters of argon plasma coagulation therapy (APC) and topical formalin treatment.

iii. Had not needed treatment intervention likely to influence anorectal function such as a constant requirement for antidiarrhoeal medication nor argon plasma coagulation therapy (APC) for rectal bleeding

iv. Had provided signed informed consent

Of the 80 patients invited to participate in the study, 48 refused, 7 were ineligible (6 had APC for rectal bleeding, 1 patient had received 2D radiotherapy).

25 age matched patients with localized prostate carcinoma in a recent randomized radiotherapy study served as control subjects [21].

2.4.2 Experimental protocol

Each subject underwent the following evaluations: (i) GI symptoms (modified LENT-SOMA scales), (ii) generic and disease specific HRQoL measures (EORTC QLQ-C30 and EORTC QLQ-PR25 questionnaires), (iii) anorectal motor and sensory function

Student's *t* test for listed parameters	Before APC	After APC	*P*	Before formalian	After formalin	*P*
Basal pressure (mm Hg)	52 ± 4	58 ± 2	NS	58 ± 5	51 ± 3	NS
Squeeze pressure (mm Hg)	95 ± 8	100 ± 9	NS	97 ± 6	89 ± 6	NS
Increased intra-abdominal pressure (mm Hg)	85 ± 4	88 ± 6	NS	87 ± 6	92 ± 6	NS
Threshold of perception pressure (mm Hg)	16 ± 1	17 ± 1	NS	18 ± 2	19 ± 2	NS
Threshold of perception volume (mL)	19 ± 2	14 ± 1	.05	17 ± 3	14 ± 1	NS
Desire to defecate (mL)	61 ± 10	48 ± 5	NS	45 ± 11	47 ± 9	NS
Rectal compliance (mm Hg/mL)	4.2 ± 0.4	3.3 ± 0.4	.01	8.1 ± 2.6	4.3 ± 0.7	NS
IAS thickness (mm)	2.4 ± 0.1	2.2 ± 0.1	NS	2.4 ± 0.1	2.4 ± 0.2	NS
EAS thickness (mm)	10.0 ± 0.5	10.5 ± 0.5	NS	11.5 ± 0.6	11.2 ± 0.6	NS

Abbreviations: *NS, not significant; EAS, external anal sphincter; IAS, internal anal sphincter; Values are mean ± SE.*
From Yeoh et al. [15], with permission.

Table 7.
Effect on anorectal function and anal sphincteric morphology parameters of argon plasma coagulation therapy (APC) and topical formalin treatment.

(manometry with a perfused sleeve and multiport assembly incorporating a highly compliant polyethylene bag in the rectum), (iv) pudendal nerve function (terminal motor nerve latency) and (v) anal sphincteric morphology (endoanal ultrasound).

The data of the 25 patients ≥2 years after 3D conformal radiotherapy for prostate cancer were compared with the before radiotherapy (baseline) data of the 25 control subjects.

The data of symptomatic (defined as patients with Total LENT-SOMA GI symptom scores ≥5, n = 13) and asymptomatic (defined as patients with Total LENT-SOMA GI symptom scores ≤4, n = 12) patients among the 25 patients ≥2 years after 3D conformal radiotherapy were also compared.

2.4.3 Data presentation and interpretation

2.4.3.1 Comparisons of modified LENT-SOMA GI symptoms and EORTC HRQoL measures

Patients in this study had significantly higher modified LENT – SOMA frequency and urgency of defaecation, rectal bleeding and mucous discharge scores ≥2 years after 3D conformal radiotherapy compared to the age matched control subjects before radiotherapy (**Table 8**). The patients also had worse (lower) EORTC QLQ-C30 cognitive functioning scores and worse (higher) EORTC QLQ-PR25 bowel symptom scores compared to the controls before radiotherapy (**Table 8**).

Symptomatic patients had significantly higher (i) modified LENT SOMA urgency of defaecation and rectal bleeding scores and (ii) EORTC QLQ-PR25 bowel and urinary symptom scores compared with asymptomatic patients (**Table 9**). Symptomatic patients also had worse (lower) EORTC QLQ-C30 social and emotional functional as well as global health scores compared to asymptomatic patients (**Table 9**).

2.4.3.2 Comparisons of anorectal and pudendal nerve function data and anal sphincter morphology measurements

All parameters of anorectal motor and sensory function except for threshold volumes for sensory perception were significantly worse ≥2 years after 3D

LENTSOMA	Whole Patient Group	Age Matched Patient Group	p value
Frequency	1 (0–3)	0 (0–1)	<0.01
Diarrhea	0 (0–2)	0 (0–1)	ns
Pain	0 (0–2)	0 (0–2)	ns
Mucous	0 (0–3)	0 (0–1)	<0.05
Urgency	2 (0–4)	1 (0–2)	<0.001
Bleeding	0 (0–3)	0 (0–0)	<0.0001
EORTC HRQoL QLQ-C30			
Physical Functioning	100 (60–100)	93 (47–100)	ns
Role Functioning	100 (50–100)	100 (17–100)	ns
Emotional Functioning	83 (58–100)	83 (67–100)	ns
Cognitive Functioning	83 (50–100)	83 (67–100)	<0.05
Social Functioning	100 (50–100)	100 (33–100)	ns
Global Health Status	83 (17–100)	83 (33–100)	ns
Dyspnoea	0 (0–33)	0 (0–100)	ns
Insomnia	33 (0–100)	33 (0–100)	ns
Appetite Loss	0 (0–33)	0 (0–33)	ns
Nausea And Vomiting	0 (0–17)	0 (0–33)	ns
Constipation	0 (0–67)	0 (0–67)	ns
Diarrhea	0 (0–100)	0 (0–33)	ns
Fatigue	22 (0–44)	22 (0–78)	ns
Pain	0 (0–100)	0 (0–100)	ns
Financial Difficulty	0 (0–33)	0 (0–67)	ns
EORTC QLQ-PR25			
Urinary Symptoms	17 (0–58)	13 (0–67)	ns
Bowel Symptoms	8 (0–42)	0 (0–17)	<0.01
Hormonal Treatment-Related Symptoms	6 (0–50)	6 (0–50)	ns

Abbreviations: *ns, not significant; LENT-SOMA, late effect normal tissue – subjective objective management analytic; EORTC, European Organization for Research and Treatment of Cancer; QLQ, quality of life questionnaire; Values are median (range).*
From Yeoh et al. [16], with permission.

Table 8.
Comparison of modified LENT-SOMA GI symptoms and EORTC generic (QOL-C30) and disease specific (QLQ-PR25) HRQoL data between whole patient group and age matched patients before radiotherapy.

conformal radiotherapy compared to age matched control subjects before radiotherapy (**Table 10**).

Unilateral and/or bilateral pudendal nerve responses were delayed in 13/24 (54%) of the patients compared to only 2/20 (10%) aged matched controls before radiotherapy ($p < 0.0001$, data not shown).

The thickness of both IAS and EAS was significantly less in the patients compared to the control subjects before radiotherapy (**Table 10**).

Fecal incontinence scores were worse in the symptomatic compared to the asymptomatic patients but no differences were detected in thickness of either IAS or EAS in the patient sub-groups (**Table 11**).

LENT-SOMA	Symptomatic patients	Asymptomatic patients	*P* Value
Frequency	1(0–3)	1(0–1)	ns
Diarrhea	1(0–2)	0(0–2)	ns
Pain	0(0–2)	0(0–2)	ns
Mucous	1(0–3)	0(0–1)	ns
Urgency	3(1–4)	1(0–4)	<.01
Bleeding	1(0–3)	0(0–1)	<.001
EORTC QLQ-C30			
Physical functioning	87(60–100)	100(73–100)	ns
Role functioning	100(50–100)	100(67–100)	ns
Emotional functioning	75(58–100)	96(67–100)	=.05
Cognitive functioning	83(50–100)	83(67–100)	ns
Social functioning	83(50–100)	100(67–100)	<.001
Global health status	67(50–83)	83(17–100)	<.05
Dyspnea	0(0–33)	0(0–33)	ns
Insomnia	33(0–100)	33(0–33)	ns
Appetite loss	0(0–33)	0(0–0)	ns
Nausea of vomiting	0(0–17)	0(0–17)	ns
Constipation	33(0–67)	33(0–33)	ns
Diarrhea	0(0–100)	0(0–33)	=.05
Fatigue	33(0–44)	11(0–33)	<.05
Pain	0(0–33)	0(0–100)	ns
Financial difficulty	0(0–33)	0(0–0)	ns
EORTC QLQ-PR25			
Urinary symptoms	25(0–58)	10(0–25)	<.05
Bowel symptoms	25(8–42)	0(0–25)	<.001
Hormonal treatment-related symptoms	11(0–50)	6(0–33)	ns

Abbreviations: *ns, not significant; LENT-SOMA, late effect normal tissue – subjective objective management analytic; EORTC, European Organization for Research and Treatment of Cancer; QLQ, quality of life questionnaire; Values are median (range).*
From Yeoh et al. [16], with permission.

Table 9.
Comparison of modified LENT-SOMA GI symptoms and EORTC generic (QOL-C30) and disease specific (QLQ-PR25) HRQoL data between symptomatic and asymptomatic patients.

Unilateral and/or bilateral pudendal nerve responses were delayed in 9/13 (69%) of symptomatic compared to only 4/11 (36%) of asymptomatic patients ($p < 0.0001$, data not shown).

Rectal and anal (i) V40Gy > 65%, (ii) Dmax >60 Gy, (iii) pudendal nerve Dmax >60 Gy and (iv) Anal V60 Gy >40% were associated with a greater prevalence of pudendal nerve function [16].

3D radiotherapy ± high dose rate brachytherapy (HDR) for localized prostate carcinoma impairs functional measures including HRQoL, anorectal and pudendal nerve function ≥2 years after treatment. Radiation dose constraints are proposed for reducing the prevalence of pudendal nerve dysfunction.

ARM	Whole patient group	Age matched patient group	*P* Value
Basal pressure (mmHg)	46 ± 4	63 ± 3	<.01
Squeeze pressure (mmHg)	105 ± 8	154 ± 8	<.0001
↑ Intra-abdominal pressure (mmHg)	82 ± 5	106 ± 5	<.01
IAS (mm)	2.1 ± 0.1	2.6 ± 0.1	<.05
EAS (mm)	8.0 ± 0.3	9.3 ± 0.3	<.01
Threshold perception (mL)	14 ± 1	16 ± 2	ns
Desire to defecate sensation (mL)	68 ± 8	97 ± 9	<.05
Rectal compliance (mL/mmHg)	3.3 ± 0.3	5.1 ± 0.4	<.01
FI score	2(0–8)	0(0–1)	<.001
Urgency score	2(0–6)	0(0–3)	<.001
Number of bowel actions/week	10.5(7–24.5)	7(3.5–21)	<.05

Abbreviations: *ns, not significant; IAS, internal anal sphincter; EAS, external anal sphincter; FI, fecal incontinence; Values are mean ± SE.*
From Yeoh et al. [16], with permission.

Table 10.
Comparison of anorectal function and anal sphincter morphology data between whole patient group and age matched patients before radiotherapy.

ARM	Symptomatic patients	Asymptomatic patients	*P* Value
Basal pressure (mmHg)	42 ± 5	51 ± 6	ns
Squeeze pressure (mmHg)	92 ± 9	119 ± 11	ns
↑ Intra-abdominal pressure (mmHg)	78 ± 7	86 ± 8	ns
IAS (mm)	2.3 ± 0.2	2.1 ± 0.2	ns
EAS (mm)	8.4 ± 0.4	7.6 ± 0.3	ns
Threshold perception (mL)	15 ± 2	13 ± 1	ns
Desire to defecate sensation (mL)	55 ± 8	81 ± 14	ns
Rectal compliance (mL/mmHg)	3.4 ± 0.4	3.2 ± 0.4	ns
FI score	3(0–8)	0(0–3)	<.01
Urgency score	3(0–6)	0(0–5)	ns
Number of bowel actions/week	14(7–24.5)	10.5(7–17.5)	ns

Abbreviations: *ns, not significant; IAS, internal anal sphincter; EAS, external anal sphincter; FI, fecal incontinence; Values are means ± SE.*
From Yeoh et al. [16], with permission.

Table 11.
Comparison of anorectal function and anal sphincter morphology data between symptomatic and asymptomatic patients.

3. Implications and summary of findings of studies and conclusion(s)

The data presented in this chapter, based on studies spanning over two decades examining gastrointestinal effects of pelvic radiotherapy for prostate and gynecological cancer, indicate that despite advances in radiotherapy technology, anorectal dysfunction persist or progressively worsen over a period of 5–10 years after treatment. The multiple deteriorations in anorectal function, consisting of weakness of the anal sphincters, stiffness of the rectal wall and consequent increase in rectal sensitivity, result in ~50% of patients being housebound and only able to go out if there is a toilet nearby. The studies also show that the prevalence of rectal bleeding is half that of urgency of defaecation. In addition, results of the first randomized trial of Argon Plasma Coagulation Therapy versus topical formalin for intractable rectal bleeding after radiotherapy for prostate cancer indicate that durable control is achieved in 94–100% of patients after a median of 2 sessions of either treatment, only 7% of patients requiring re-treatment after a median follow-up of 9 years [15]. In contrast, therapeutic options for anorectal dysfunction are limited to medications such as loperamide and nicardipine based on pathophysiological evaluation of bowel disorders which include chronic radiation proctitis. For example, nicardipine which increases the rectal threshold for desire to defecate in patients with irritable bowel syndrome and reported to be effective in the treatment of urgency of defecation has been proposed for the treatment of urgency of defecation associated with chronic radiation proctitis since threshold volumes for desire to defecate are also reduced in CRP [14]. Similarly, loperamide, by increasing basal anal and squeeze pressures in patients with fecal incontinence of diverse aetiologies including radiation bowel disease, has been proposed for the treatment of fecal incontinence associated with CRP [14]. However, loperamide reduces stool bulk potentially increasing the risk of rectal bleeding and a lower dose than that prescribed for other bowel disorders is recommended [2]. Whilst the most advanced radiation treatment technique of intensity modulated radiation therapy (IMRT) was not used in the studies here, the prevalence of anorectal toxicity after IMRT for prostate cancer has been reported to be 65%, worse or no different from that reported in studies using less advanced treatment techniques including those reported here [1, 2, 6, 14, 16]. A likely explanation for the failure of IMRT to reduce anorectal dysmotility after treatment is that its underlying pathogenesis is damage to neural tissue in the bowel wall and/or the pudendal nerves [2, 16]. As discussed in the editorial accompanying

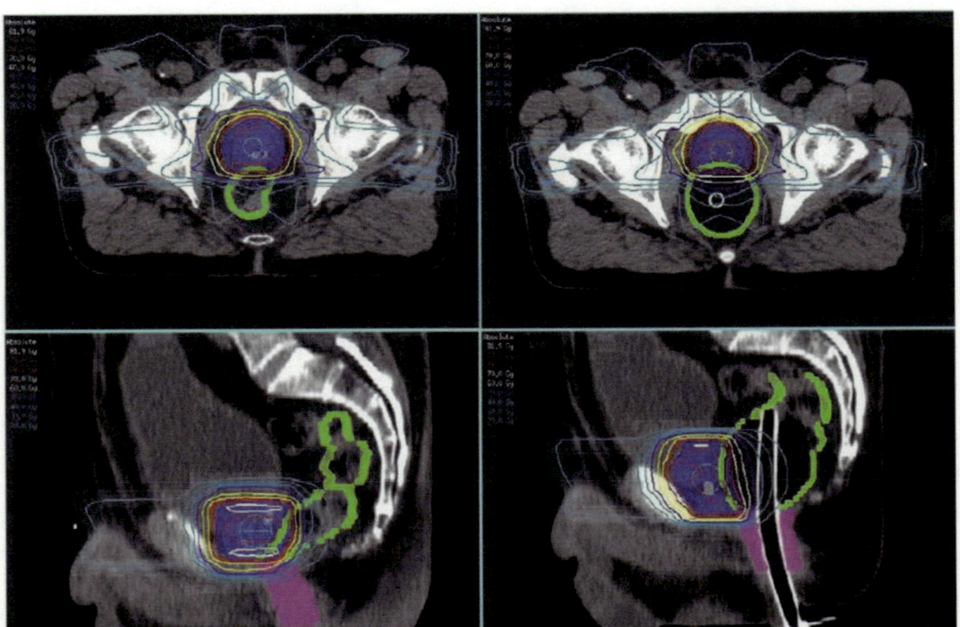

Figure 6.
Transverse (top) and sagittal dose distributions of IMRT plans for prostate cancer without (left) and with (right) endorectal balloon in place. Contours: Rectal wall (green), anal wall (purple). (From Smeenk et al. [5], with permission).

the published findings of the final study of this chapter [19], the pudendal nerves are not considered as normal tissues at risk of radiation damage and therefore could potentially receive the same if not higher doses of radiation as the prostate target of irradiation. Radiation dose constraints for normal tissues at risk including the pudendal nerves have been proposed (Section 2.4 above) and if applied now that IMRT has been adopted almost universally, patients who need pelvic radiotherapy for urological and gynecological cancer can look forward to a future free of distressing bowel morbidity. Furthermore, the daily insertion of endorectal balloons during radiotherapy (**Figure 6**), which have been shown to be very well tolerated and to further reduce radiation exposure of the rectal and anal wall (and the anatomically closely related pudendal nerves) by IMRT [5] means a bowel complication free cure of pelvic malignant disease can be realistically achieved in the foreseeable future.

Acknowledgements

The work reported in this chapter is based on 4 published studies of the effect of radiotherapy for prostate and gynecological cancer on anorectal function. All studies were performed in the Departments of Radiation Oncology, Gastroenterology and Colorectal Surgery, Royal Adelaide Hospital, Australia, affiliated with the University of Adelaide with substantial technical expertise for the performance of pudendal nerve terminal motor latency provided by the Department of Gastroenterology and Surgery, Flinders Medical Centre, Australia, affiliated with Flinders University.

The names of the contributors to the 4 published studies, listed as co-authors in the references section, are acknowledged although none of these co-authors contributed to the writing of this chapter.

Author details

Eng (Eric) Kiat Yeoh
Adelaide Medical School, Faculty of Health and Medical Sciences, University of Adelaide, SA, Australia

*Address all correspondence to: eric.ek.yeoh@gmail.com

References

[1] Andreyev HJN. Gastrointestinal problems after pelvic radiotherapy: Th past, the present and the future. Clin Oncol (R Coll Radiol) 2007; 19:790-799.

[2] Yeoh EK, Holloway RH, Fraser RJ et al. Pathophysiology and natural history of anorectal sequelae following radiation therapy for carcinoma of the prostate. Int J Radiat Oncol Biol Phys 2012; 84(5):e593-e599.

[3] Krol R, Smeenk RJ, van Lin ENJT, Hopman WPM. Impact of late anorectal dysfunction on quality of life after pelvic radiotherapy. Int J Colorectal Dis 2013; 28(4):519-526.

[4] Lawton CA, Won M, Pilepich MV et al. Long term treatment sequelae following external beam radiation for adenocarcinoma of the prostate: analysis of RTOG studies 7506 and 7706. Int J Radiat Oncol Biol Phys 1991; 21:935-939.

[5] Smeenk RJ, Teh BS, Butler B, van Lin ENJT, Kaanders JHAM. Is there a role for endorectal balloons in prostate radiotherapy? A systematic review. Radiother Oncol 2010; 95:277-282.

[6] Putta S, Andreyev HJN. Faecal Incontinence: A late side-effect of pelvic radiotherapy. Clin Oncol (R Coll Radiol) 2005; 17:469-477.

[7] Denham JW, O'Brien PC, Dunstan RH et al. Is there more than one late radiation proctitis syndrome? Radiother Oncol 1999; 51:43-53.

[8] Franklin CIV, Parker CA, Morton KM. Late effects of radiation therapy for prostate carcinoma: the patient's perspective of bladder, bowel and sexual morbidity. Aust Radiol 1998; 42:58-65.

[9] Widmark A, Fransson P, Tavelin B. Self-assessment questionnaire for evaluating urinary and intestinal late side effects after pelvic radiotherapy in patients with prostate cancer compared with an age-matched control population. Cancer 1994; 74:2520-2532.

[10] Varma JS, Smith AN, Busuttil A. Function of the anal sphincters after chronic radiation injury. Gut 1986; 27: 528-533.

[11] Yeoh EK, Holloway RH, Fraser RJ et al. Anorectal function after three versus two-dimensional radiation therapy for carcinoma of the prostate. Int J Radiat Oncol Biol Phys 2009; 73: 46-52.

[12] Yeoh EK, Holloway RH, Fraser RJ et al. Anorectal dysfunction increases with time following radiation therapy for carcinoma of the prostate. Am J Gastroenterol 2004; 99:361-369.

[13] Yeoh EK, Holloway RH, Fraser RJ et al. Hypofractionated versus conventionally fractionated radiation therapy for prostate carcinoma: updated results of a Phase III randomized trial. Int J Radiat Oncol Biol Phys 2006; 66: 1072-1083.

[14] Yeoh E, Sun WM, Russo A, Ibanez L, Horowitz M. A retrospective study of pelvic irradiation for gynaecological cancer on anorectal function. Int J Radiat Oncol Biol Phys 1996; 35(5):1003-1010.

[15] Yeoh E, Tam W, Schoeman M et al. Argon Plasma Coagulation Therapy versus Topical Formalin for intractable rectal bleeding and anorectal dysfunction after radiation therapy for prostate carcinoma. Int J Radiat Oncol Biol Phys 2013; 87(5):954-959.

[16] Yeoh E, Botten R, Di Matteo A et al. Pudendal nerve injury impairs anorectal function and health related quality of life measures ≥2 years after 3D

conformal radiotherapy for prostate cancer. Acta Oncologica 2018; 57(4): 456-464.

[17] Krol R, Hopman WPM, Smeenk RJ, van Lin ENJT. Increased recta wall stiffness after prostate radiotherapy: relation with faecal urgency. Neurogastroenterol Motil 2011; 24(4): 339-E166.

[18] Yeoh EK, Bartholomeusz, Holloway RH et al. Disturbed colonic motility contributes to anorectal symptoms and dysfunction after radiation therapy for prostate carcinoma. Int J Radiat Oncol Biol Phys 2010; 78:773-780.

[19] Steineck G, Bull C, Sjoberg F. Contouring pudendal nerves. Editorial. Acta Oncologica 2018; 57(4):438-439.

[20] Yeoh EK, Horowitz M, Russo A et al. Effect of pelvic irradiation on gastrointestinal function: A prospective longitudinal study. Am J Med 1993; 95: 397-406.

[21] Botten RJ, Di Matteo AC, Sharma KG et al. Endorectal balloon during image guided radiation therapy for carcinoma of the prostate reduces long term radiation induced rectal bleeding and subsequent Argon Plasma Coagulation Treatment. Gastroenterology 2019; 156(6):S353-S354.

Section 3

Inflammatory Bowel Disease

Chapter 5

Current Elective Surgical Treatment of Inflammatory Bowel Disease

Enio Chaves Oliveira, Mauro Bafutto, Alexandre Augusto Ferreira Bafutto, Salustiano Gabriel Neto and Jarbas Jabur Bittar Neto

Abstract

The incidence of inflammatory bowel disease (IBD) is increasing world-wide and most patient will require some surgical treatment once in life. IBD surgical patients are a challenge to surgeons. Main goals of surgical treatment are (1) to preserve the small bowel integrity because many resections may lead the patient to a small bowel short syndrome and (2) restore normal function as they have absorption disturbances. IBD patients may present mal-nutrition status and/or immunosuppression at the time of surgery. Types of surgery range from a simple plasty in Crohn disease to a total procto-colectomy in Ulcerative Colitis. For Crohn disease most procedures avoid resection and use diseased segments to prevent disabsorption. Herein we describe the most currently used techniques to treat IBD patients, when to indicate surgery and how to prepare them to less outcomes. Patients with Crohn disease with high risk for short bowel syndrome and intestinal failure should be submitted to Strictureplasty otherwise, Bowel Resection is the favored surgical technique for the management of fibrostenotic. Bowel Resection is associated with lower recurrence rate and longer recurrence-free survival.

Keywords: inflammatory bowel disease, strictureplasty, bowel resection, Crohn's disease, ulcerative colitis, surgical outcomes

1. Introduction

1.1 Epidemiology

Many epidemiologic studies report an increase in incidence and prevalence of Crohn's disease [CD] and Ulcerative Colitis (UC) in a global proportion. It is more evident in countries that going through an industrialization process, e.g., Asia, South America and Middle East [1–3]. The incidence follows the country industrialization and people living in urban areas has a greater incidence of IBD [4, 5]. The global prevalence of IBD has increased from 79.5 to 84.3 per 100,000 persons in recent years. IBD has been considered a disease of high-income regions. The USA had the highest age-standardized prevalence rate globally; approximately a quarter of total global patients with IBD living there in 2017. The UK had the highest age-standardized prevalence in Europe. The prevalence of IBD range from 252 to 439 cases per 100 000 population in the USA and 373 per 100 000 population in UK [6].

1.2 Pathogenesis

The complete mechanism of pathogenesis of IBD still unclear. IBD has a complex immune-mediated inflammatory disease that affects primarily the digestive tube. Those individuals with a genetic predisposition when exposed to different environmental factors may initiate an inflammatory response that is influenced by gut microbiome (**Figure 1**) [7]. The process is characterized by chronic relapsing and remitting inflammation for life.

Many diet components were reported to be protective factors to IBD as fiber, short-chain fatty acids, wheat, gluten, zinc, vitamin D. On the other hand some kind of food may worsen the disease: FODMAPs, red meat, emulsifiers and sugar [8].

The interaction of diet components with the microbiome is not so simple: more fiber, less flares. Some patients complain worsening of symptoms with fibers consumption. One hypothesis is that altered microbiome may produce incomplete fermentation and then, originating pro-inflammatory byproducts as succinate [9].

The microbiome is the group of all organisms found in the whole gut and includes bacteria, fungi, viruses and protozoa. Most of them are found in the colon. Many studies showed that IBD patients have altered microbiome and pro-inflammatory bacteria. When you treat a patient with Crohn disease and make an ostomy avoid intestinal transit in affected bowel segment it result in decreased inflammation [10–13].

Another evidence of environmental factor is the impairment in Peroxisome proliferator-activated receptors-γ (PPARγ) activity. Environmental pollutants can block the PPARy signaling pathway while mesalazine enhances its expression [14].

The Hippo pathway is an evolutionarily conserved pathway that controls organ size and homoeostasis through modulating cell proliferation, survival, apoptosis, and stemness. Hippo pathway is involved in the IBD pathogenesis, including intestinal cell regeneration, gut microbiota, and angio- genesis of the intestines [15, 16].

Crohn disease (CD) and Ulcerative Colitis (UC) are grouped as inflammatory bowel diseases but each one has distinct clinical characteristics (**Table 1**). These differences have to be in mind when a bowel resection and anastomosis is done in a patient with Crohn disease.

Clinically CD may be classified into three phenotypes: inflammatory, penetrating (fistulizing) and stricturing [17]. During the diagnosis evaluation 10% may be

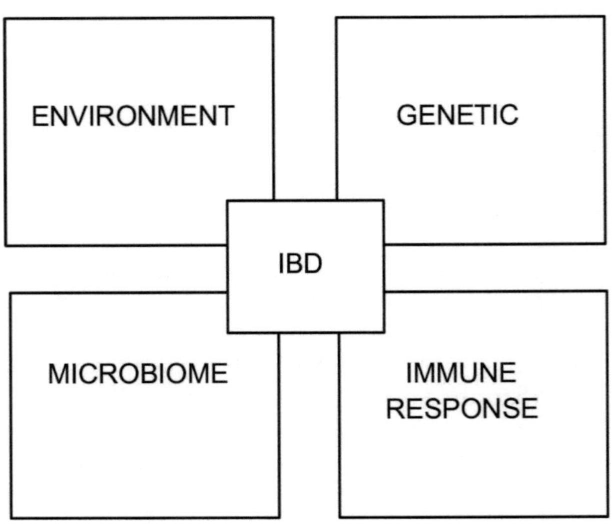

Figure 1.
Pathogenesis of IBD.

in the stricturing group and one decade later up to one third of patients may present stricturing **Figure 2** [18, 19].

The treatment of strictures may be done by endoscopy (endoscopic balloon dilatation, strictureplasty or surgical resection of bowel segment.

According to Cosnes et al. [18] the site of lesions is the most important factor to determine the disease behavior and progression to complication:

- Small bowel and anoperineal > stricture and penetrating complications;
- Esphagogastroduodenal and colon > inflammation.

In general, 75% of patients with strictures may require surgery once during lifetime but it may range from 70–90%. Right timing in indication of surgery for CD

Differences	Crohn disease	Ulcerative colites
Histopathology	Full thickness inflammation of bowel wall	Compromise mucosa
Organs	All gastrointestinal segments; Generally ilium and colon; Non-continuous pattern.	Rectum and/or entire colon; Continuous pattern.
Complications	Abscesses, fistulas, strictures.	Bleeding, perforation, toxic megacolon.

Table 1.
Characteristics of n disease (CD) and Ulcerative Colites (UC).

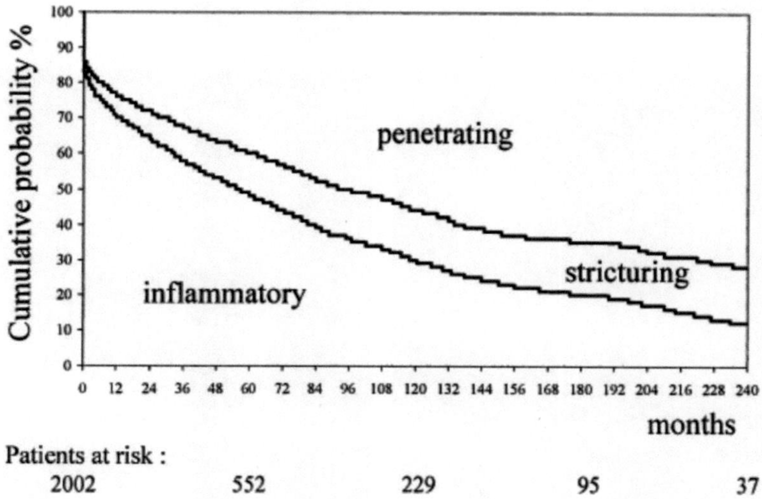

Figure 2.
Natural progression of Crohn disease. (From Jacques Cosnes et al. [18].)

- Refractory to medical therapy
- Fibrostenosing
- Growth retardation
- Fistulizing disease and related complications
- Neoplasia and dysplasia

Table 2.
Indications for surgery in CD.

may reduce complication rates, diminish operative technical difficulties and stoma indication, less emergency surgeries and also better mortality rates [18, 20, 21].

As CD does not have cure, surgery has a well-defined hole in therapeutic armamentarium. The aim of surgery is to treat complications, control symptoms, to try to preserve bowel length and keep to bowel function (**Table 2**).

2. Preoperative exams

2.1 Endoscopy and enteroscopy

Endoscopy may confirm the IBD diagnosis in most cases up to 90% of patients with Crohn disease or Ulcerative colitis. It allows a detailed examination of the mucosa of terminal ilium, colon and rectum. It is considered the gold standard exam for IBD diagnosis. Enteroscopy is indicated in patients with normal colonoscopy and gastroscopy but present suspection of Crohn disease. Enteroscpy may be diagnostic or therapeutic with dilation of strictures areas (**Figure 3**) [22].

2.2 Enterography CT and MR

Both radiological methods CT or MR Enterography have been the best non-invasive exams to evaluate the small bowel in Crohn disease. Enterography may identify affected segments, disease activity and complications (abscess and fistula). Enterography may help to differentiate inflammatory or fibrotic areas of stenosis (**Figure 4–6**). Stricture is defined as a bowel segment with luminal narrowing and unequivocal upstream bowel dilation (**Table 3**) [23].

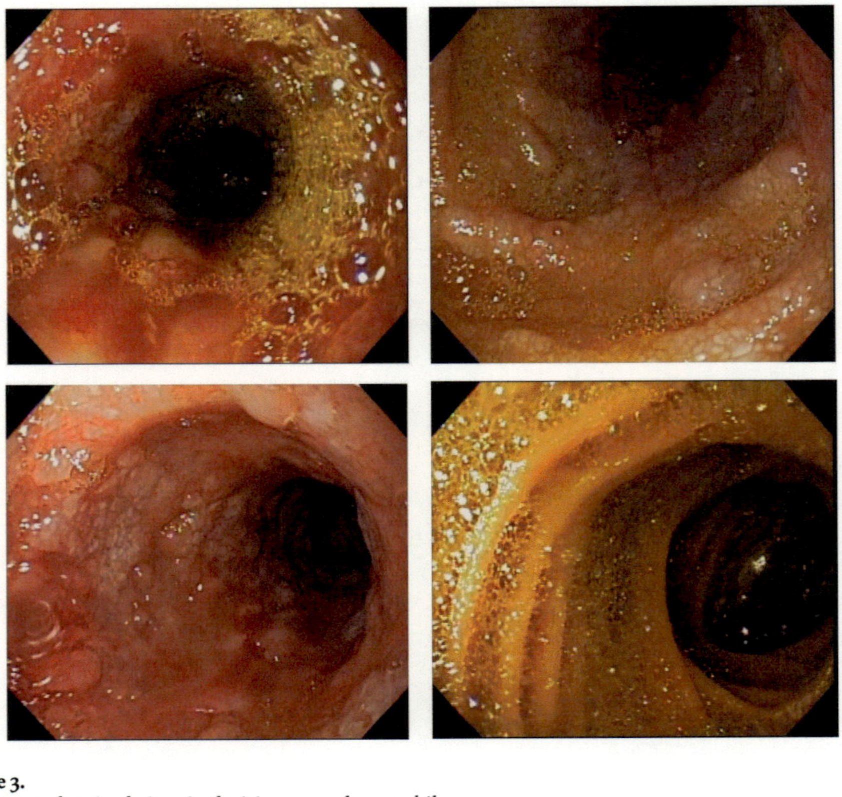

Figure 3.
Enteroscopy showing lesions in the jejunum and normal ileum.

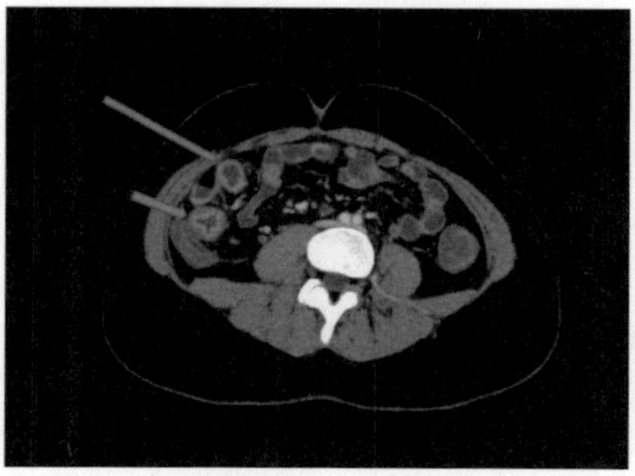

Figure 4.
Axial contrast- enhanced CT enterography: homogeneous mural hyperenhancement (long arrow) and stratified mural hyperenhacement (short arrow).

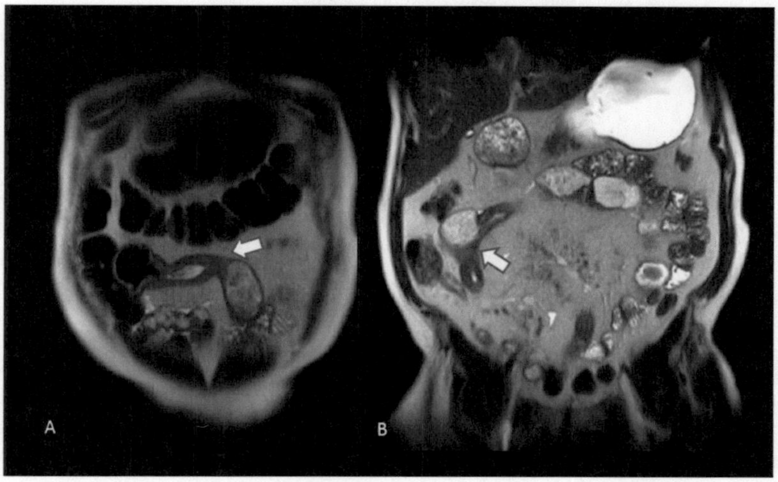

Figure 5.
A – Coronal T2 sequence MR enterography: homogeneous small bowel wall thickening and sacculations (arrow); B - Coronal T2 sequence MR enterography: small bowel wall thickening with stratified (bilaminar) mural hyperenhancement (arrow).

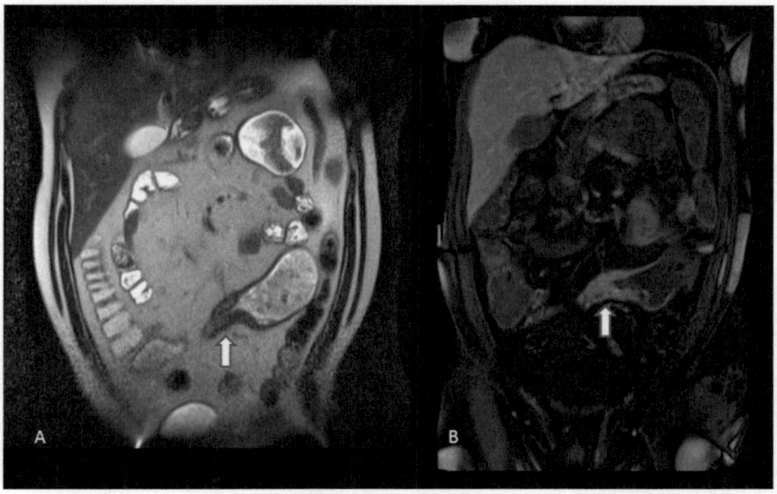

Figure 6.
A – Coronal T2 sequence MR enterography: homogeneous small bowel wall thickening (arrow); B - Coronal contrast-enhanced fat-suppressed T1-weighted MR enterography: small bowel wall thickening with stratified (bilaminar) mural hyperenhancement (arrow).

Segmental mural hyperenhancement
• asymemetric • stratified – bilaminar or trilaminar • homogeneous, symmetric
Wall thickening
• mild – 3 -5 MM • moderate –>5–9 MM • severe - >10 mm
Stricture
• probable stricture without upstream dilation (< 3 cm) • stricture with mild upstream dilation (3–4 cm) • stricture with moderate to severe upstream dilation (> 4 cm)

Table 3.
Radiological findings in CT or MR enterography in Crohn disease.

3. Crohn disease

3.1 Surgical options

3.1.1 Resection

The primary approach is to resect the small bowel stricture. Resection is associated to lower rates of recurrence. Patients submitted do strictureplasty alone may present a higher rate of disease recurrence [24]. The patient should have a small length stricture and no prior resection (**Table 4**).

Surgery may be done by laparotomy or laparoscopy with same good results and 2 cm margins of normal tissue is advised to make an anastomosis. Both anastomosis may be used: hand-sewn or stapled.

When a ileocolic resection is done the mesentery should be removed. When mesentery is left it is associated with higher recurrence rates and reoperations [25].

3.1.2 Bypass

Bypass surgery has been rarely employed due to the risk of neoplasia in the excluded segment [26, 27]. It may be an option to treat duodenal disease. There are two types of bypass: simples bypass and exclusion bypass [28]. Exclusion bypass

Crohn's disease is a panintestinal disease, with intermittent activity and the potential of focal exacerbations throughout the patient's life
It is impossible to cure Crohn's disease by excision. The surgeon is required only to treat the complications
The essence of surgical treatment is to make the operation as safeas possible. If the operation becomes safe and patients survive, they will inevitably have recurrences and so repeated operations may be required.
Therefore, it is important to conserve as much gut as possible All diseased bowels need not be excised, only that part with complications
If only stenotic complications are being treated, perhaps the stenosis can be simply widened by strictureplasty or dilatation

Table 4.
Five "Golden Rules" of surgical management of Crohn's disease.

is used when you cannot remove the affected segment because adherences to the retroperitoneum (**Figure 7**).

3.1.3 Strictureplasty

Strictureplasty is indicated to prevent small bowel syndrome in those patients after repeated resections or extensive bowel resections. Strictures are identified by palpation of the small bowel or alternatively introducing a 20 mm ball into the

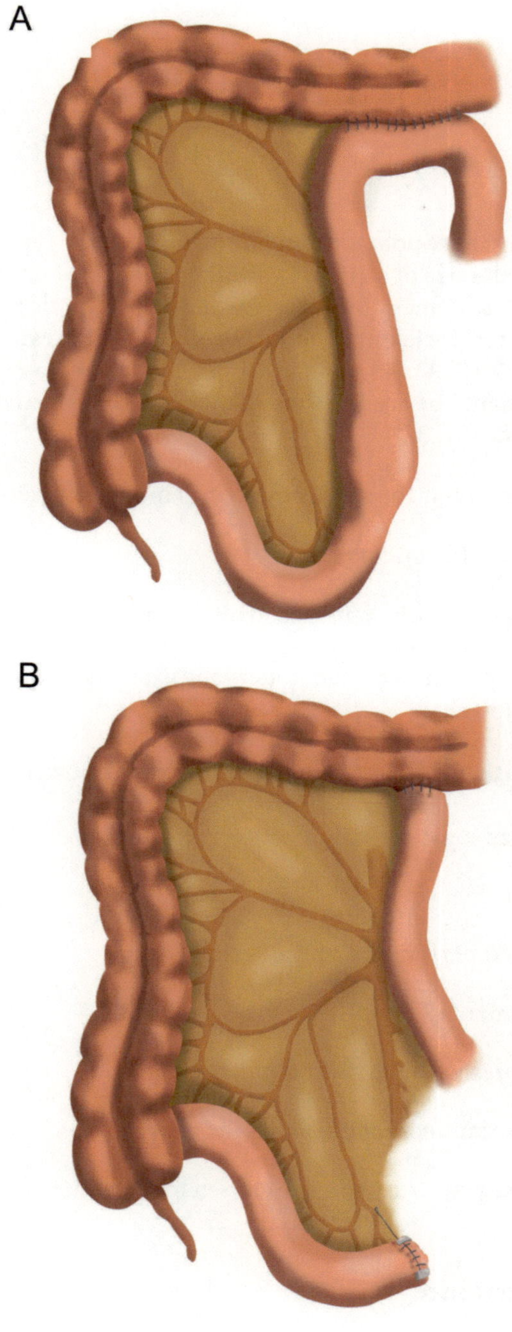

Figure 7.
Bypass surgery: simples bypass (A) and exclusion bypass (B).

Size of stricture	Techniques
Short-length (<10 cm)	Heineke-Mikulicz
	Moskel-Walske-Neumayer
	Judd
Medium-length (10–20 cm)	Finney
	Jaboulay
Long-length (>20 cm)	Michelassi
	Poggioli
	Sasaki
	Hotokezaka

Table 5.
Techniques of strictureplasty.

intestine and locating those points where the ball stops. The type of surgery is chosen according to the size of stricture (**Table 5**). The most used techniques are Heineke-Mikulicz 81%, Finney 10%, side-to-side isoperistaltic 5%, others 4%. The segments more affected are jejunum and/or ileum (94%), previous ileocolonic or ileorectal anastomosis (IRA) (4%), duodenum (1%), and colon (1%) [29, 30].

Strictureplasty should be used in those patients with concern for development of short bowel syndrome [31, 32].

- Diffuse involvement of the small bowel with multiple strictures.
- Non phlegmonous fibrotic stricture.
- Rapid recurrence of Crohn's disease manifested as obstruction.
- Stricture(s) in a patient who had undergone previous major resection(s) of small bowel (>100 cm).
- Stricture in a patient with intestinal failure or short bowel syndrome.

Strictureplasty has some contraindications [29, 32]:

- Colonic strictures.
- Free or contained perforation of the small bowel.
- Hypoalbuminemia (<2.0 g/dL).
- Multiple strictures within a short segment.
- Phlegmonous inflammation involving the affected site.
- Stricture in close proximity to a site chosen for resection.

4. Short-lenght stricture

The technique of Heineke-Mikulicz (**Figure 8**) [33, 34] is the most used one and is similar to that used for pyloroplasty. A small incision over the stricture is extended

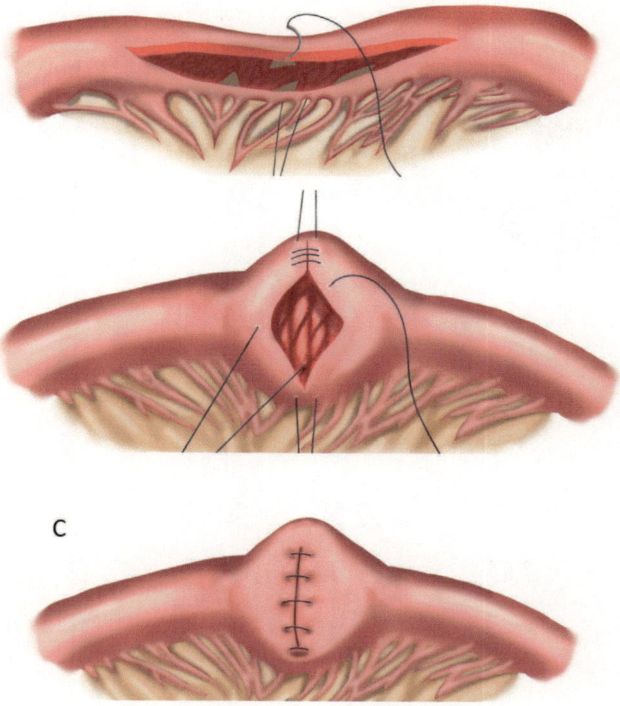

Figure 8.
The Heineke-Mikulicz technique. A - Longitudinal incision; B - transverse suture; C - final aspect.

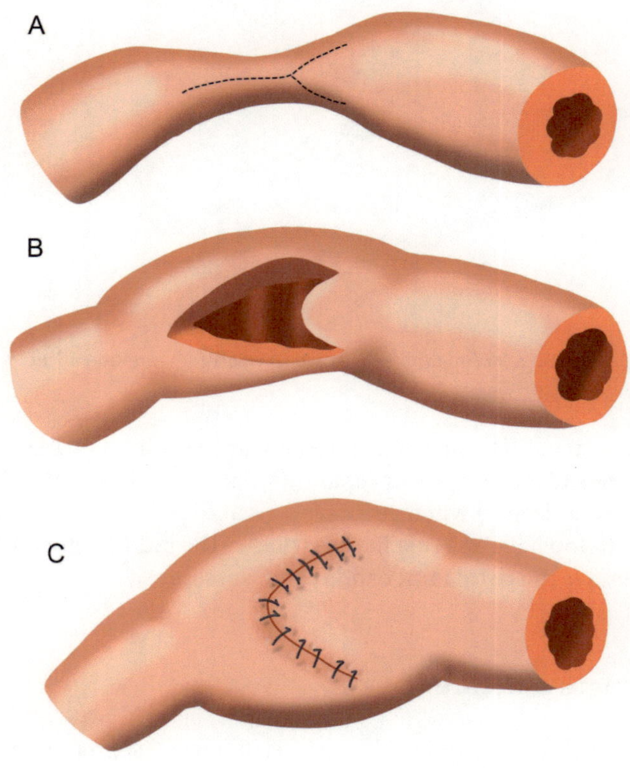

Figure 9.
The Moskel-Walske-Neumayer technique. A-Stenosis between segments with different diameters; B - It is made an Y shape incision; C - A free-tension suture is made.

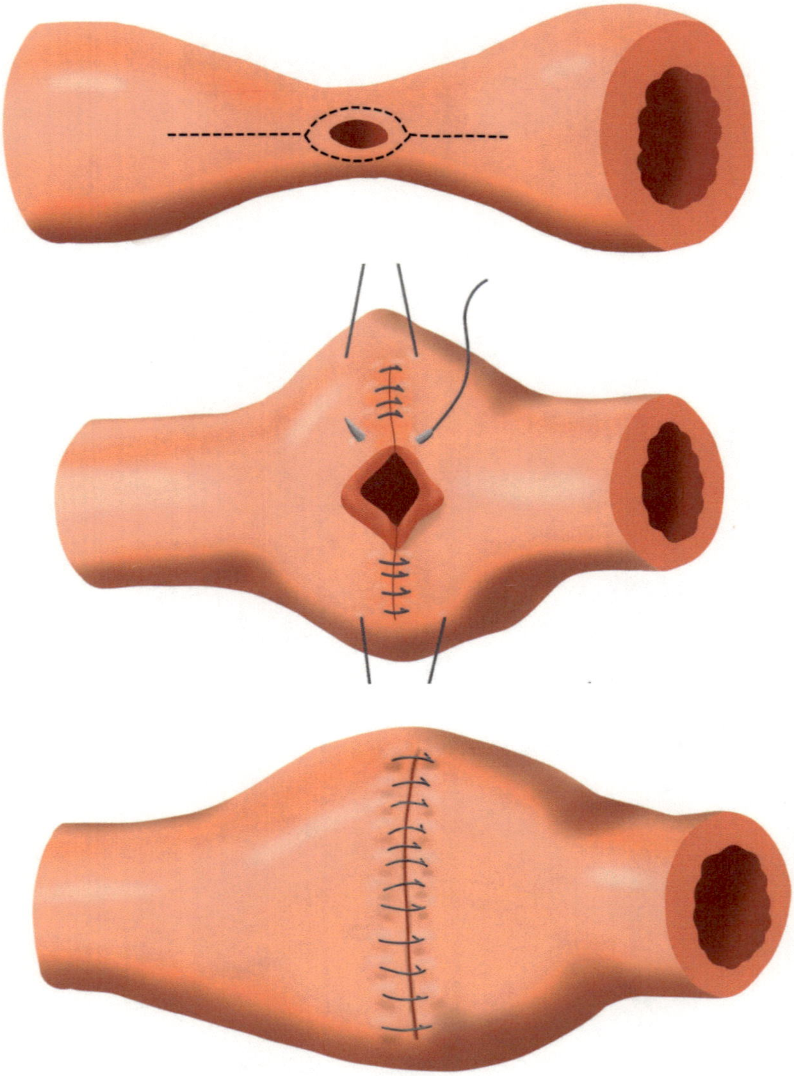

Figure 10.
The Judd technique. A- stenosis with fistula; B - the fistula is removed; C - end-to-end anastomosis.

to 2 cm in normal tissue. The incision is closed transversally: 1 or 2 layers with absorbable suture and continuous or separate stitch. The Moskel-Walske-Neumayer technique (**Figure 9**) is used when you have a great difference in the width of bowel to anastomosis. If you have a fistula in the stricture the Judd (**Figure 10**) technique is preferable to remove the fistula tract and repair the stenosis.

5. Medium-length stricture

The Jaboulay technique requires 2 incisions in normal segments avoiding the center of the stenosis (**Figure 11**).

The Finney technique (**Figure 11**) consist in one incision along the stenosis reaching up the normal tissue and them the bowel is folded in a U shape to be closed.

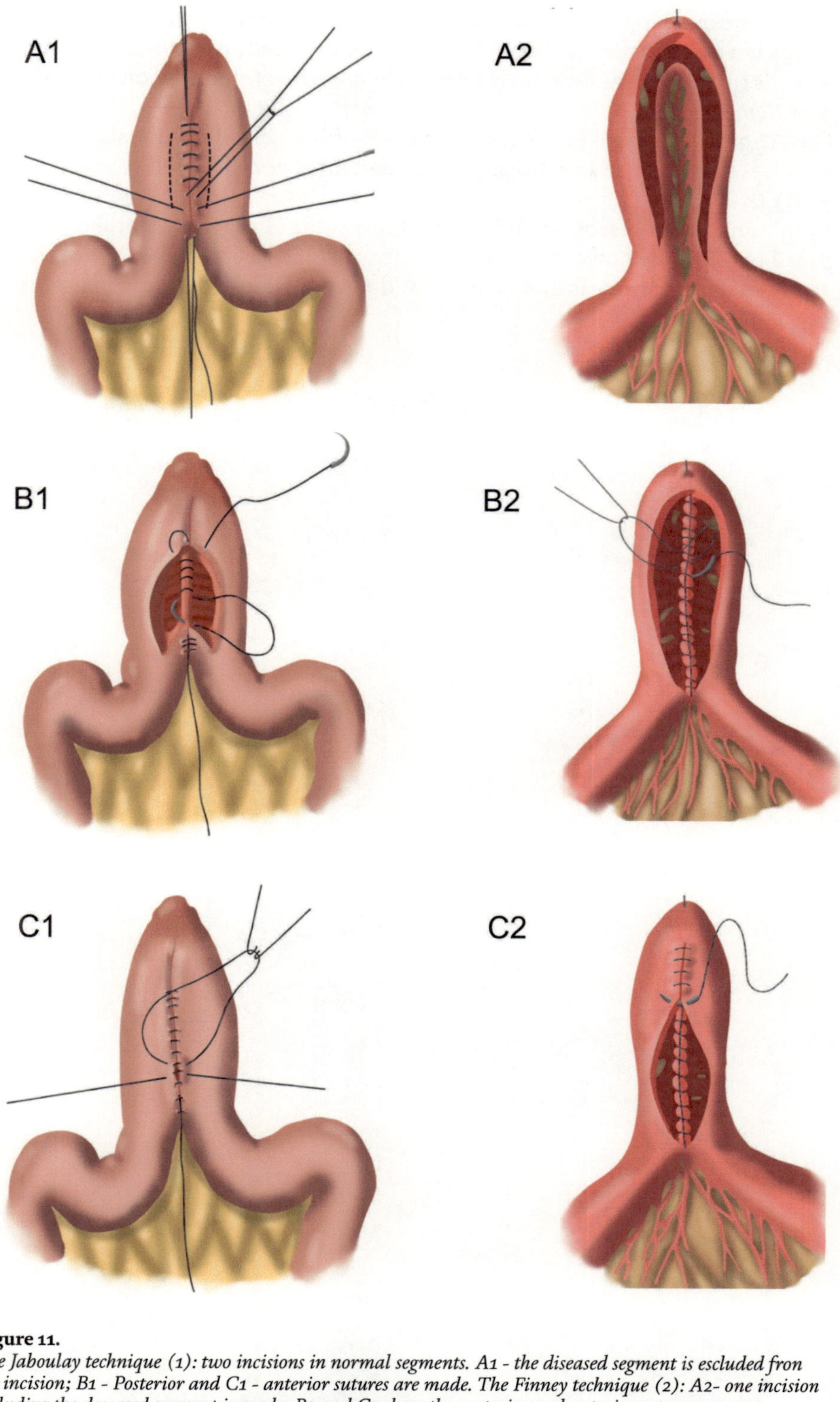

Figure 11.
The Jaboulay technique (1): two incisions in normal segments. A1 - the diseased segment is escluded fron the incision; B1 - Posterior and C1 - anterior sutures are made. The Finney technique (2): A2- one incision including the deseased segment is made; B2 and C2 show the posterior and anterior sutures.

6. Long-length stricture

In the Michelassi technique [35] the stenotic segment is divided in the middle and a longitudinal incision is made in both segments. A restoring anastomosis is made with the overlapping of both diseased segments (**Figure 12**). The Sasaki technique is a modification of Michelassi technique with the use of nonspatulated bowel ends to create an additional Heineke-Mikulicz strictureplasty on both ends (**Figure 12**) [36].

The Poggioli technique [37] is a modification of Michelassi technique and the difference is that we overlap a diseased segment with a non-diseased segment (**Figure 13**).

A combination of resection and enterostomy was described by Hotokezaka (**Figure 14**) [38]. The bowel segment with severe stenosis is removed. The remaining segment with stenosis is divide in the midpoint. A side-to-side antimesenteric

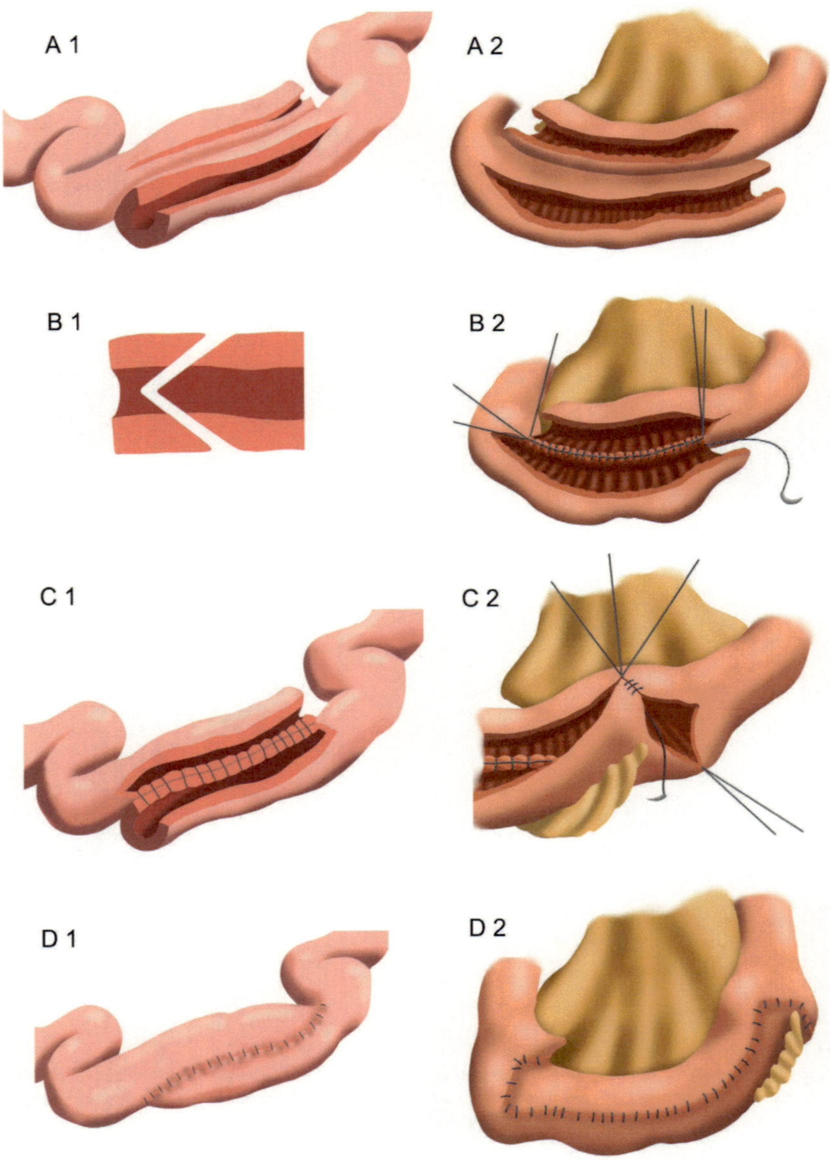

Figure 12.
The Michelassi technique (1): A1 - anastomosis of two stenotic segments B1 - the edges of bowel can be trimmed to allow better approximation; C1 - latero-lateral anastomosis; D1- final aspect. The variation is the Sasaki technique (2): A2 - anastomosis of two diseased segments; B2 - the edges of bowels are mantained; C2 - the end of the anastomosis is then transversely closed; D2 - final aspect.

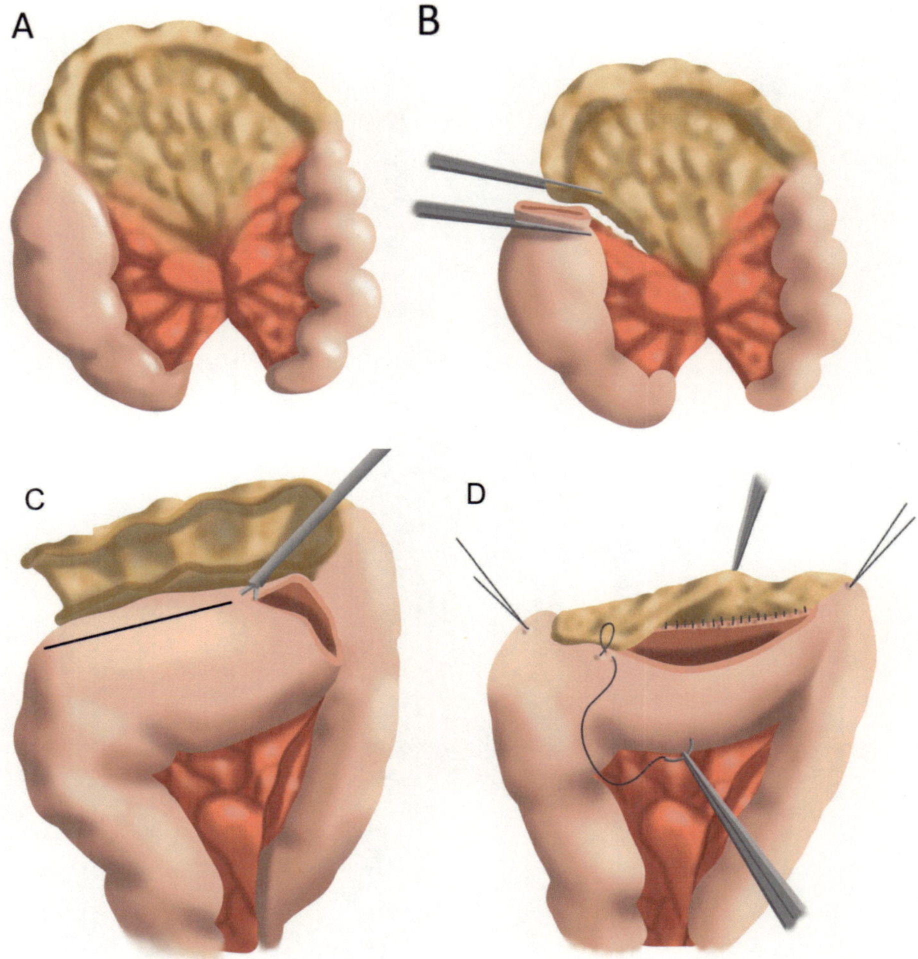

Figure 13.
The Poggioli technique. A - long diseased segment; B - the diseased segment is separated from normal segment; C - a longitudinal incision is made in both segments; D - lateral enterostomy with overlap of affected and normal segments.

enterostomy with the 2 bowel segments are made and them and end-to-end anastomosis are made between the strictureplasty and the resection site.

Results Strictureplasty vs. Resection.

The rate of complication for strictureplasty is about 4% to abscess, fistula and leakage [31]. Bowel resection is associated with lower recurrence rate (25.1%) compared to structureplasty (35.9%; p = 0.04). Recurrence-free survival was longer for bowel resection vs. strictureplasty (p = 0.02) [39, 40].

Surgical recurrence was higher for bowel resection (29.4%) vs. strictureplasty (39.7%; p = 0.002). No difference was observed for medical recurrence for bowel resection (12.4%) vs. strictureplasty (18.0%; p = 0.82) and also for overall morbidity between bowel resection (18.1%) vs. strictureplasty (10.7%; p = 0.65) [39, 40].

In fact, most cases a combination of techniques are used: resection for the severe lesion and plasty for the other. This approach seems to have the same rate of complications. This approach may decrease the risk of intestinal failure because patients may need future interventions and additional resection. Young age may be a risk for recurrent stricture. The 5-year reoperation rate for recurrent obstruction was 22%

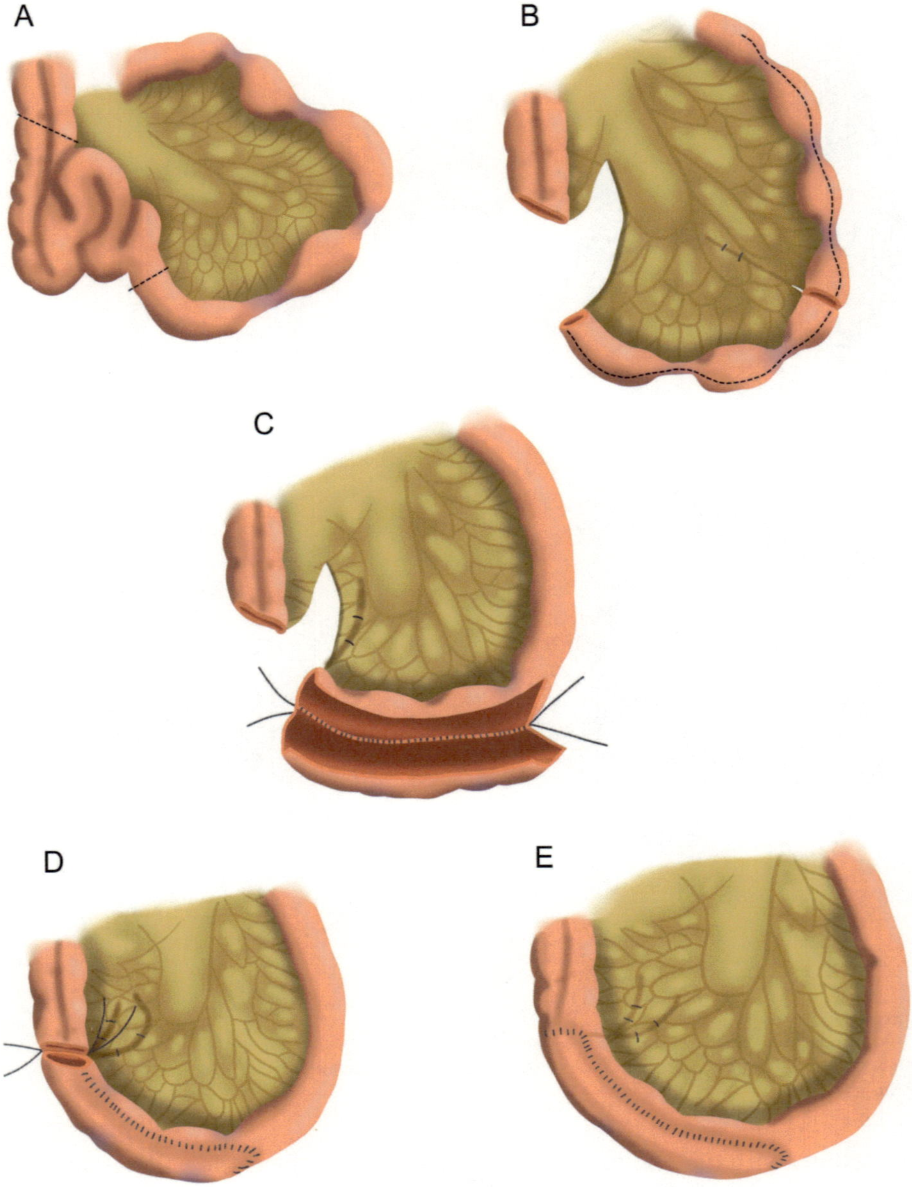

Figure 14.
The Hotokezaka technique. A - cecum and terminal ilium are resectes; B - a less affected segment is used to strictureplasty; C - Diseased segment is divide at the midle; D - side-to-side antimesenteric enterostomy with the 2 bowel segments is made; E - final aspect.

for resection alone, 30% for strictureplasty alone and 42% for strictureplasty and resection (P = 0.038) [39, 40].

7. Kono-S anastomosis

Kono et al. [41] reported a new technique of anchored anastomosis that could prevent recurrence. After resection of a severe stenosis with linear staple both end are put together with suture and a Jaboulay like side-to-side anastomosis is performed (**Figure 15**) [42].

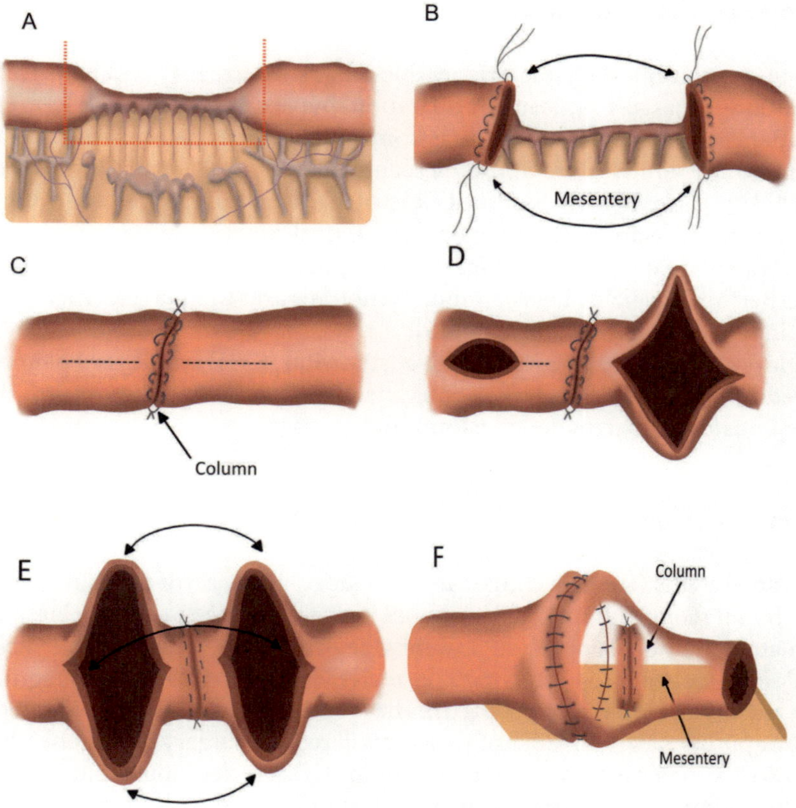

Figure 15.
Kono-S anastomosis: A - stenosis is removed; B - the ends of both segments are closed; C - both ends are put send-to-end; D - longitudinal incisions are made in both segments; E - the suture column beside the laterallateral anastomosis may sustain the lumen open and prevent stenosis; F - final aspect.

8. Fecal diversion

The use of fecal diversion is not common but in some clinical conditions may be indicated [31]:

- long-term and/or high-dose steroid use,
- recent use of biologics,
- malnutrition with hypoalbumenia (<2 g/dL).

9. Colonic disease

Colonic Crohn disease may be treated by segmental or total colectomy with ileorectal anastomosis. Total proctocolectomy with definitive ileostomy are indicated in those patients with severe perineal disease. Ileal pouch–anal anastomosis is less indicated due to pouch complications.

Strictureplasty should not be used in large bowel because the risk of malignization. Chronic inflammation is a risk factor for colon cancer and dysplasia is considered to be the precursor of most colorectal cancer in IBD patients [43].

10. Duodenal Crohn disease

Due to its anatomical characteristics duodenal stricture may require different therapeutic alternatives: endoscopic dilatation, bypass, resection or strictureplasty. The incidence of duodenal or upper gastrointestinal tract by Crohn disease varies according to age: adults 0.3 to 5%, adolescents 28% and 43% in pediatric patients with CD [44]. Patients with duodenal CD may present more aggressive evolution with high rates of recurrence and needs for surgical treatments [45].

Clinically patient complain: Epigastric pain, nausea, anorexia, early satiety, blation and belching, weight, Less common symptoms are: anemia, diarrhea, feculent vominiting, hematemesis or melena [46].

Surgical treatment indication: outlet obstruction (83%), refractory pain (11%), and bleeding (5%) [47]. Surgical options are: resection, gastrojejunostomy, duodeno- jejunostomy, gastroduodenostomy and by-pass.

11. Ulcerative Colitis

Ulcerative colitis (UC) is a chronic inflammatory condition of the colon and rectum. Initial therapeutic approach is based in different classes of medicine: anti-inflammatory, immunosuppressant (aminosalicylates, corticosteroids, thiopurines) and biological treatment as anti-tumor necrosis factor (anti-TNF), anti-integrins, anti-jak and other. However, most patients have successful clinical control and good evolution approximately 20–30% of patients will require surgery during their life [48].

However, surgery is a curative treatment for UC, the decision about an elective surgery is preference-sensitive. Generally, the indications for surgery are: medically refractory disease, dysplasia and carcinoma.

The surgery basically is total proctocolectomy with anastomosis or end ileostomy. The proctocolectomy with anastomosis is the ileal pouch–anal anastomosis (IPAA).

Total abdominal colectomy with ileorectal anastomosis is not indicated to patients with UC. The reasons are: half of patients will have a worsen disease in the rectum that will need protectomy and the risk of rectal cancer is 7–8% [49].

Proctocolectomy and ileal pouch–anal anastomosis (IPAA)

IPAA procedure may be done in stages:

- Three-stage operation: (1) total colectomy with end ileostomy and rectal stump, (2) proctectomy with IPAA and loop ileostomy, and (3) ileostomy closure;

- Two-stage operation: (1) total proctocolectomy with IPAA and loop ileostomy and (2) ileostomy tclosure;

- One-stage operation: total proctocolectomy with IPAA and no diversion.

There are different types of pouch and most surgeons favor the J pouch due to the simplicity to construct and good outcomes. The procedure may be done by laparotomy, laparoscopy, robotic or associated approaches.

12. Continent ileostomy or Kock pouch

It is indicated for those patients who does not meet the criteria for IPAA. It is contraindicated in obese patients. The patient has to be able to handle the ostomy and do self-intubation.

13. Conclusion

Surgery for bowel Crohn disease is not curative and procedures hat to be as less aggressive as possible. Surgery is indicated only in those cases with complication as obstruction and fistula. Resection approach is preferable to patients without risk to develop short bowel syndrome. Strictureplasty may be used to preserve bowel integrity. Different techniques are used depend upon the length of the stenosis. Bowel Resection is associated with lower recurrence rate and longer recurrence-free survival.

Acknowledgements

Dr. Carlos Alberto Ximenes Filho for providing CT and MR figures.

Conflict of interest

The authors declare no conflict of interest.

Author details

Enio Chaves Oliveira[1,2,3]*, Mauro Bafutto[4,5,6], Alexandre Augusto Ferreira Bafutto[6], Salustiano Gabriel Neto[1,8] and Jarbas Jabur Bittar Neto[7,8]

1 Surgery Department, School of Medicine, Universidade Federal de Goiás, Goiânia, Brazil

2 Digestive Unit, Hospital das Clínicas, Universidade Federal de Goiás, Goiânia, Brazil

3 Brazilian College of Surgeons, Brazilian College of Digestive Surgery and Brazilian Society of Coloproctology, Brazil

4 Gastroenterology, Internal Medicine Department, School of Medicine, Universidade Federal de Goiás, Goiânia, Brazil

5 Federação Brasileira de Gastroenterologia, Brazil

6 Instituto Goiano de Gastroenterologia e Endoscopia Digestiva, Goiânia, Brazil

7 Hospital do Coração de Goiás, Goiânia, Brazil

8 Brazilian College of Surgeons, Brazilian College of Digestive Surgery, Brazil

*Address all correspondence to: eco1.br@gmail.com

References

[1] Khalili H. The Changing Epidemiology of Inflammatory Bowel Disease: What Goes Up May Come Down. Inflamm Bowel Dis, 2020;26(4):591-592. doi: 10.1093/ibd/izz186.

[2] Ng SC, Shi HY, Hamidi N, et al. Worldwide incidence and prevalence of inflam- matory bowel disease in the 21st century: a systematic review of population-based studies. Lancet. 2017;390:2769-2778.

[3] Selvaratnam S, Gullino S, Shim L, Lee E, Lee A, Paramsothy S, Leong RW. Epidemiology of inflammatory bowel disease in South America: A systematic review. World J Gastroenterol. 2019;25(47):6866-6875. doi: 10.3748/wjg.v25.i47.6866.

[4] Park J, Cheon JH. Incidence and Prevalence of Inflammatory Bowel Disease across Asia. Yonsei Med J. 2021;62(2):99-108. doi: 10.3349/ymj.2021.62.2.99.

[5] Mak WY, Zhao M, Ng SC, Burisch J. The epidemiology of inflammatory bowel disease: east meets west. J Gastroenterol Hepatol. 2020;35:380-389.

[6] The global, regional, and national burden of inflammatory bowel disease in 195 countries and territories, 1990-2017: a systematic analysis for the Global Burden of Disease Study 2017. Lancet Gastroenterol Hepatol. 2020;5(1):17-30.

[7] Cleynen I, Boucher G, Jostins L, Schumm LP, Zeissig S, Ahmad T, Andersen V, et al. Inherited determinants of Crohn's disease and ulcerative colitis phenotypes: a genetic association study. Lancet. 2016;387(10014):156-67. doi: 10.1016/S0140-6736(15)00465-1

[8] Wark G, Samocha-Bonet D, Ghaly S, Danta M. The role of diet in the pathogenesis and management of inflammatory bowel disease: a review. Nutrients. 2020;13(1):135. doi: 10.3390/nu13010135.

[9] Armstrong H, Mander I, Zhang Z, Armstrong D, Wine E. Not all fibers are born equal; variable response to dietary fiber subtypes in IBD. Front Pediatr. 2021;8:620189. doi: 10.3389/fped.2020.620189.

[10] Zheng L, Wen XL. Gut microbiota and inflammatory bowel disease: The current status and perspectives. World J Clin Cases. 2021;9(2):321-333. doi: 10.12998/wjcc.v9.i2.321.

[11] Tarris G, de Rougemont A, Charkaoui M, Michiels C, Martin L, Belliot G. Enteric viruses and inflammatory bowel disease. Viruses. 2021;13(1):104. doi: 10.3390/v13010104.

[12] Di Sabatino A, Lenti MV, Giuffrida P, Vanoli A, Corazza GR. New insights into immune mechanisms underlying autoimmune diseases of the gastrointestinal tract. Autoimmun Rev. 2015;14:1161-1169 DOI: 10.1016/j.autrev.2015.08.004]

[13] Caioni G, Viscido A, d'Angelo M, Panella G, Castelli V, Merola C, Frieri G, Latella G, Cimini A, Benedetti E. Inflammatory Bowel Disease: new insights into the interplay between environmental factors and PPARγ. Int J Mol Sci. 2021;22(3):985. doi: 10.3390/ijms22030985.

[14] Dubuquoy L, Rousseaux C, Thuru X, Peyrin-Biroulet L, Romano O, Chavatte P, Chamaillard M, Desreumaux P. PPARgamma as a new therapeutic target in inflammatory bowel diseases. Gut. 2006;55:1341-1349.

[15] Ma, S., Meng, Z., Chen, R. & Guan, K. L. The Hippo pathway: biology and pathophysiology. Annu. Rev. Biochem. 2019;88:577-604.

[16] Xie Z, Wang Y, Yang G, Han J, Zhu L, Li L, Zhang S. The role of the hippo pathway in the pathogenesis of inflammatory bowel disease. Cell Death Dis. 2021;12(1):79. doi: 10.1038/s41419-021-03395-3.

[17] Silverberg MS, Satsangi J, Ahmad T, Arnott ID, Bernstein CN, Brant SR, Caprilli R, Colombel JF, Gasche C, Geboes K, Jewell DP, Karban A, Loftus EV Jr, Peña AS, Riddell RH, Sachar DB, Schreiber S, Steinhart AH, Targan SR, Vermeire S, Warren BF. Toward an integrated clinical, molecular and serological classification of inflammatory bowel disease: report of a Working Party of the 2005 Montreal World Congress of Gastroenterology. Can J Gastroenterol 2005; 19 Suppl A: 5A- 36A DOI: 10.1155/2005/269076]

[18] Cosnes J, Cattan S, Blain A, Beaugerie L, Carbonnel F, Parc R, Gendre JP. Long-term evolution of disease behavior of Crohn's disease. Inflamm Bowel Dis 2002;8:244-250 [PMID: 12131607 DOI: 10.1097/00054725-200207000-00002]

[19] Collyer R, Clancy A, Agrawal G, Borody TJ. Crohn's strictures open with anti-mycobacterial antibiotic therapy: A retrospective review. World J Gastrointest Endosc. 2020 Dec 16;12(12):542-554. doi: 10.4253/wjge.v12.i12.542.

[20] Bednarz W, Czopnik P, Wojtczak B, Olewiński R, Domosławski P, Spodzieja J. Analysis of results of surgical treatment in Crohn' s disease. *Hepatogastroenterology* 2008; 55: 998-1001

[21] Toh JW, Stewart P, Rickard MJ, Leong R, Wang N, Young CJ. World indications and surgical options for small bowel, large bowel and perianal Crohn's disease. J Gastroenterol. 2016; 22(40):8892-8904. doi: 10.3748/wjg.v22.i40.8892.

[22] Klinger AL, Kann, BR. Endoscopy in inflammatory bowel disease. Surg Clin N Am 2019; 99:1063-1082. doi.org/10.1016/j.suc.2019.08.005

[23] Guglielmo FF, Anupindi SA, Fletcher JG, et al. Small bowel Crohn disease at CT and MR enterography: imaging atlas and glossary of terms. Radiographics 2020; 40:354-375. doi.org/10.1148/rg.2020190091

[24] Butt WT, Ryan ÉJ, Boland MR, McCarthy EM, Omorogbe J, Hazel K, Bass GA, Neary PC, Kavanagh DO, McNamara D, O'Riordan JM. Strictureplasty versus bowel resection for the surgical management of fibrostenotic Crohn's disease: a systematic review and meta-analysis. Int J Colorectal Dis. 2020; 35(4):705-717. doi: 10.1007/s00384-020-03507-z.

[25] Coffey CJ, Kiernan MG, Sahebally SM, et al. Inclusion of the Mesentery in Ileocolic resection for Crohn's disease is associated with reduced surgical recurrence. J Crohn's Colitis, 2018, 1139-1150

[26] Greenstein AJ, Sachar D, Pucillo A, Kreel I, Geller S, Janowitz HD, Aufses A, Jr, Cancer in Crohn's disease after diversionary surgery. A report of seven carcinomas occurring in excluded bowel. Am J Surg 1978;135(1):86-90.

[27] Yamamoto T, Watanabe T. Surgery for luminal Crohn's disease. World J Gastroenterol 2014; 20(1): 78-90

[28] Homan WP, Dineen P. Comparison of the results of resection, bypass, and bypass with exclusion for ileocecal Crohn' s disease. Ann Surg 1978;187:530-535 [PMID: 646491 DOI: 10.1097/00000658-197805000-00011]

[29] Yamamoto T, Fazio VW, Tekkis PP. Safety and efficacy of strictureplasty for Crohn's disease: a systematic review and meta-analysis. Dis *Colon Rectum*. 2007;50:1968-1986 [PMID: 17762967 DOI: 10.1007/s10350-007-0279-5]

[30] Alexander-Williams J, Haynes IG. Up-to-date management of small-bowel Crohn's disease. Adv Surg. 1987;20:245-264

[31] Feinberg AE, Valente MA. Elective abdominal surgery for inflammatory bowel disease. Surg Clin N Am. 2019;99:1123-1140

[32] Strong AS. Strictureplasty in Complex Crohn's Disease: Beyond the Basics. Clin Colon Rectal Surg. 2019;32(4):243-248

[33] Katariya RN, Sood S, Rao PG, Rao PL. Stricture-plasty for tubercular strictures of the gastro-intestinal tract. Br J Surg. 1977;64:496-498

[34] Lee EC, Papaioannou N. Minimal surgery for chronic obstruction in patients with extensive or universal Crohn's disease. Ann R Coll Surg Eng. 1982;64:229-233

[35] Michelassi F. Side-to-side isoperistaltic strictureplasty for multiple Crohn's strictures. Dis *Colon Rectum*. 1996;39:345-349

[36] Sasaki I, Shibata C, Funayama Y, Fukushima K, Takahashi K, Ogawa H, Ueno T, Hashimoto A, Nagao M, Watanabe K, Haneda S, Shiiba K, Rikiyama T, Naito H. New reconstructive procedure after intestinal resection for Crohn's Disease: modified side-to-side isoperistaltic anastomosis with double Heineke–Mikulicz procedure. Dis *Colon Rectum*. 2004;47:940-949. doi: 10.1007/s10350-004-0517-z

[37] Poggioli G, Laureti S, Pierangeli F, Ugolini F. A new model of strictureplasty for multiple and long stenoses in Crohn's ileitis: side-to-side diseased to diseasefree anastomosis. Dis *Colon Rectum*. 2003;46:127-130

[38] Hotokezaka M, Ikeda T, Uchiyama S, Hayakawa S, Tsuchiya K, Chijiiwa K. Side-to-side-to-end strictureplasty for Crohn's disease. Dis *Colon Rectum*. 2009;52:1882-1886

[39] Butt WT, Ryan EJ, Boland MR, et al. Strictureplasty versus bowel resection for the surgical management of fibrostenotic Crohn's disease: a systematic review and meta-analysis. International Journal of Colorectal Dis. 2020;35:705-717 doi.org/10.1007/s00384-020-03507-z

[40] Landerholm K, Reali C, Mortensen NJ, et al. Short- and long-term outcomes of strictureplasty for obstructive Crohn's disease. Colorectal Dis. 2020;22(9):1159-1168. doi: 10.1111/codi.15013.

[41] Kono T, Ashida T, Ebisawa Y, et al. A new antimesenteric func- tional end-to-end handsewn anastomosis: surgical prevention of anastomotic recurrence in Crohn's disease. Dis *Colon Rectum*. 2011;54:586-592.

[42] Kono T, Fichera A, Maeda K, et al. Kono-S anastomosis for surgical prophylaxis of anastomotic recurrence in Crohn's disease: an international multicenter study. J Gastrointest Surg. 2016;20(4):783-790.

[43] Kim KO, Chiorean MV. Advanced neoplasia detection using chromoendoscopy and white light colonoscopy for surveillance in patients with inflammatory bowel disease. Intest Res. 2020;18(4):438-446. doi: 10.5217/ir.2019.00090.

[44] Saadah OI, Fallatah KB, Baumann C, et al. Histologically confirmed upper gastrointestinal Crohn's disease: is it rare or are we just not searching hard enough? Intest Res. 2020;18(2):210-218. doi: 10.5217/ir.2019.00091.

[45] Song XM, Gao X, Li MZ, et al. Clinical features and risk factors for primary surgery in 205 patients with

Crohn's disease: analysis of a South China cohort. Dis *Colon Rectum*. 2011;54:1147-1154.

[46] Schwartzberg DM, Brandstetter S, Grucela AL. Crohn's disease of the esophagus, duodenum, and stomach. Clin Colon Rectal Surg. 2019;32(4):231-242. doi: 10.1055/s-0039-1683850

[47] Reynolds HL Jr, Stellato TA. Crohn's disease of the foregut. Surg Clin North Am. 2001;81(1):117-135, viii

[48] Baker DM, Folan AM, Lee MJ, Jones GL, Brown SR, Lobo AJ. A systematic review and meta-analysis of outcomes after elective surgery for ulcerative colitis. Colorectal Dis. 2021;23(1):18-33. doi: 10.1111/codi.15301.

[49] Ng KS, Gonsalves SJ, Sagar PM. Ileal-anal pouches: A review of its history, indications, and complications. World J Gastroenterol. 2019;25(31):4320-4342. doi: 10.3748/wjg.v25.i31.4320.

Chapter 6

Restorative Proctocolectomy: When to Propose and When to Avoid

Marisa D. Santos

Abstract

Restorative proctocolectomy with ileal pouch-anal anastomosis (RPC-IPAA) is a surgical procedure performed when excising the entire colon and rectum is need and reconstitution of the intestinal transit through an ileal pouch is made with anastomosis to the anus. It is mainly used to treat patients with familial adenomatous polyposis (FAP) and ulcerative colitis (UC). It is a complex surgery with potential complications, and the functional outcomes can be worse over time. So, it is essential to select the appropriate patient, proceed to a correct surgical technique, and know-how to deal with and solve the main ileal pouch complications. This chapter intends to be a reflection on this subject.

Keywords: restorative proctocolectomy, ileal pouch-anal anastomosis, ileal-anal pouch complications, ileal-anal pouch failure, ileal-anal pouch results, familial adenomatous polyposis, ulcerative colitis, Crohn's disease

1. Introduction

Restorative proctocolectomy with ileal pouch-anal anastomosis (RPC-IPAA) is a complicated colorectal surgical procedure. It is mainly used to treat patients with familial adenomatous polyposis (FAP) and ulcerative colitis (UC). It is also performed to treat selected patients with Crohn's disease (CD), indeterminate colitis, and synchronous colorectal cancer (CRC) [1]. Among these pathologies, ulcerative colitis is the primary postoperative histopathological diagnosis, as Fazio data show, in 2013 [2].

IPAA surgery, first described by Parks and Nicholls in 1978 [3], aims to definitively cure disease and prevent malignant degeneration while providing adequate continence and avoiding a permanent stoma.

The majority of patients experience long-term success but are not absent from significant surgical complications. The main ones are pelvic sepsis, pouchitis, pouch failure, fecal incontinence, female infertility, and sexual dysfunction. Others, like stenosis, pouch dysplasia/cancer, IPAA prolapse, preileal IPAA pouchitis, and anemia, are rare [4].

IPAA results depend on several factors, such as the pathology underlying and specific features, gender, age, IBM, patient comorbidities, surgical techniques, and surgeon experience.

IntechOpen

So, before to propose or avoid RPC with IPAA, there are aspects to take into account:

- What is the underlying pathology, and if the RPC indication is absolute or relative;
- if the patient needs a total proctocolectomy or if it is possible to spare part of the rectum;
- rule out the presence of relative or absolute contraindication for IPAA and also,
- evaluation of all elements that increase the risk of IPAA failure.

2. Indications for proctocolectomy: the underlying pathology and specific features

There is specific colorectal pathology that, during its natural development, requires a colectomy or a proctocolectomy, with or without restorative gest. Let us analyze the characteristics of the different underlying pathology and how they can influence the surgical decision.

2.1 Familial adenomatous polyposis

FAP is an inherited disease classically characterized by the development of hundreds to thousands of adenomas in the rectum and colon during the second decade of life (**Figure 1**). A less aggressive variant of FAP is the so-called attenuated FAP (aFAP), where the rectum is frequently spared.

Although FAP is responsible for less than 1% of colorectal malignancies, untreated individuals with FAP carry a 100% risk of colorectal cancer by 40–50 years.

Thus, for patients with FAP, the single way to prevent colorectal cancer is surgery.

Nowadays, it is widely accepted that RPC-IPAA is the procedure of choice to treat patients with classical FAP.

We can choose for aFAP, total abdominal colectomy with ileorectal anastomosis (TAC-IRA), or proctocolectomy with stapled ileal pouch distal rectal anastomosis (CP-IPDRA).

FAP highlights:

- young population; absolute indication for surgery; if present rectal involvement, proctocolectomy is required; higher risk of desmoid in some family; RPC-IPAA is the procedure of choice to treat patients with classical FAP; RPC-IPAA easier in FAP than in UC [5].

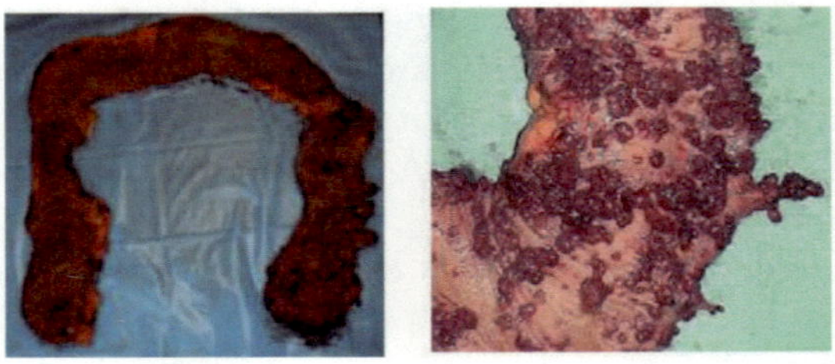

Figure 1.
Familial adenomatous polyposis – colon details.

2.2 Ulcerative colitis

UC is a chronic inflammatory condition characterized by continuous mucosal inflammation of the colon and rectum.

Nowadays, surgery is required in a limited number of patients with UC, either in an elective or in an emergency setting.

In patients with UC and indication for surgery, RPC is widely considered the gold standard surgical procedure. However, TAC-IRA is justified for some particular cases.

Emergent colectomy in UC is indicated in acute severe UC, not responding to medical therapy, or when complications occur such as severe bleeding, toxic megacolon, and colon perforation [6].

2.2.1 Acute severe ulcerative colitis, not responding to medical therapy

Acute UC is considered severe when the patient has at least 10 stools per day, tachycardia, fever, anemia, and increased erythrocyte sedimentation rate (ERS)/C reactive protein (CRP). The severity of ulcerative colitis classification by Truelove and Witts distinguishes acute severe ulcerative colitis from fulminant ulcerative colitis [7]. All authors do not recognize this division, but it makes it possible to infer the probability of failure with corticosteroid therapy and the need for a total colectomy (**Table 1**).

Acute severe UC, not responding to medical therapy, is one of the few cases that require emergent colectomy in UC. As shown in the management of flowchart in ASUC situations (**Figure 2**), about 30% of cases do not respond to corticosteroid therapy, and 50% of the ASUC will require surgery during the following year [8].

According to Saha et al., the policy of early colectomy, within 7 days, in patients with ASUC who fail to respond to intensive steroid-based therapy improves perioperative outcomes with significantly low inhospital mortality and morbidity [9].

Disease severity	Features
Slight	<4 stools/day with +/− blood, normal ESR, Without sepsis signs
Mild	4–6 stools/day with occasional blood loss, minimal signs of sepsis, CRP ≤30 mg/L
Severe	≥6 bloody stools/day with any of the following parameters: • temperature > 37.8°C • tachycardia > 90 ppm • anemia, Hgb < 10.5 g/dL • ERS > 30 mm/h, • CRP > 30 mg/L
Fulminant	10 stools/day with continued bleeding, abdominal distension and tenderness, need of blood transfusions, toxic megacolon in X-ray.

CRP = C reactive protein; ERS = erytrocyte sedimentation rate; Hgb = hemoglobin.

Table 1.
Ulcerative colitis severity classification. Adapted from Truelove and Witts criteria.

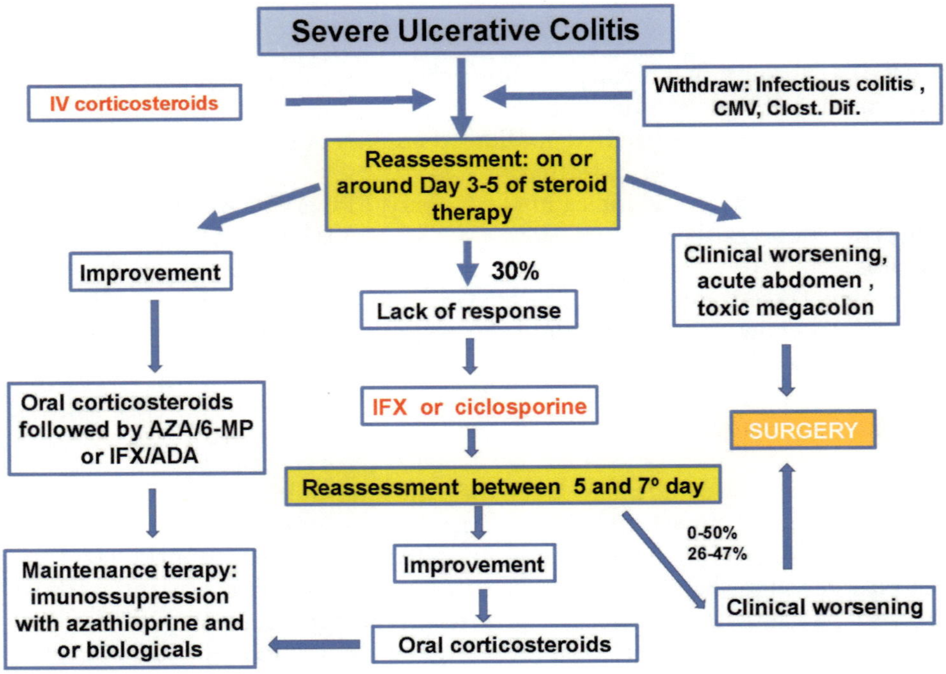

Figure 2.
Management of flowchart in acute severe ulcerative colitis.

On the other hand, when complications occur in severe ASUC, such as severe bleeding, toxic megacolon, and perforation, emergency surgery is mandatory. In these particular situations, the timing of colectomy is of utmost importance to reduce the postoperative complication rates.

2.2.2 Complications of acute severe ulcerative colitis

Severe bleeding, toxic megacolon, and perforation are the main complications of ASUC (**Figures 3** and **4**).

They are rare, but their presence increases surgery morbidity and mortality. If the UC surgery is urgent or emergent, the decision to perform surgery should be made in a multidisciplinary team, including the gastroenterologist and colorectal surgeon. In those cases, surgery is usually performed in three-step. Total colectomy, the first step, is made in an emergency room. The other steps electively, after confirmed diagnosis in the resected specimen.

2.2.3 Chronic refractory UC

Elective RPC for UC is indicated in chronic refractory UC (**Figure 5**) and also in the presence of high-grade dysplasia (HGD) or colorectal malignancies.

The introduction of biologic therapy has added further complexity to medical management decisions, surgery, and the relative timing of these choices. Appropriate medical management of UC may induce and maintain remission and may prevent surgery. However, medical management also carries risks of adverse effects, and recent data suggest that delay of surgery during ineffective medical therapy can increase the chances of adverse surgical outcomes. To make individualized, timely treatment decisions, early collaboration between gastroenterologists and surgeons is essential, and more data on predictors of treatment response and

DOI: http://dx.doi.org/10.5772/intechopen.98987

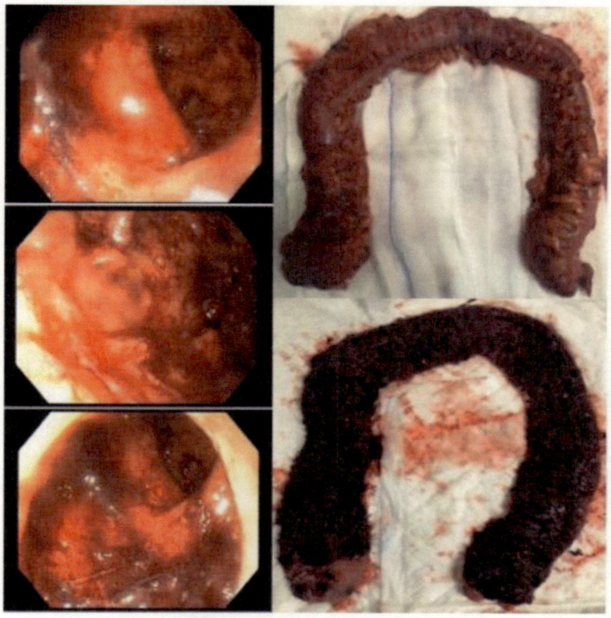

Figure 3.
Severe bleeding in acute severe ulcerative colitis not a responder to corticosteroids and infliximab. Surgery was performed in the emergency room.

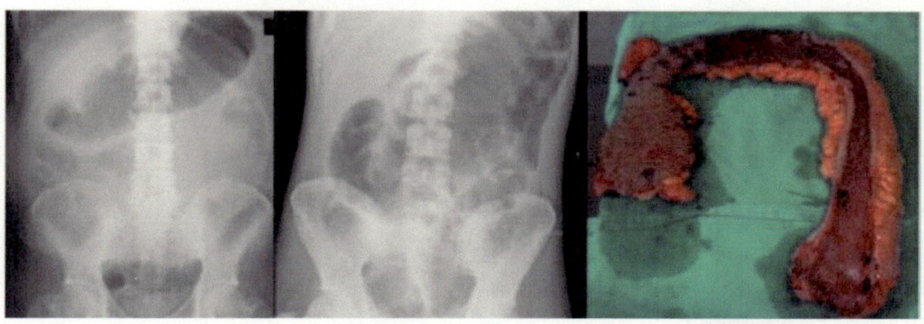

Figure 4.
X-ray and surgical specimen of toxic megacolon reports. There are more frequent in extensive ulcerative colitis than in ulcerative proctosigmoiditis. Surgical mortality is 1–8% that rises to 40% in colon perforation with peritonitis.

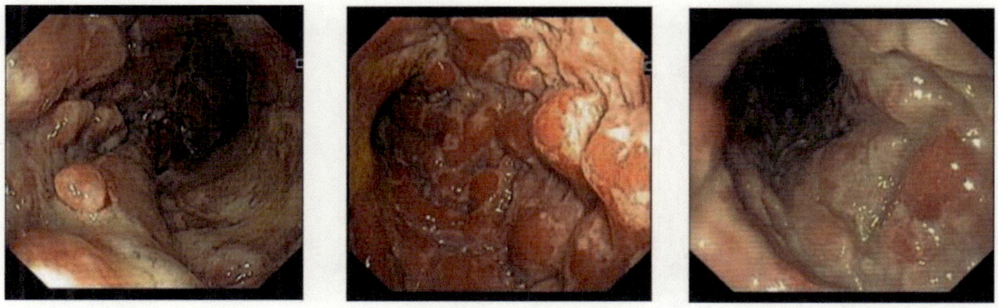

Figure 5.
Endoscopic images of chronic refractory ulceratice colitis.

positive outcomes are needed. Early identification of patients who would benefit from biologic therapy or surgery is challenging, and the definition of chronic refractory ulcerative colitis (CRUC) difficult. In CRUC (**Figure 4**), several therapeutic options have already been tried, such as infliximab, adalimumab, cyclosporine, azathioprine with 6-mercaptopurine, tacrolimus, or fecal transplantation, without success. When the therapeutic side effects are unbearable, or despite treatment, the patient has no quality of life, and RPC with IPAA may be the best solution.

2.3 Presence of high-grade dysplasia or colorectal malignancies

The presence of high-grade dysplasia (HGD) or colorectal cancer is another indication for elective RPC with IPAA in IC.

Colorectal surveillance in UC obeys specific rules (**Figure 6**) [10], and chromoendoscopy has an essential role in dysplasias identification (**Figure 7**) [11, 12]. In UC surveillance, the chromoendoscopy allows to split the cases in visible dysplasia and invisible dysplasia (**Figure 7**) [13, 14].

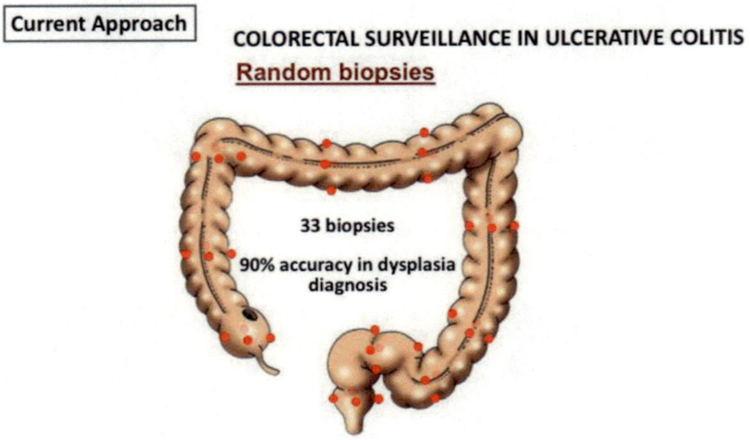

Figure 6.
Colorectal surveillance in UC (33 biopsies allow 90% accuracy in dysplasia diagnosis).

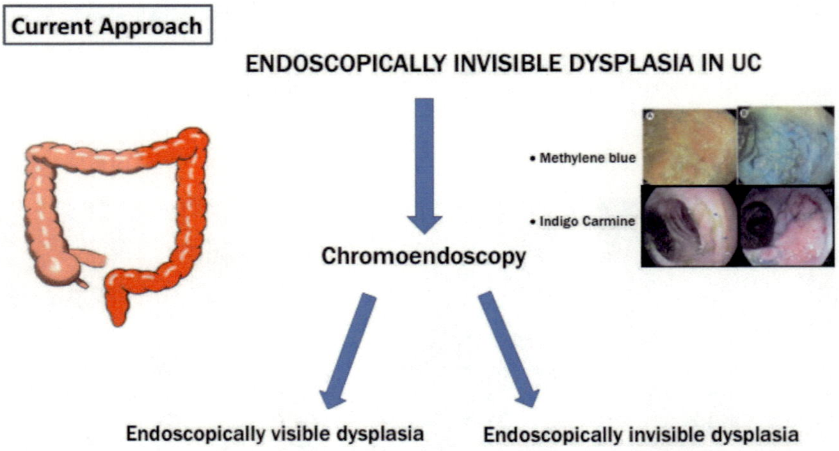

Figure 7.
Role of chromoendoscopy in dysplasia endoscopic visiblility.

Nowadays, dysplasia management in UC takes into account the grade and number of dysplasia, whether visible or not, and the presence of primary sclerosing cirrhosis (PSC) (**Figures 8** and **9**) [11, 15, 16].

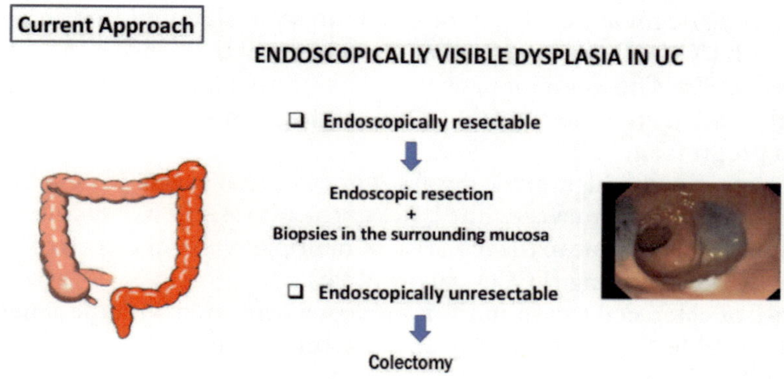

Figure 8.
Management of visible dysplasia in ulcerative colitis.

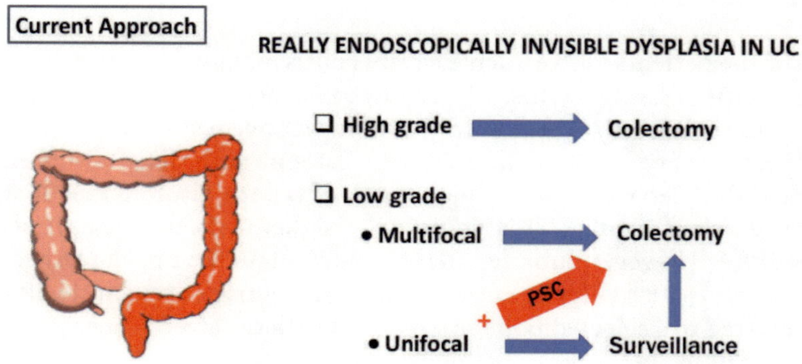

Figure 9.
Management of invisible dysplasia in ulcerative colitis.

Risk factor	Magnitude of the risk	References
Primary sclerosing cholangitis	OR: 4.0	Soetikno RM et al. *Gastrointestinal Endoscoc* 2002 [19]
Disease duration		
Cumulative incidence 20 years	2.5–8.0%	Eaden et al. [20]
Cumulative incidence 30 years	7.5–18.0%	Lakatos PL et al. *World J Gastroenterol* [21]
Extent of inflammation		
Pancolitis	SIR: 5.1–14.8	Eaden et al. [20]
Left-sided colitis	SIR: 2.1–2.8	Soderlund S et al. *Gastroenterology* 2009 [22]
Pseupolyposis	OR: 2.1–2.5	Velayos FS *et al. World J Gastroenterol.* 2013 [23] Rutter MD *et al. Gut.* 2004 [24]
Family history of CRC	RR: 2.4–9.2	Velayos FS *et al. World J Gastroenterol.* 2013 [23] Rutter MD *et al. Gut.* 2004 [24]
Degree of inflammation		
Endoscopy	OR: 2.5	Rutter MD *et al. Gut.* 2004 [24]
Histology	OR: 5.1	

Table 2.
CRC risk factors in ulcerative colitis.

In a systematic review of the literature, Fumery et al. found that among patients with UC-LGD under surveillance, the annual incidence of progression to CRC was 0.8%. Concomitant primary sclerosing cholangitis, invisible dysplasia, distal location, and multifocal LGD are high-risk features associated with dysplasia progression [17].

In UC patients with high-grade dysplasia or colorectal cancer (CRC), the colon and rectum should be removed with *en bloc* oncologic resection of lymph nodes in all colonic segments due to the high risk of multiple synchronous tumors and preoperative under staging (ECCO statement 9A) [18].

The risk of colorectal cancer in UC is increased compared with the general population (**Table 2**) [19–24]. Moreover, it is estimated to be around 18% after 30 years of UC duration [20].

Occasionally, total abdominal colectomy with ileorectal rectal anastomosis (TAC-IRA) can be considered.

2.4 Colitis in Crohn disease

Some of the patients with an acute severe colitis inaugural picture have indeterminate colitis or Crohn colitis. When they indicate emergency surgery, the first step is the colectomy. The realization of an elective restorative proctectomy with an IPAA must be individually analyzed. Patients with CD after IPAA, when compared with UC, have a fivefold higher risk of failure, twofold risk of strictures, and a sixfold risk of fistulae. This risk is much higher if the diagnosis is performed only after IPAA. However, function in those who retain the pouch seemed similar to that of patients with UC. CD does not increase the risk of pouchitis. IPAA could be offered to a selected population of CD patients after proper preoperative counseling (**Figure 10**).

Ileal pouch rectal anastomosis seems to be another viable alternative to permanent ileostomy in Crohn's proctocolitis patients. IPRA offers durable preservation

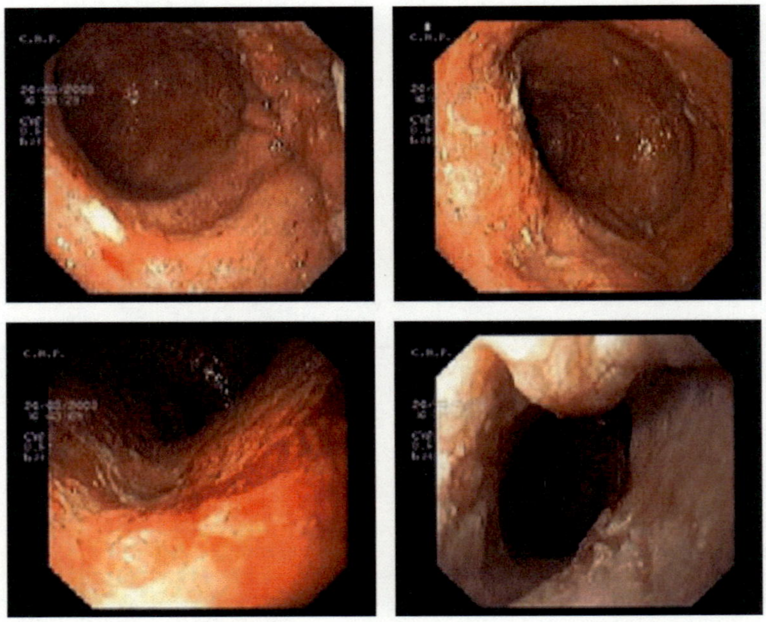

Figure 10.
Nine years after IPAA in a patient with Crohn's disease.

of bowel continuity and proper function and quality of life (QOL) in selected CC patients who might otherwise require a permanent ileostomy [25].

3. When the rectum can be partially spare

When the rectum can be partially spare, total abdominal colectomy with ileorectal anastomosis (TAC-IRA), a less complicated colorectal surgical procedure than RCP-IPAA, is an option. These solutions must be considered in attenuated familial adenomatous polyposis (aFAP) and synchronous colorectal cancer, and infrequently in UC and Crohn's disease.

The assessment of the rectum state is a parameter to consider when the surgical plan procedure is made. In FAP, behind the number of polyps present in the rectum (less than 10), the aggressiveness and development of extracolonic symptoms of the disease are other aspects to take into account. The mutation site on the APC gene is associated with the FAP phenotype, including desmoid tumor (DT) development. The more distal the mutation (closer to 3′ end), the higher the risk of the patient being affected by the desmoid tumor [1, 9, 17]. Typical disease symptoms were observed in families who harbored mutations between exon 4 (codon 169) and codon 1393 of exon 15. Mutations beyond codon 1403 were associated with a more varied phenotype concerning the development of extracolonic symptoms, namely desmoid tumor (DT). Their presence is related to aggressiveness disease and usually dictates the outcome of the patient. Despite the possibility of DT arising in any location, DT related to FAP is mostly on the abdominal region: intra-abdominal, on the abdominal wall, and transabdominal. Some of them take a benign course, with slow evolution, stabilization of growth, or even remission. Others show aggressive behavior with rapid growth and mass effect on surrounding structures, particularly in intra-abdominal DT. Possible complications of intra-abdominal DT are intestinal obstruction, ischemia, hemorrhage, and perforation or ureteric obstruction [1, 4, 8]. When DT develops in FAP patients, they can be the reason for the pouch failure case, and they are the second most common cause of mortality [20].

In synchronous CRC, the rectal tumor stage and location define the surgery to perform. If the rectum can be spare, TAC-AIR is the choice. RPC-IPAA with total mesorectum excision and with or without neoadjuvant chemoradiotherapy may be the solution in selected patients with medium or distal rectal cancer, depending on if the tumor is localized or locally advanced.

In IBD with proctocolitis involvement, rectum spare is controversial, mainly is ulcerative colitis. The decision-based in the absence of activity in the rectal mucosa.

4. When the rectum cannot be spare

When the rectum cannot be spare, it is mandatory to rule out the presence of relative or absolute contraindication for IPAA. There are absolute contraindications for IPAA: They are the presence of poor anal sphincter function with fecal incontinence in all pathologies, the distance between the tumor and pectin line inferior to 1 cm or sphincter involvement in distal rectal cancer, and the presence of perianal disease beyond proctocolitis in Crohn disease. The aggressive phenotype in FAP, indeterminate proctocolitis, and Crohn's disease, with involvement limited to the colon and rectum, are the relative contraindications. Morbid obesity increased technical difficulties and can be considered a relative contraindication, as the willingness in young women to get pregnant.

4.1 Evaluation of factors that increase the risk of IPAA failure when rectum cannot be spared

RCP with IPAA is, in fact, a complicated colorectal surgical procedure even in the hands of experienced high-volume surgeons. In an extensive series of 1789 patients undergoing proctocolectomy, IPAA was attempted but abandoned intraoperatively in 4.1% [26].

So, the relative indication for that type of elective surgery must be carefully considered. Several aspects must take into account for surgery plan mainly in UC cases:

- the pathology underlying and specific features;
- if the surgery is elective or urgent;
- patient age;
- patient comorbidities;
- patient anal sphincter and rectum status;
- and the experience of the surgeon.

Moreover, weigh the risk and frequency of IPAA morbidity and the patient is will after informed consent, which are also factors that influence the surgical decision.

5. Surgical alternatives to IPAA after a proctocolectomy/total colectomy

RPC-IPAA is "the gold standard" procedure to treat patients with classical FAP and elective surgery in UC, although other surgical solutions are possible (**Table 3**).

Operation	Advantages	Disadvantages
Rectal mucosectomy with ileal pouch-anal canal Anastomosis	Complete excision of large intestinal disease Transanal defecation and fecal continence preserved No ileostomy	Two operations required At risk for pouchitis Nocturnal fecal spotting present
Stapled ileal pouch-distal rectal anastomosis	Transanal defecation and fecal continence preserved No ileostomy Easier technically	At risk for pouchitis and cancer from residual rectal mucosa
Continent ileostomy	Complete excision of large intestinal disease Fecal continence preserved No external appliance	Stoma present Intubation of pouch required At risk for pouchitis and need for valve revision
Brooke ileostomy	Complete excision of large intestinal disease One operation	Stoma present, risk of parastomal hernia Incontinent for feces Need of external appliance
Ileorectal anastomosis	Transanal defecation and fecal continence preserved No ileostomy	Diseased rectum remains to produce symptoms, require treatment, and predispose to cancer

Table 3.
Bowel transit reconstruction types after a proctocolectomy/total colectomy.

6. IPAA surgical procedure and technical aspects that interfere in pouch results

RPC-IPAA is a complex procedure that pouch results also depend on technical surgical details and surgeon experience.

6.1 RPC-IPAA procedure

RPC with IPAA is a procedure that can be made in one, two, or three stage, by laparoscopic or open surgery.

The laparoscopic approach, if feasible, allows better cosmetics and outcomes.

One-stage or two-stage procedure is recommended for elective surgery and three-stage for emergent surgery.

Stage 1—An ileal pouch is made, and anastomosed to the anus is made after de proctocolectomy without a protective ileostomy. The operation is made in elective surgery and completed in a single stage (one surgery).

Stage 2—After a PC and IPAA confection, the anastomosis is protected by a loop ileostomy, and ileostomy closure is posterior realized (two surgeries).

Stage 3—At the emergency room, the first step is the total abdominal colectomy and ileostomy. The second step is the IPAA with the anastomosis protected by a loop ileostomy. The third surgery is the ileostomy closure (three surgeries).

Due to anastomotic complications (infection, fistulization, development of Crohn's disease, disease recurrence, or poor function), an ileostomy may be required (stage 2) to prevent complications or if the pouch fails postoperatively. The authors are not unanimous about the need to do a derivative ileostomy by routine during IPAA construction (stage 1 vs. stage 2).

Lovegrove et al. found to be associated with ileostomy omission: stapled anastomosis (odds ratio [OR], 6.4), no preoperative corticosteroid use (OR, 3.2), familial adenomatous polyposis diagnosis (OR, 2.6), cancer diagnosis (OR, 3.4), female sex (OR, 1.6), and age at surgery younger than 26 years (OR, 2.1) ($p < 0.01$ for all). They are convinced that incorporating a five-point nomogram in the preoperative assessment of patients undergoing RPC might help clinicians identify a select group of patients who may be candidates for ileostomy omission during RPC [27]. Karjalainen et al. showed in their study that a diverting ileostomy is associated with considerable morbidity, and it does not seem to prevent later failure of the pouch. Therefore, they suggest that a diverting ileostomy should only be constructed for high-risk patients [28]. On the other hand, Rottoli et al. demonstrated that closure of ileostomy after three-stage IPAA is associated with a low rate of serious complications, despite the higher number of previous abdominal surgeries, supporting the construction of routine ileostomy during IPAA to reduce the risk of pelvic sepsis [29].

6.2 IPAA pouch confection

The most used pouch configurations are the J-pouch and de S-pouch, wherein most centers opt for J-pouch. S-pouch is usually reserved for patients with high IBM, short mesentery, or handsewn anastomosis necessity. Wu et al. recommend using an S-pouch when constructing an IPAA with a handsewn technique. A total of 502 patients included 169 patients with an S-pouch (33.7%). The frequencies of short-term complications in the two groups were similar ($p > 0.05$), but pouch fistula or sinus ($p = 0.047$), pelvic sepsis ($p = 0.044$), postoperative partial small-bowel obstruction ($p = 0.003$), or postoperative pouch-related hospitalization ($p = 0.021$) occurred in fewer patients with an S-pouch. At a median follow-up of 12.2 (range, 4.3–20.1) years, patients with an S-pouch were found to have fewer bowel movements ($p < 0.001$), less frequent pad use ($p = 0.001$), and a lower fecal incontinence severity index score ($p = 0.015$). The pouch failed in 62 patients (12.4%), but neither univariate nor multivariate analysis showed a significant association with pouch configuration IPAA surgery stage [30].

6.3 IPAA-mucosectomy vs. anal transactional zone mucosa and handsewn vs. stapled anastomosis

The IPAA can be made with transanal mucosectomy and handsewn anastomosis or preserving the anal transitional zone mucosa in a small rectal cuff and stapled anastomosis.

Dafni et al. refer that stapled IPAA and younger age at the onset of UC correlated with better functional results, and the HRQOL scores were high [31].

Kirat et al. studied the influence of stapler size used at IPAA on the anastomotic leak, stricture, long-term functional outcomes, and quality of life. They analyzed the stapled IPAA performed between 1983 and 2007: A (stapler size 28–29 mm) ($n = 1.221$) and B (stapler 31–33 mm) ($n = 899$). They did not found a significant difference in rates of leak (4.5% vs. 6.2%, $p = 0.08$) or stricture (1.9% vs. 2.7%, $p = 0.1$) for groups A and B. There was no significant association between the size of the stapler used at IPAA and long-term complications [32].

7. Main surgical complications in restorative proctocolectomy with ileal pouch anal anastomosis (RPC-IPAA)

Surgical complications in RPC with IPAA are not unusual as functional deterioration of pouch and quality of life (QOL). Fazio et al. encountered in their data early perioperative complications in 33.5% of patients with a mortality rate of 0.1%. On the other hand, he refers to good functional outcomes and QOL in 95% [2]. Nevertheless, these results by Fazio, mainly the functional outcomes of the IPAA, are not reached in all centers, probably depending on the surgeon experience and the high patient volume. The most leading and frequent IPAA complications are described as follows:

7.1 Pelvic sepsis

Pelvic sepsis occurs in 9% of the procedure, and its presence increases the risk of pouch failure. Pelvic sepsis is a common early complication with far-reaching consequences of long-term pouch dysfunction, but prompt intervention (either radiological or surgical) reduces the risk of pouch failure. According to Lavryk et al., 4031 patients who underwent IPAA in 1983–2014 (patients with Crohn's disease or cancer were excluded), 357 (8.8%) developed IPAA-related pelvic sepsis with or without anastomotic dehiscence [33].

7.2 Acute pouchitis

The inflammation of the IPAA can appear in acute (60%) or chronic (60%) form.

Kayal et al. state 53% that acute pouchitis occurred in 205 patients (53%), 60 of whom (30%) progressed to chronic pouchitis [34].

Hashavia et al. followed prospectively 201 UC patients who underwent IPAA (1981–2009 for a mean of 108 months). A total of 138 (69%) of these had either a regular pouch or episodes of acute pouchitis and 63 (31%) developed chronic pouchitis [35].

7.3 Pouch failure rate

Pouch failure rates range from 5.5 to 8.5%, depending upon the length of follow-up [36]. In Fazio data, 3707 patients underwent primary pouch, and 328 (8.1%) redo pouch surgery (primary surgery in other centers). Pouch failure occurred in 197 (5.5%) of the 3707. During a median follow-up of 84 months, 119 patients (3.2%) required excision of the pouch, 32 (0.8%) had a nonfunctioning pouch, and 46 patients (1.2%) had redo IPAA [2].

7.4 Fecal incontinence: mild – 17%; severe – 3.7%

Mild fecal incontinence is a common complication of IPAA and seems to worsen with time [37].

Mild and severe fecal incontinence during the day: 17 and 3.7% of patients, respectively.

(Incontinence during the night: 13.1 and 4.5%; urge incontinence during the day: 7.3%).

At 12 months post-IPAA, it has been reported that 19% of patients suffered occasional daytime incontinence, and 49% suffered nocturnal incontinence [7]. Consequently, this can have a significantly negative impact on the quality of life of patients. The evidence to support the use of SNS for fecal incontinence after IPAA remains very limited.

7.5 Female infertility

Studies have shown that fertility in women with UC is comparable to the background population but drops following restorative proctocolectomy [38].

This problem can be restricted, opting for a laparoscopic approach and using *in vitro* fertilization.

Laparoscopy was associated with a significantly reduced time to conceive compared with the open approach [39].

Females with RPC for UC have an increased incidence of *in vitro* fertilization by more than a factor of three. The odds that a treatment results in live birth are similar, and six times more children are born due to *in vitro* fertilization compared with females without restorative proctocolectomy [40].

7.6 Sexual dysfunction: 1.5–4%

Sexual dysfunction can appear after RCP with IPAA. Postoperative impotence and retrograde ejaculation have been observed in approximately 1.5–4% of men, respectively. Transient dyspareunia occurs in about 7% of women [41].

7.7 Pouch dysplasia/cancer: 1%

About 1% of patients develop dysplasia or carcinoma after surgery, which occurs in the retained rectum, anal transitional zone, or ileal pouch, depending upon the procedure performed.

Mark-Christensen et al. analyzed 1723 patients with IPAA operated for ulcerative colitis in the period 1980–2010 that matched to 8615 individuals from the background population. They concluded that pouch cancer following IPAA is sporadic, questioning the need for general, rather than selective, surveillance. The overall cancer risk is comparable to that of the background population (**Figure 11**).

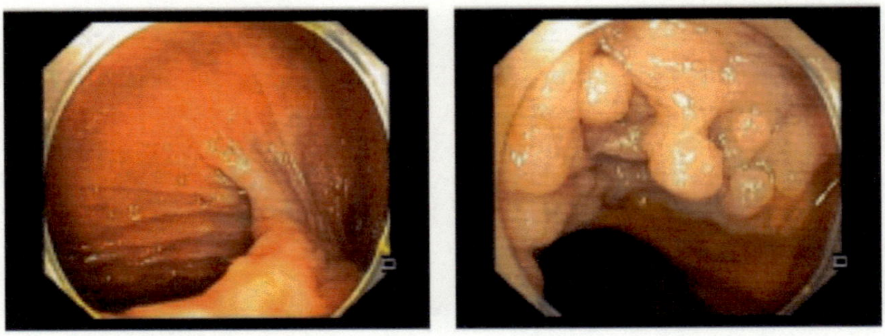

Figure 11.
Nine years passed between RCP with IPAA for FAP. The residual polyps were appearing in IPAA, easily handled by endoscopic surveillance with polypectomy.

The increased risk of hepatobiliary cancer is likely an effect of coexisting liver disease and not causally related to IPAA [42].

8. Conclusion

RCP with IPAA in the hands of experienced high-volume surgeons is a safe procedure associated with good functional results, provided that the risk-benefit is appropriately weighted.

9. Take-home messages

- RPC with IPAA is the golden standard procedure for FAP and selected UC when the rectum cannot be spared, and the patient has a normal anal sphincter function.
- RPC with IPAA can also be performed in some patients with indeterminate colitis, Crohn's disease, and synchronous CRC.
- IPAA has morbidity and functional results that worsen with time, mainly if the underlying pathology is Crohn's disease or indeterminate colitis.

To propose an RPC with IPAA, it is necessary:

- to confirm a normal anal sphincter function and the need for total proctocolectomy;
- know the underlying pathology and specific features;
- assess the risk of pouch morbidity and disfunction taking into account beyond the underlying pathology:
    - patient age, gender, IBM, and comorbidities.
    - indication for the surgery.
    - the time between the onset of the disease and surgery.
    - experience of the center in RPC with IPAA and patient's will.

Author details

Marisa D. Santos
Unit of Colorectal Surgery, University Hospital Center of Oporto (Centro Hospitalar Universitário do Porto—CHUP), Oporto, Portugal

*Address all correspondence to: marisadsantos@gmail.com

References

[1] Melton GB, Fazio VW, Kiran RP, et al. Long-term outcomes with ileal pouch-anal anastomosis and Crohn's disease: Pouch retention and implications of delayed diagnosis. Annals of Surgery. 2008;**248**:608-616

[2] Fazio VW, Kiran RP, Remzi FH, et al. Ileal pouch anal anastomosis: Analysis of outcome and quality of life in 3707 patients. Annals of Surgery. 2013;**257**: 679-685

[3] Parks AG, Nicholls RJ. Proctocolectomy without ileostomy for ulcerative colitis. British Medical Journal. 1978;**2**:85-88

[4] Magro F, Gionchetti P, Eliakim R, et al. Third European evidence-based consensus on diagnosis and management of ulcerative colitis. Part 1: Definitions, diagnosis, extra-intestinal manifestations, pregnancy, cancer surveillance, surgery, and ileo-anal pouch disorders. Journal of Crohn's and Colitis. 2017;**11**:649-670

[5] Moslein G. Surgical considerations in FAP-related pouch surgery: Could we do better? Familial Cancer. 2016;**15**: 457-466

[6] Holubar SD, Larson DW, Dozois EJ, et al. Minimally invasive subtotal colectomy and ileal pouch-anal anastomosis for fulminant ulcerative colitis: A reasonable approach? Diseases of the Colon & Rectum. 2009;**52**: 187-192

[7] Truelove SC. Medical management of ulcerative colitis and indications for colectomy. World Journal of Surgery. 1988;**12**:142-147

[8] Mowat C, Cole A, Windsor A, et al. Guidelines for the management of inflammatory bowel disease in adults. Gut. 2011;**60**:571-607

[9] Saha SK, Panwar R, Kumar A, et al. Early colectomy in steroid-refractory acute severe ulcerative colitis improves operative outcome. International Journal of Colorectal Disease. 2018;**33**:79-82

[10] Itzkowitz SH, Present DH, Crohn's, Colitis Foundation of America Colon Cancer in IBDSG. Consensus conference: Colorectal cancer screening and surveillance in inflammatory bowel disease. Inflammatory Bowel Diseases. 2005;**11**:314-321

[11] Kaminski MF, Hassan C, Bisschops R, et al. Advanced imaging for detection and differentiation of colorectal neoplasia: European Society of Gastrointestinal Endoscopy (ESGE) Guideline. Endoscopy. 2014;**46**:435-449

[12] Aaij R, Adeva B, Adinolfi M, et al. Observation of B (s)0-->J/psi f1(1285) decays and measurement of the f1(1285) mixing angle. Physical Review Letters. 2014;**112**:091802

[13] Rutter MD, Riddell RH. Colorectal dysplasia in inflammatory bowel disease: A clinicopathologic perspective. Clinical Gastroenterology and Hepatology. 2014;**12**:359-367

[14] Laine L, Kaltenbach T, Barkun A, et al. SCENIC international consensus statement on surveillance and management of dysplasia in inflammatory bowel disease. Gastrointestinal Endoscopy. 2015; **81**:489-501

[15] Shah SA, Rubin DT, Farraye FA. Chromoendoscopy for colorectal cancer surveillance in patients with inflammatory bowel disease. Current Gastroenterology Reports. 2014;**16**:407

[16] Bae SI, Kim YS. Colon cancer screening and surveillance in

inflammatory bowel disease. Clinical Endoscopy. 2014;**47**:509-515

[17] Fumery M, Dulai PS, Gupta S, et al. Incidence, risk factors, and outcomes of colorectal cancer in patients with ulcerative colitis with low-grade dysplasia: A systematic review and meta-analysis. Clinical Gastroenterology and Hepatology. 2017;**15**:665-674

[18] Oresland T, Bemelman WA, Sampietro GM, et al. European evidence based consensus on surgery for ulcerative colitis. Journal of Crohn's Colitis. 2015;**9**:4-25

[19] Soetikno RM, Lin OS, Heidenreich PA et al. Increased risk of colorectal neoplasia in patients with primary sclerosing cholangitis and ulcerative colitis: A meta-analysis. Gastrointest Endosc. 2002;**56**:48-54

[20] Eaden JA, Abrams KR, Mayberry JF. The risk of colorectal cancer in ulcerative colitis: A meta-analysis. Gut. 2001;**48**:526-535

[21] Lakatos PL, Lakatos L. Risk for colorectal cancer in ulcerative colitis: changes, causes and management strategies. World J Gastroenterol. 2008;**14**:3937-3947

[22] Soderlund S, Brandt L, Lapidus A et al. Decreasing time-trends of colorectal cancer in a large cohort of patients with inflammatory bowel disease. Gastroenterology. 2009;**136**: 1561-1567; quiz 1818-1569

[23] Velayos FS, Ullman TA. Looking forward to understanding and reducing colorectal cancer risk in inflammatory bowel disease. Gastroenterology. 2013;**145**:47-49

[24] Rutter MD, Saunders BP, Wilkinson KH et al. Cancer surveillance in longstanding ulcerative colitis: endoscopic appearances help predict cancer risk. Gut. 2004;**53**:1813-1816

[25] Kariv Y, Remzi FH, Strong SA, et al. Ileal pouch rectal anastomosis: A viable alternative to permanent ileostomy in Crohn's proctocolitis patients. Journal of the American College of Surgeons. 2009;**208**:390-399

[26] Browning SM, Nivatvongs S. Intraoperative abandonment of ileal pouch to anal anastomosis—The Mayo Clinic experience. Journal of the American College of Surgeons. 1998;**186**:441-445

[27] Lovegrove RE, Tilney HS, Remzi FH, et al. To divert or not to divert: A retrospective analysis of variables that influence ileostomy omission in ileal pouch surgery. Archives of Surgery. 2011;**146**:82-88

[28] Karjalainen EK, Renkonen-Sinisalo L, Mustonen HK, Lepisto AH. Morbidity related to diverting ileostomy after restorative proctocolectomy in patients with ulcerative colitis. Colorectal Disease. 2019;**21**:671-678

[29] Rottoli M, Casadei B, Vallicelli C, et al. Morbidity associated with closure of ileostomy after a three-stage ileal pouch-anal anastomosis. Updates in Surgery. 2019;**71**:533-537

[30] Wu XR, Kirat HT, Kalady MF, Church JM. Restorative proctocolectomy with a handsewn IPAA: S-pouch or J-pouch? Diseases of the Colon & Rectum. 2015;**58**:205-213

[31] Dafnis G. Functional outcome and quality of life after ileal pouch-anal anastomosis within a defined population in Sweden. Digestive Diseases. 2019;**37**:1-10

[32] Kirat HT, Kiran RP, Lian L, et al. Influence of stapler size used at ileal pouch-anal anastomosis on anastomotic leak, stricture, long-term functional outcomes, and quality of life. The American Journal of Surgery. 2010;**200**:68-72

[33] Lavryk OA, Hull TL, Duraes LC, et al. Outcomes of ileal pouch-anal anastomosis without primary diverting loop ileostomy if postoperative sepsis develops. Techniques in Coloproctology. 2018;**22**:37-44

[34] Kayal M, Plietz M, Rizvi A, et al. Inflammatory pouch conditions are common after ileal pouch anal anastomosis in ulcerative colitis patients. Inflammatory Bowel Diseases. 2020;**26**(7):1079-1086

[35] Hashavia E, Dotan I, Rabau M, Klausner JM, Halpern Z, Tulchinsky H. Risk factors for chronic pouchitis after ileal pouch-anal anastomosis: A prospective cohort study. Colorectal Disease. 2012;**14**:1365-1371

[36] Kiely JM, Fazio VW, Remzi FH, et al. Pelvic sepsis after IPAA adversely affects function of the pouch and quality of life. Diseases of the Colon & Rectum. 2012;**55**:387-392

[37] Silva AC, Sampaio M, Marcos-Pinto R, et al. Functional outcomes in patients submitted to restorative proctocolectomy with ileal pouch anal anastomosis in a single tertiary center. Journal of Coloproctology. 2018;**38**:30-36

[38] Galloway R, Dusch E, Elder L, et al. Women's perceptions of iron deficiency and anemia prevention and control in eight developing countries. Social Science & Medicine. 2002;**55**:529-544

[39] Gorgun E, Cengiz TB, Aytac E, et al. Does laparoscopic ileal pouch-anal anastomosis reduce infertility compared with open approach? Surgery. 2019;**166**:670-677

[40] Pachler FR, Toft G, Bisgaard T, Laurberg S. Use and Success of in vitro fertilisation following restorative proctocolectomy and ileal pouch-anal anastomosis. A nationwide 17-year cohort study. Journal of Crohn's and Colitis. 2019;**13**:1283-1286

[41] Bauer JJ, Gelernt IM, Salky B, Kreel I. Sexual dysfunction following proctocolectomy for benign disease of the colon and rectum. Annals of Surgery. 1983;**197**:363-367

[42] Mark-Christensen A, Erichsen R, Brandsborg S, et al. Long-term risk of cancer following ileal pouch-anal anastomosis for ulcerative colitis. Journal of Crohn's and Colitis. 2018;**12**:57-62

Section 4

Colorectal Cancer – Basic Sciences

Chapter 7

Pelvic Anatomy for Distal Rectal Cancer Surgery

Sanghyun An and Ik Yong Kim

Abstract

Worldwide, colorectal cancer is the third most common cancer and one of the leading causes of cancer-related deaths. Currently, total mesorectal excision (TME) is considered as the gold standard surgical procedure for rectal cancer. To achieve a good oncologic outcome and functional outcome after TME in distal rectal cancer, exact knowledge regarding the pelvic anatomy including pelvic fascia, pelvic floor, and the autonomic nerve is essential. Accurate TME along the embryologic plane not only reduces local recurrence rate but also preserves urinary and sexual function by minimizing nerve damage. In the past, pelvic floor muscles and autonomic nerves could not be visualized clearly, however, the development of imaging studies and improvements of minimally invasive surgical techniques such as laparoscopic and robotic surgery can clearly show the anatomy of the pelvic region. In this chapter, we will provide accurate anatomy of the rectum and the anal canal, pelvic fascia, and the pelvic autonomic nerve. This anatomical information will be an important indicator for performing an adequate operation for distal rectal cancer.

Keywords: rectal neoplasms, anatomy, colorectal surgery, autonomic nervous system, pelvic floor

1. Introduction

Colorectal cancer is the third most common cancer and the fourth leading cause of cancer-related deaths worldwide [1]. Especially, rectal cancer accounts for 30–40% of colorectal cancer, and the treatment strategy is different and more complicated compared to colon cancer because of its anatomical features. Although the treatment outcome of rectal cancer has greatly improved with the development of multimodality treatment including neoadjuvant radiotherapy, cytotoxic chemotherapy, and target agents, surgery remains the mainstay of therapy. Since the concept of total mesorectal excision (TME) was first described by Richard Heald in 1979, this procedure became the gold standard technique for rectal cancer surgery until now [2]. The fundamental principle of TME is en bloc resection of the rectum with its surrounding fatty tissue complex which contains the blood vessels and lymphatics down to the pelvic floor. To achieve complete TME and sphincter preserving surgery in low-lying rectal cancer, knowledge for regarding the pelvic fascia (mesorectal, parietal) and autonomic nerves, a thorough understanding of the pelvic floor anatomy is essential.

2. Pelvic anatomy

2.1 Basic anatomy of the rectum and mesorectum

The rectum is the most distal part of the large intestine that exists from the sacral promontory level to the anorectal ring. The anterior and lateral portion of the upper one-third of the rectum is covered with peritoneum, and the middle one-third of the rectum is covered with peritoneum on its anterior portion. The lower one-third cannot be observed in the intraperitoneal space because it is located in the extraperitoneal space. The taenia coli disappears in the rectum, forming one longitudinal muscle layer surrounding the rectum. The length of the rectum is approximately 12-15 cm and has three curvatures, which is related to Houston's valves. The upper and lower part are convex to the right, and the middle portion is convex to the left. The middle valve is the most prominent and is located approximately equal to the level of peritoneal reflection [3].

The rectum is surrounded by a fatty tissue complex called the mesorectum, which corresponds to the mesentery of the rectum. Mesorectum contains abundant blood vessels, lymphatics, and lymph nodes, and it is enveloped by thin visceral pelvic fascia [4]. It is developed thickest in the posterolateral side and the anterior part is formed relatively thin. In addition, the volume of the mesorectum decreases as it approaches the pelvic floor, and disappears approximately 2 cm above the levator ani muscle (**Figure 1**). A number of studies have revealed that the mesorectum is an important structure for tumor spreading, and en bloc resection through sharp dissection of mesorectum is very important in improving treatment outcomes [2, 5, 6].

2.2 Fascia structures around the rectum

Dissecting the correct anatomical plane can lead to good oncological outcomes and preserve the autonomic nerves to prevent postoperative urinary, sexual, and defecatory dysfunction. If pelvic dissection is performed along the exact embryologic fascial plane, the operation can be done without bleeding. To perform precise total mesorectal excision, a thorough understanding of the fascia around the rectum and pelvic cavity is essential. **Figure 2** shows the anatomical relationship of the fascia around the rectum.

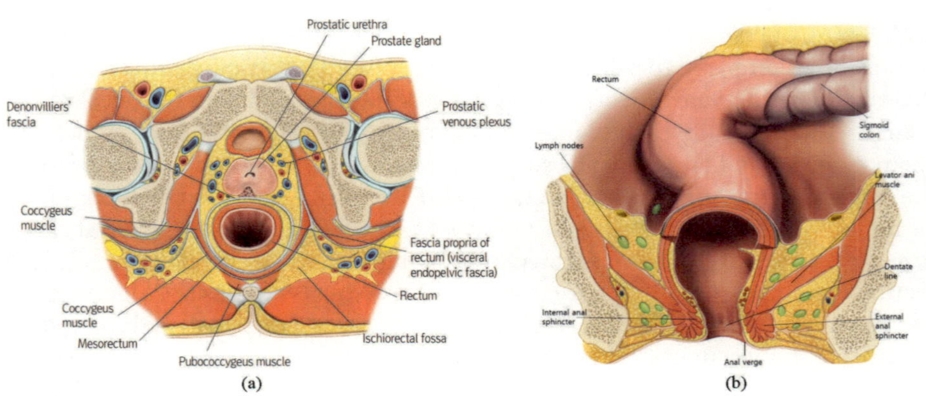

Figure 1.
Anatomy of the rectum and mesorectum. (a) Structures around the rectum. The rectum is surrounded by mesorectum, and the rectum and mesorectum are enveloped by the fascia propria of the rectum. (b) Total mesorectal excision (TME). En bloc resection of mesorectum is important.

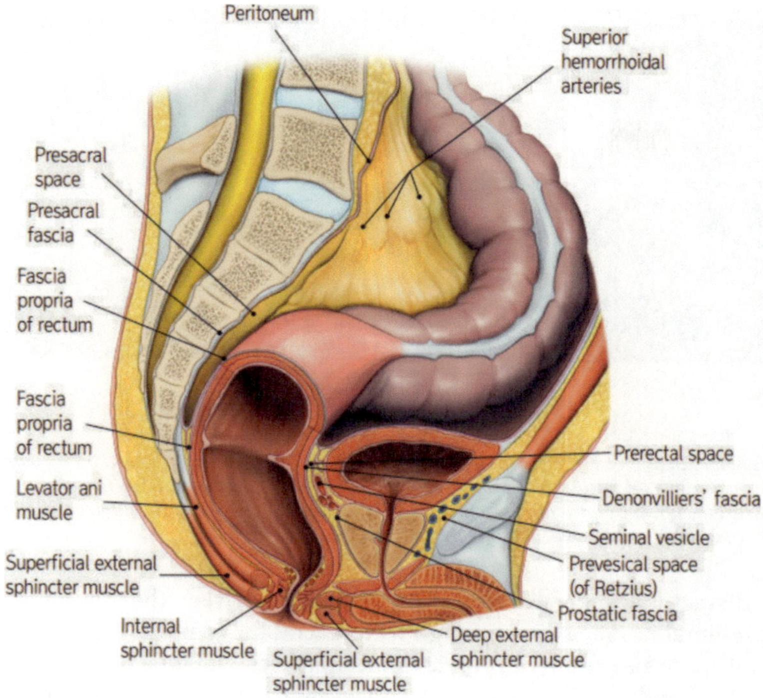

Figure 2.
Anatomy of fascia around the rectum. The fascia propria of the rectum covers the rectum and mesorectum. The presacral fascia covers the anterior surface of the sacrum. It combines with the fascia propria of the rectum at the S4 level (recto-sacral fascia = Waldeyer's fascia). Denonvilliers' fascia is a dense membrane between the rectum and seminal vesicles.

2.2.1 Fascia propria of the rectum and presacral fascia

The rectum and mesorectum are enveloped by the fascia propria of the rectum, also called as mesorectal fascia. The mesorectal fascia corresponds to the visceral fascia of the rectum. Caudally, it ends at the internal sphincter and laterally ends at the internal iliac artery, and is connected to the parietal pelvic fascia [7]. A magnetic resonance image scan (MRI) can clearly show the boundaries of these mesorectum and mesorectal fascia (**Figure 3**). During total mesorectal excision, it is important to completely excise this mesorectal fascia without damage to obtain optimal oncologic outcome [6, 8, 9].

The presacral fascia, also called as parietal pelvic fascia, covers the anterior surface of the sacrum and encloses the sacral vessels and nerves. It combines with the mesorectal fascia at the S4 level and became part of the anococcygeal ligament at the level of anorectal junction. The presacral venous plexus is formed by the two lateral sacral veins, the middle sacral vein, and the communicating veins, and it runs underneath the presacral fascia. If the dissection plane is too deep to damage the presacral fascia during the posterior dissection, life-threatening massive bleeding can occur and it often is difficult to control. Therefore, dissection should be done along with the space between the mesorectal fascia and the presacral fascia until the recto-sacral fascia is encountered [10, 11].

2.2.2 Recto-sacral fascia (Waldeyer's fascia)

Recto-sacral fascia, also known as Waldeyer's fascia, is a dense connective tissue linking the presacral fascia to the mesorectal fascia at the S4 level. As the

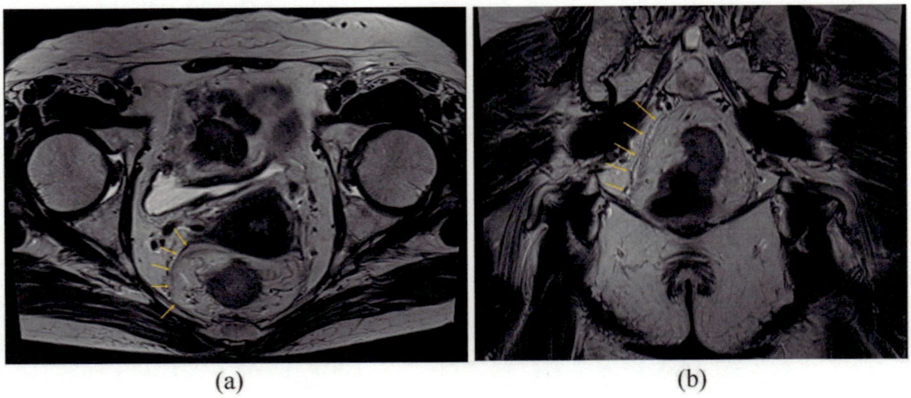

Figure 3.
Magnetic resonance image scan. Magnetic resonance image scan (MRI) can clearly show the boundaries of these mesorectum and mesorectal fascia. (a) T2 weighted image on MRI. Axial view. The rectum and mesorectum are enveloped by the fascia propria of the rectum (mesorectal fascia). (b) T2 weighted image on MRI. Coronal view. Mesorectum, mesorectal fascia, and puborectalis muscle.

posterior dissection proceeds down along the plane between the mesorectal fascia and the presacral fascia, a dense, tough recto-sacral fascia is identified. To enter the retro-rectal space and reach the pelvic floor, this fascia must be incised and dissected further caudally. This fascia has a different thickness from individuals, it is not visible when it is too thin. Because the presacral artery and venous plexus and autonomic nerves pass behind this fascia, it is important to perform sharp division to avoid excessive bleeding due to presacral vein injury (**Figure 4**) [8, 12].

2.2.3 Denonvilliers' fascia

During the anterior dissection of the rectum, a thin, dense connective tissue layer known as the Denonvilliers' fascia presents between the seminal vesicles and

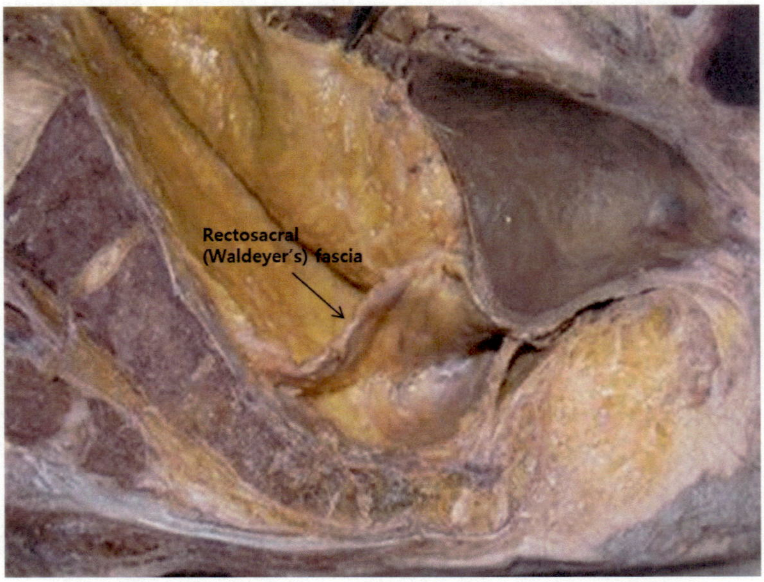

Figure 4.
Recto-sacral fascia (Waldeyer's fascia). Recto-sacral fascia (Waldeyer's fascia) is a dense connective tissue linking the presacral fascia to the mesorectal fascia at the S4 level. It is important to perform sharp dissection [11].

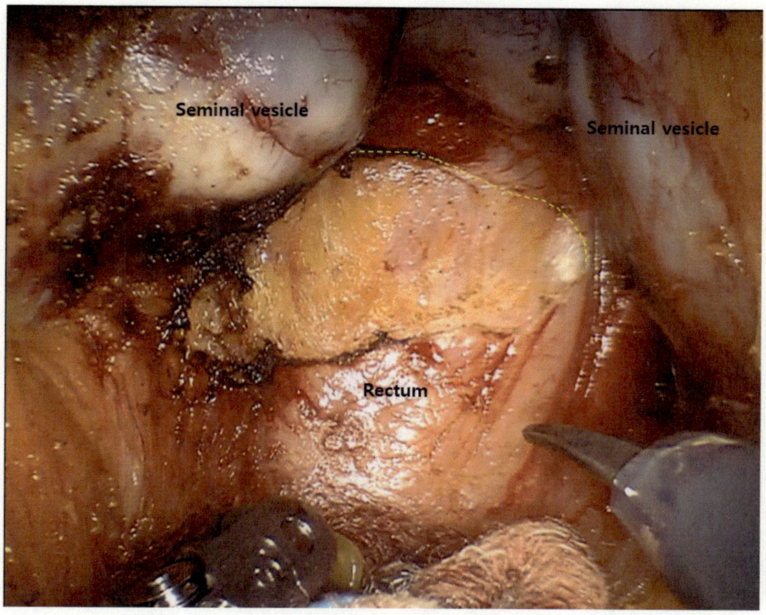

Figure 5.
Denonvilliers' fascia. During anterior dissection of the rectum. The dense connective tissue between rectum and seminal vesicles can be seen. The dissection should be performed below the Denonvilliers' fascia.

rectum [13]. The rectum can be separated from the seminal vesicles and prostate by opening this membrane at the level of anterior peritoneal reflection. After incising the fascia and entering the embryologic plane between the rectum and the seminal vesicles, the dissection should be performed below the Denonvilliers' fascia [14]. It is because there were neurovascular bundles running from the pelvic plexus to the ventral side of the Denonvilliers' fascia, especially in the directions of 10 and 2 o'clock, and these neurovascular bundles were related to urogenital function (**Figure 5**) [15]. However, if the deeply infiltrative tumor is located on the anterior wall of the rectum, the dissection should be performed in front of the Denonvilliers' fascia for curative resection. In females, there is a thin membranous structure that separates the rectum and vagina, which is called the rectovaginal septum. Although Denonvilliers reported that the Denonvilliers' fascia was not present in females, many researchers considered that the rectovaginal septum was consistent with the Denonvilliers' fascia in males (**Figure 6**) [16–19]. During the anterior dissection of the rectum in female, care must be taken not to perforate the vagina since this septum is very thin.

2.3 Anal canal

The rectum enters the pelvic floor and becomes the anus. The anal canal is defined as from the dentate line to the anal verge by anatomists, but most surgeons consider the anal canal from the anorectal ring to the anal verge [20]. The anorectal ring is where the rectum enters the pelvic floor and is angled by the puborectalis muscle. This ring can be palpated by a meticulous digital rectal exam. The dentate line, which divides the upper two-thirds and lower third of the anal canal, is an anatomically important landmark of the anal canal, and there are 6–14 longitudinal folds on the dentate line known as columns of Morgagni (**Figure 7**). The upper and lower part of the anal canal differs in venous and lymphatic drainage, innervation, and the epithelial surface based on the dentate line. Above the dentate line, the blood drains into the portal venous system, and lymphatics drains to the superior

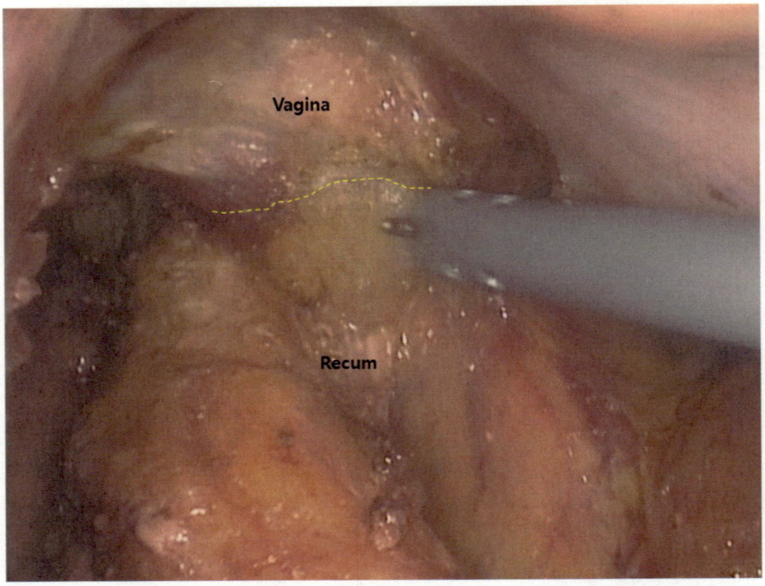

Figure 6.
Rectovaginal septum. In female, the rectovaginal septum was consistent with the denonvilliers' fascia in male.

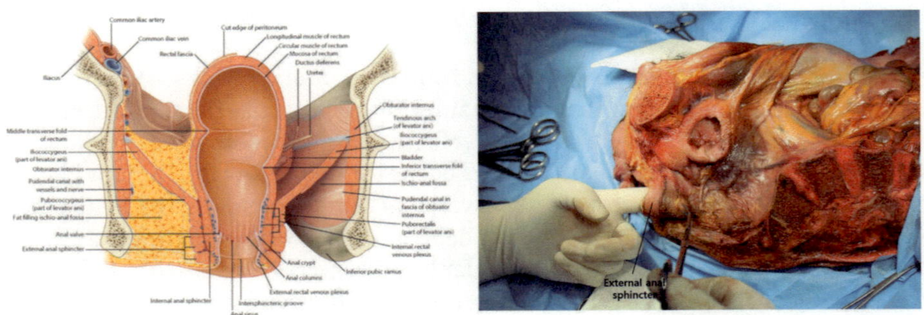

(a) (b)

Figure 7.
Anal canal and anal sphincter complex. (a) The dentate line divides the upper two thirds and lower third of the anal canal, and there are longitudinal folds known as columns of Morgagni. The external sphincter consists of three separate parts: Subcutaneous, superficial, and deep part [21]. (b) External anal sphincter. Lt. Hemipelvis.

rectal and iliac lymphatic chains. Below the dentate line, the blood drains into the caval system, and lymphatics drain into the inguinal lymph nodes.

There are two sphincter muscles surrounding the anus, the internal sphincter and the external sphincter. The internal sphincter is connected from the inner circular smooth muscle of the rectum and descends to 1–1.5 cm below the dentate line. Its length is about 2.5–4 cm and the mean thickness is about 0.5 cm. It is an involuntary smooth muscle and plays an important role in the maintenance of fecal incontinence because it contributes a majority of the resting pressure of the anal canal. The outer longitudinal muscle of the rectum conjoins the fibers from the puborectalis muscle and is located between the external and internal sphincter. The external sphincter muscle is a striated muscle surrounding the internal sphincter in the shape of a cylinder, and it extends slightly below the internal sphincter. The external sphincter consists of three separate parts: subcutaneous, superficial, and deep part. The subcutaneous external sphincter attaches to the perianal skin encircling the anus. The external anal sphincter is innervated by the rectal branch of the pudendal nerve and is under voluntary control [20, 22, 23]. The intersphincteric groove between the internal and external sphincter is an important landmark in surgery for patients with distal rectal cancer such as intersphincteric resection (ISR) [24].

2.4 Pelvic floor

The pelvic floor is a structure that forms the bottom of the pelvis, and plays an important role in supporting the pelvic organs. In the past, pelvic floor muscles could not be visualized clearly, however, the development of magnetic resonance imaging assessments and improvements in minimally invasive surgery techniques such as laparoscopy and robotic surgery can clearly show the anatomy of this region It is mainly composed of the levator ani muscle complex: pubococcygeus, iliococcygeus, and puborectalis muscle. The levator ani muscle received direct innervation from sacral nerve roots (S3-S5) and play an important role in cooperative action through coordinated contraction and relaxation during defecation [25]. The pubococcygeus is located in the most anterior portion of the levator ani muscles, and from both pubic bone to the coccyx. The iliococcygeus is the posterior part of the levator ani muscle and extends from the ischial spine to the anococcygeal raphe and coccyx. The puborectalis muscle, which is located below the pubococcygeus, forms a U-shaped ring around the rectum and makes an anorectal angle to prevent fecal incontinence. The coccygeus muscle, which is also a part of the pelvic floor, is located posterior portion of the levator ani muscle and reinforces the posterior pelvic floor (**Figure 8**) [20]. The pelvic floor has two hiatuses: the urogenital hiatus and the rectal hiatus. The rectal hiatus is located in the posterior of the pelvic floor through which the anal canal passes. The perineal body, a pyramidal fibromuscular mass, is located between the urogenital hiatus and the anal canal, strengthens the pelvic floor [26]. During distal rectal cancer surgery for sphincter preservation such as ISR, the intersphincteric space between the puborectalis muscle and the rectal wall should be identified, and the dissection continues down to the deep part of the anal canal through the intersphincteric space (**Figure 9**) [24]. On the other hand, during an abdominoperineal resection, the levator ani muscles must be cut [27].

2.4.1 Anococcygeal ligaments

The anococcygeal ligament is a fibrous membrane, which extends between the coccyx and the margin of the anal canal. In an anatomical study, the anococcygeal

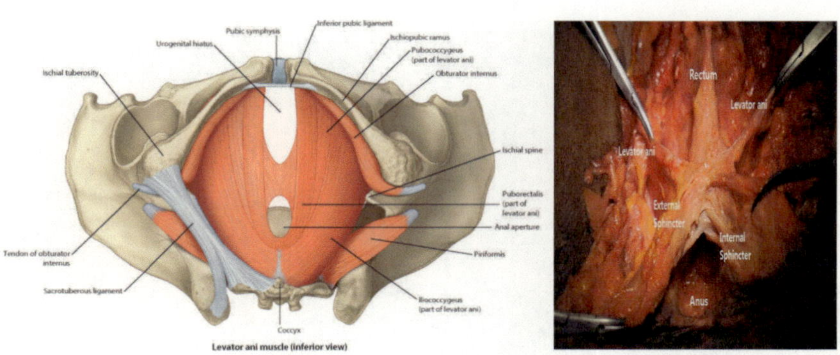

(a) (b)

Figure 8.
Anatomy of the pelvic floor. (a) Inferior view. The levator ani muscle consists of pubococcygeus, iliococcygeus, and puborectalis muscle [21]. (b) Pelvic floor muscles and anal sphincter complex [20].

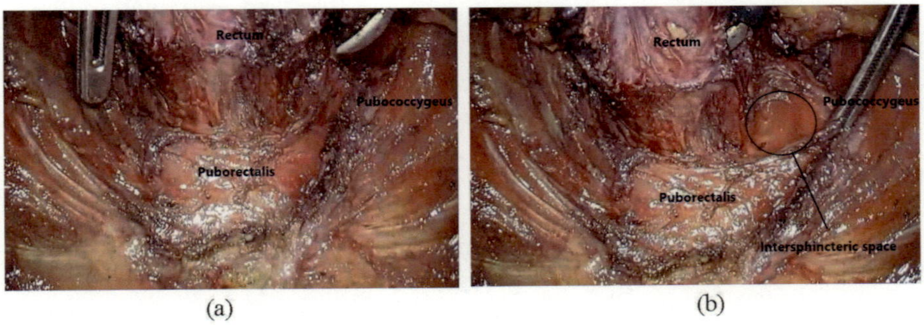

Figure 9.
Levator ani muscles and intersphincteric space. (a) Puborectalis and pubococcygeus muscle. (b) Intersphincteric space between rectum and puborectalis muscle.

ligament was divided into two layers. The ventral layer of the ligament was loose and rich in small and fragile vessels and extended from the presacral fascia to the conjoint longitudinal muscle layer of the anal canal. The dorsal layer of the ligament was thin and dense and extended between the coccyx and external anal sphincter (**Figure 10**) [28]. To fully mobilize the rectum from the pelvic floor at the final stage of total mesorectal excision, the anococcygeal ligament must be divided. If the anococcygeal ligament cannot be seen in the final step, it can be visualized after the mesorectum is completely mobilized from the pelvic floor.

2.5 Surgical plane for very low-lying rectal cancer

In case of very low-lying rectal cancer, several surgical options can be considered (**Figure 11**). If the tumor did not invade the anal sphincter complex, the ultra-low anterior resection with coloanal anastomosis could be considered. If the tumors are located close to the dentate line, the intersphincteric resection (ISR) could be considered. The ISR is the partial or complete resection of the internal anal sphincter along the intersphincteric plane. However, if the tumor invades the external sphincter complex, the abdominoperineal resection (APR) should be performed. For invasive low rectal cancer which invades the levator ani muscle, extralevator APR (ELAPE) should be considered to achieve adequate resection margin. The ELAPE is the cylindrical anorectal excision and removes more tissue around the tumor including levator ani muscle (**Figure 12**). This procedure has the advantage of reducing the risk of tumor perforation during operation and acquiring sufficient

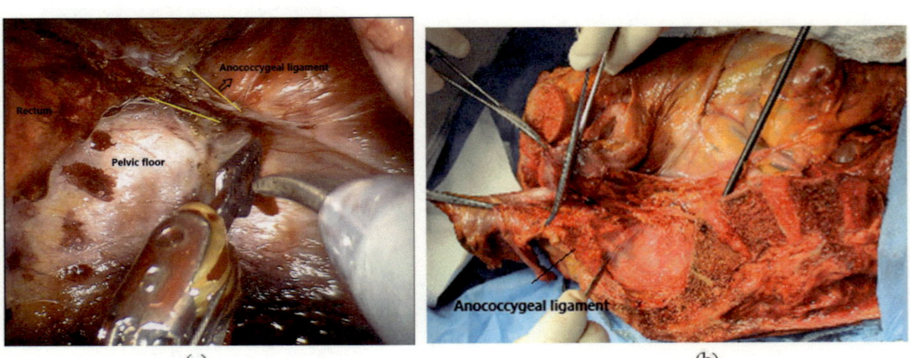

Figure 10.
Anococcygeal ligament. (a) Anococcygeal ligament and pelvic floor. During posterior dissection of the rectum. (b) Anococcygeal ligament during cadeveric dissection. Lt. hemipelvis.

DOI: http://dx.doi.org/10.5772/intechopen.99120

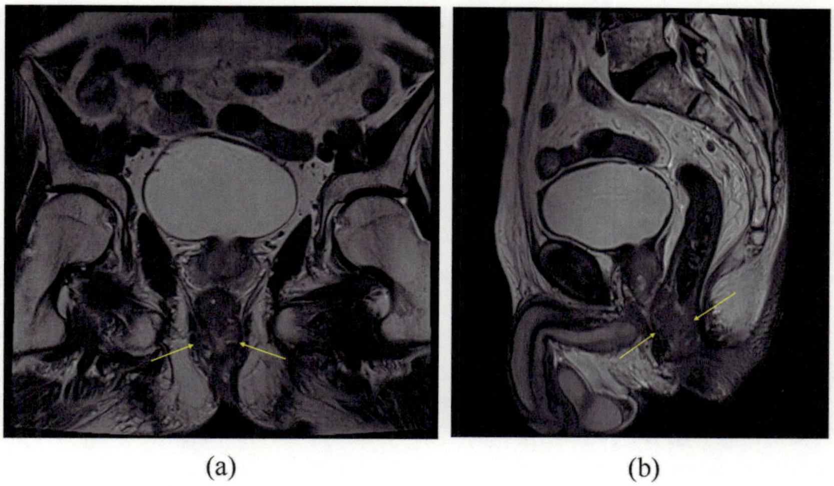

Figure 11.
Low-lying rectal cancer. (a) T2 weighted image on MRI. Coronal view. The low-lying rectal cancer invades internal anal sphincter. (b) T2 weighted image on MRI. Sagittal view.

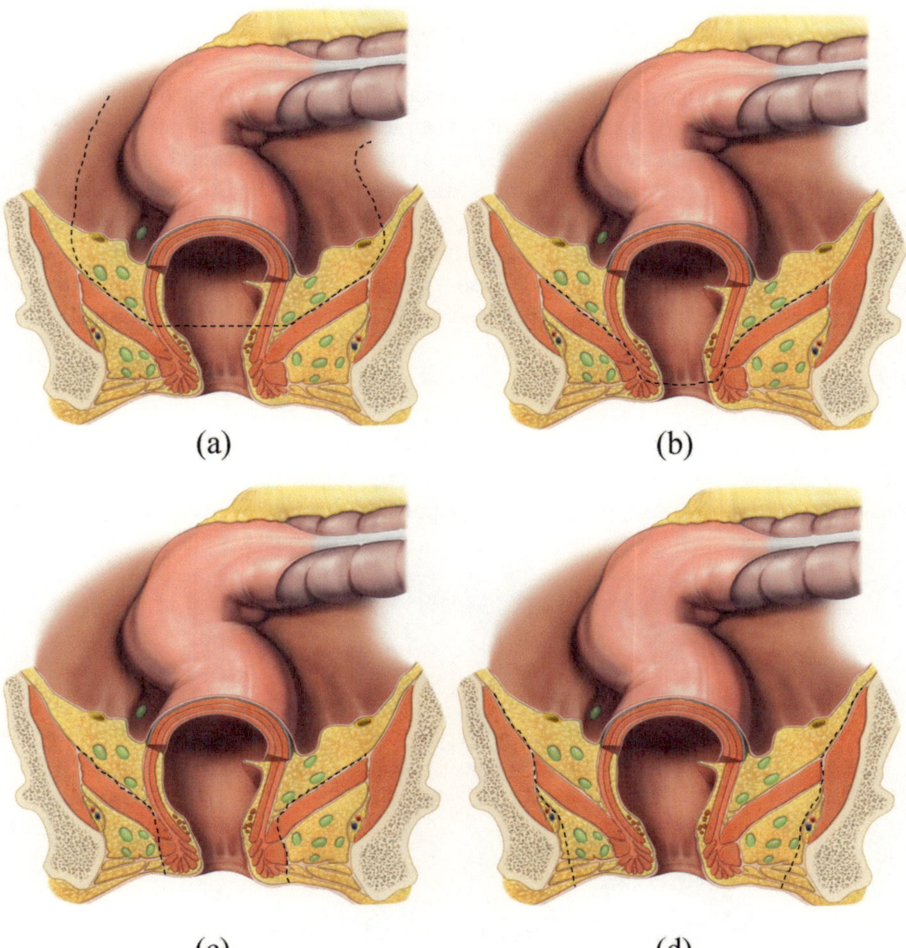

Figure 12.
Sugical plane for low-lying rectal cancer. (a) Low anterior resection (LAR). (b) Intersphincteric resection (ISR). (c) Abdominoperineal resection (APR). (d) Extralevator APR.

safety resection margin, but there is still controversy about the long-term oncologic outcome [29]. In addition, the postoperative complications can be increased due to the wide resection range.

2.6 Pelvic autonomic nerve system

In terms of quality of life, the importance of not only oncological outcomes but also functional outcomes such as urinary function, sexual function, and defecatory function after rectal cancer surgery have been emphasized. Urinary dysfunction after rectal surgery occurs in approximately 27%, and it includes difficulty emptying the bladder and incontinence [30, 31]. Sexual dysfunction for males consists of erectile dysfunction, absence of ejaculation, or retrograde ejaculation. For females, it causes sexual dysfunction such as impaired ability to achieve orgasm, decreased vaginal secretion, or dyspareunia [15]. The major cause of postoperative urogenital dysfunction is autonomic nerve damage that occurs during surgery. As minimally invasive surgery such as laparoscopy and robotic approach develops, meticulous nerve preserving surgery became possible with good visualization of the pelvic autonomic nerves [32–34]. To preserve the postoperative urogenital function, a thorough understanding of the anatomy of the pelvic autonomic nerve is crucial.

2.6.1 Superior hypogastric plexus and hypogastric nerves

The superior hypogastric plexus, which is a collection of sympathetic nerve bundles arising from T10-L3, forms a dense nerve plexus at the anterior area to the body of L5 and bifurcates into hypogastric nerves at the level of the sacral promontory (**Figure 13**). The superior hypogastric plexus runs around the inferior mesenteric artery. Therefore, this nerve can be damaged during dissection around the origin of the inferior mesenteric artery, and it results in retrograde ejaculation, urinary incontinence [35]. The hypogastric nerve crosses the left common iliac artery at the level of the first sacrum and descends to the pelvic cavity along the lateral pelvic wall.

2.6.2 Pelvic splanchnic nerves

The pelvic splanchnic nerves are considered to be parasympathetic nerves that arise from the second to fourth sacral spinal nerves. These nerves enter the pelvis through the sacral foramen, posterior to the parietal fascia that covers the piriformis

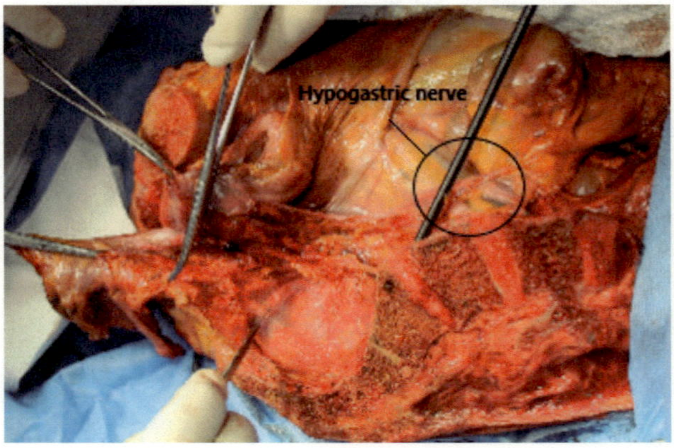

Figure 13.
Hypogastric nerves. The hypogastric nerves run from the superior hypogastric plexus and descend to the pelvic cavity and meet the pelvic splanchnic nerves.

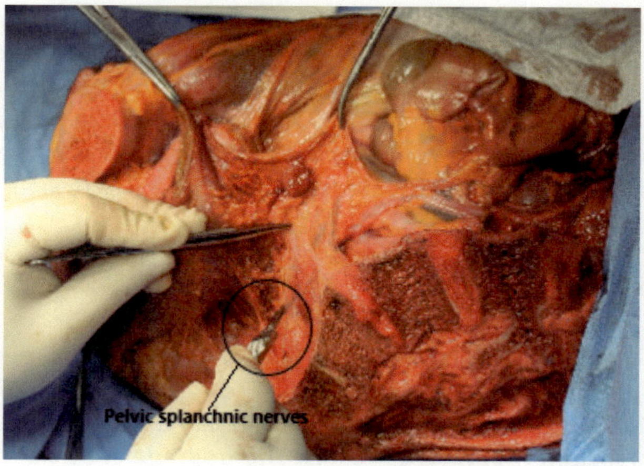

Figure 14.
Pelvic splanchnic nerves. The pelvic splanchnic nerves arise from the S2 to S4 spinal nerves. Small branches of the pelvic splanchnic nerves run medially and enter the mesorectum.

muscle and crosses the retrorectal space, to enter the visceral compartment through the visceral fascia about 4 cm from the midline. Small branches of the pelvic splanchnic nerves run medially and enter the mesorectum (**Figure 14**). These nerves regulate the emptying of the urinary bladder and influence erectile functions and motility of the rectum. Therefore, damage to these nerves causes erectile dysfunction and decreased blood flow to the vagina and vulva, which can reduce vaginal lubrication.

2.6.3 Inferior hypogastric (pelvic) plexus

The pelvic splanchnic nerves meet the hypogastric nerves and form the inferior hypogastric plexus at the lateral pelvic wall. It lies outside the fascia propria in the superficial layer of the parietal fascia. The inferior hypogastric plexus can be observed as a mesh-like structure at the posterolateral pelvic wall close to the prostate and seminal vesicles. Because the inferior hypogastric plexus consists of both sympathetic and parasympathetic efferent fibers, any damage to this plexus may cause severe disturbances in urogenital and sexual function including erection and ejaculation. It extends forward to form neurovascular bundles running down the seminal vesicle at 2 o'clock and 10 o'clock direction (**Figure 15**).

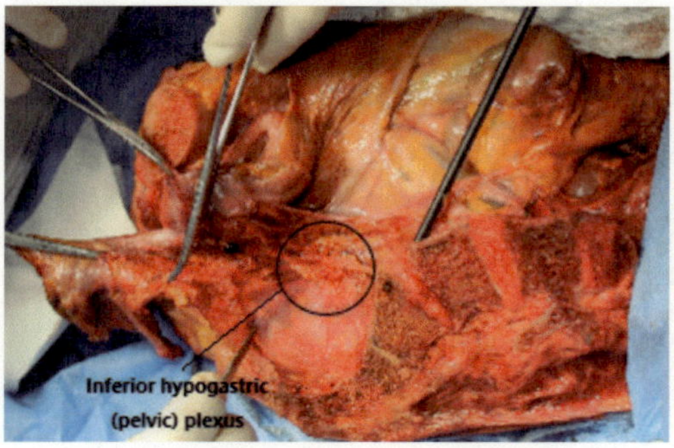

Figure 15.
Inferior hypogastric (pelvic) plexus. The inferior hypogastric (pelvic) plexus is a network of sympathetic and parasympathetic fibers arising from the hypogastric nerves and the pelvic splanchnic nerves. It can be observed as a mesh-like structure at the posterolateral pelvic wall. It extends forward to form neurovascular bundles running down the seminal vesicle on both sides.

These neurovascular bundles run through the posterolateral border of the prostate and continue to the periprostatic plexus, which supplies to the prostate, seminal vesicles, corpi cavernosi, and the vas deferens [15, 36]. Injury to the neurovascular bundles during anterior dissection may cause urinary and sexual dysfunction. Meticulous dissection is required because nerve damage may occur when surgery is performed along the wrong plane or excessive traction is performed.

3. Conclusion

The rectum is surrounded by a fatty tissue complex called the mesorectum, which contains abundant blood vessels, lymphatics, and lymph nodes. The rectum and mesorectum are enveloped by the mesorectal fascia. During total mesorectal excision, it is important to completely excise this mesorectal fascia without damage. The mesorectal fascia conjoins with the recto-sacral fascia, which extends forward from the presacral fascia at the level of S4, and descends to the pelvic floor. To enter the retro-rectal space and reach the pelvic floor, this fascia must be incised and sharp dissection should be performed to prevent severe bleeding due to injury to the presacral plexus. During the anterior dissection of the rectum, it is important to recognize Denonvillers' fascia located between the rectum and seminal vesicles, and dissection should be performed below the Denonvilliers' fascia. The pelvic floor is a structure that forms the bottom of the pelvis and is mainly composed of the levator ani muscle complex: pubococcygeus, iliococcygeus, and puborectalis muscle. The levator ani muscle received direct innervation from sacral nerve roots (S3-S5) and play an important role in cooperative action during defecation. To reach the deep part of the anal canal, the dissection should be performed between the puborectalis muscle and the rectal wall. During the whole process of TME, surgeons should take care to identify and preserve the autonomic nerve in order to avoid postoperative urogenital dysfunction. Care should be taken not to damage the superior hypogastric nerve during IMA ligation, and not to damage the pelvic plexus during posterolateral pelvic dissection. In addition, during anterior dissection of the rectum, it is important to perform meticulous dissection so as not to injure small numerous neurovascular bundles running in the 2 o'clock and 10 o'clock directions of the seminal vesicle. Based on a sufficient understanding of pelvic anatomy, precise surgical techniques using advanced surgical tools will give favorable oncologic and functional outcomes for rectal cancer patients.

Conflict of interest

The authors declare no conflict of interest.

Notes/thanks/other declarations

None.

Author details

Sanghyun An and Ik Yong Kim*
Department of Surgery, Yonsei University Wonju College of Medicine, Wonju, Korea

*Address all correspondence to: iykim@yonsei.ac.kr

References

[1] Ferlay J, Colombet M, Soerjomataram I, Parkin DM, Pineros M, Znaor A, et al. Cancer statistics for the year 2020: An overview. International Journal of Cancer. 2021. DOI:10.1002/ijc.33588

[2] Heald RJ, Husband EM, Ryall RDH. The mesorectum in rectal cancer surgery—the clue to pelvic recurrence? British Journal of Surgery. 1982;69:613-616. DOI:10.1002/bjs.1800691019

[3] Engin O. Colon polyps and the prevention of colorectal cancer: Springer; 2015. 249 p. DOI:10.1007/978-3-319-17993-3

[4] Culligan K, Walsh S, Dunne C, Walsh M, Ryan S, Quondamatteo F, et al. The mesocolon: a histological and electron microscopic characterization of the mesenteric attachment of the colon prior to and after surgical mobilization. Annals of Surgery. 2014;260:1048-1056. DOI:10.1097/SLA.0000000000000323

[5] Bokey EL, Öjerskog B, Chapuis PH, Dent OF, Newland RC, Sinclair G. Local recurrence after curative excision of the rectum for cancer without adjuvant therapy: role of total anatomical dissection. British Journal of Surgery. 1999;86:1164-1170. DOI:10.1046/j.1365-2168.1999.01216.x

[6] Silva-Velazco J, Stocchi L, Valente MA, Church JM, Liska D, Gorgun E, et al. The relationship between mesorectal grading and oncological outcome in rectal adenocarcinoma. Colorectal Disease. 2019;21:315-325. DOI:10.1111/codi.14535

[7] Stelzner S, Heinze T, Nikolouzakis TK, Torge Mees S, Witzigmann H, Wedel T. Perirectal fascial anatomy: New insights into an old problem. Diseases of the Colon and Rectum. 2021;64:91-102. DOI:10.1097/DCR.0000000000001778

[8] Kim NK, Kim HS, Alessa M, Torky R. Optimal complete rectum mobilization focused on the anatomy of the pelvic fascia and autonomic nerves: 30 years of experience at Severance Hospital. Yonsei Medical Journal. 2021;62:187-199. DOI:10.3349/ymj.2021.62.3.187

[9] Heald RJ, Santiago I, Pares O, Carvalho C, Figueiredo N. The perfect total mesorectal excision obviates the need for anything else in the management of most rectal cancers. Clinics in Colon and Rectal Surgery. 2017;30:324-332. DOI:10.1055/s-0037-1606109

[10] Lou Z, Zhang W, Meng RG, Fu CG. Massive presacral bleeding during rectal surgery: from anatomy to clinical practice. World Journal of Gastroenterology : WJG. 2013;19:4039-4044. DOI:10.3748/wjg.v19.i25.4039

[11] Kim NK. Anatomic basis of sharp pelvic dissection for curative resection of rectal cancer. Yonsei Medical Journal. 2005;46:737-749. DOI:10.3349/ymj.2005.46.6.737

[12] Açar Hİ, Kuzu MA. Anatomical planes in rectal cancer surgery. Turkish Journal of Colorectal Disease. 2019;29:165-170. DOI:10.4274/tjcd.galenos.2019.2019-10-2

[13] Lindsey I, Guy RJ, Warren BF, Mortensen NJ. Anatomy of Denonvilliers' fascia and pelvic nerves, impotence, and implications for the colorectal surgeon. British Journal of Surgery. 2000;87:1288-1299. DOI:10.1046/j.1365-2168.2000.01542.x

[14] Zhu XM, Yu GY, Zheng NX, Liu HM, Gong HF, Lou Z, et al. Review of Denonvilliers' fascia: the controversies and consensuses. Gastroenterology Report. 2020;8:343-348. DOI:10.1093/gastro/goaa053

[15] Nagpal K, Bennett N. Colorectal surgery and its impact on male sexual function. Current Urology Reports. 2013;14:279-284. DOI:10.1007/s11934-013-0341-x

[16] Kim JH, Kinugasa Y, Hwang SE, Murakami G, Rodriguez-Vazquez JF, Cho BH. Denonvilliers' fascia revisited. Surgical and Radiologic Anatomy : SRA. 2015;37:187-197. DOI:10.1007/s00276-014-1336-0

[17] Kraima AC, West NP, Treanor D, Magee DR, Rutten HJ, Quirke P, et al. Whole mount microscopic sections reveal that Denonvilliers' fascia is one entity and adherent to the mesorectal fascia; implications for the anterior plane in total mesorectal excision? European Journal of Surgical Oncology. 2015;41:738-745. DOI:10.1016/j.ejso.2015.03.224

[18] Ludwikowski B, Hayward IO, Fritsch H. Rectovaginal fascia: An important structure in pelvic visceral surgery? About its development, structure, and function. Journal of Pediatric Surgery. 2002;37:634-638. DOI:10.1053/jpsu.2002.31624

[19] Aigner F, Zbar AP, Ludwikowski B, Kreczy A, Kovacs P, Fritsch H. The rectogenital septum: morphology, function, and clinical relevance. Diseases of the Colon and Rectum. 2004;47:131-140. DOI:10.1007/s10350-003-0031-8

[20] Lee JM, Kim NK. Essential anatomy of the anorectum for colorectal surgeons focused on the gross anatomy and histologic findings. Annals of Coloproctology. 2018;34:59-71. DOI:10.3393/ac.2017.12.15

[21] Richard L. Drake, A. Wayne Vogl and Adam W.M. Mitchell. Gray's Atlas of Anatomy, 5, 213-292

[22] Kim NK, Sugihara K, Liang J-T. Surgical treatment of colorectal cancer: Asian perspectives on optimization and standardization; : Springer Singapore 2018. 414 p. DOI:10.1007/978-981-10-5143-2

[23] Fritsch H, Brenner E, Lienemann A, Ludwikowski B. Anal sphincter complex: reinterpreted morphology and its clinical relevance. Diseases of the Colon and Rectum. 2002;45:188-194. DOI:10.1007/s10350-004-6144-x

[24] Rullier E, Zerbib F, Laurent C, Bonnel C, Caudry M, Saric J, et al. Intersphincteric resection with excision of internal anal sphincter for conservative treatment of very low rectal cancer. Diseases of the Colon and Rectum. 1999;42:1168-1175. DOI:10.1007/Bf02238569

[25] Eickmeyer SM. Anatomy and physiology of the pelvic floor. Physical Medicine and Rehabilitation Clinics of North America. 2017;28:455-460. DOI:10.1016/j.pmr.2017.03.003

[26] Siccardi MA, Bordoni B. Anatomy, Abdomen and Pelvis, Perineal Body [Internet]. 2021. Available from: https://www.ncbi.nlm.nih.gov/books/NBK537345/ [Accessed: 2021-04-01]

[27] Stelzner S, Holm T, Moran BJ, Heald RJ, Witzigmann H, Zorenkov D, et al. Deep pelvic anatomy revisited for a description of crucial steps in extralevator abdominoperineal excision for rectal cancer. Diseases of the Colon and Rectum. 2011;54:947-957. DOI:10.1097/DCR.0b013e31821c4bac

[28] Kinugasa Y, Arakawa T, Abe S, Ohtsuka A, Suzuki D, Murakami G, et al. Anatomical reevaluation of the anococcygeal ligament and its surgical relevance. Diseases of the Colon and Rectum. 2011;54:232-237. DOI:10.1007/DCR.0b013e318202388f

[29] Tao Y, Han JG, Wang ZJ. Extralevator abdominoperineal excision for advanced low rectal cancer: Where to go. World

Journal of Gastroenterology : WJG. 2020;26:3012-3023. DOI:10.3748/wjg.v26.i22.3012

[30] Kim NK, Kim YW, Cho MS. Total mesorectal excision for rectal cancer with emphasis on pelvic autonomic nerve preservation: Expert technical tips for robotic surgery. Surgical Oncology. 2015;24:172-180. DOI:10.1016/j.suronc.2015.06.012

[31] Chew MH, Yeh YT, Lim E, Seow-Choen F. Pelvic autonomic nerve preservation in radical rectal cancer surgery: changes in the past 3 decades. Gastroenterology Report. 2016;4:173-185. DOI:10.1093/gastro/gow023

[32] Luca F, Valvo M, Ghezzi TL, Zuccaro M, Cenciarelli S, Trovato C, et al. Impact of robotic surgery on sexual and urinary functions after fully robotic nerve-sparing total mesorectal excision for rectal cancer. Annals of Surgery. 2013;257:672-678. DOI:10.1097/SLA.0b013e318269d03b

[33] Garbarino GM, Canali G, Tarantino G, Costa G, Ferri M, Balducci G, et al. Laparoscopic versus open rectal resection: a 1:2 propensity score-matched analysis of oncological adequateness, short- and long-term outcomes. International Journal of Colorectal Disease. 2021;36:801-810. DOI:10.1007/s00384-021-03841-w

[34] Hur H, Bae SU, Kim NK, Min BS, Baik SH, Lee KY, et al. Comparative study of voiding and male sexual function following open and laparoscopic total mesorectal excision in patients with rectal cancer. Journal of Surgical Oncology. 2013;108:572-578. DOI:10.1002/jso.23435

[35] Mari GM, Crippa J, Cocozza E, Berselli M, Livraghi L, Carzaniga P, et al. Low ligation of inferior mesenteric artery in laparoscopic anterior resection for rectal cancer reduces genitourinary dysfunction: Results from a randomized controlled Trial (HIGHLOW Trial). Annals of Surgery. 2019;269:1018-1024. DOI:10.1097/SLA.0000000000002947

[36] Hollabaugh Jr RS, Steiner MS, Sellers KD, Samm BJ, Dmochowski RR. Neuroanatomy of the pelvis: Implications for colonic and rectal resection. Diseases of the Colon and Rectum. 2000;43:1390-1397. DOI:10.1007/BF02236635

Chapter 8

Lipoxygenase and Colon Cancer

Muslim Abas Abed AlAdlee and Sahar Ghazi Imran

Abstract

The enzymes involved in the oxidative metabolism of n-6 polyunsaturated fatty acids, such as lipoxygenase (LOX) and cyclooxygenase (COX), are significant in the pathogenesis of colorectal cancer. The aim of this study is to estimate the effectiveness and partial purification of LOX and measure gamma-glutamyl transferase (GGT) activity in the serum of patients with colon cancer in Baghdad. The study included samples from 80 male patients with colon cancer and 50 samples of apparently healthy males (control) as the comparison group. The result displayed a noteworthy increase in lipoxygenase effectiveness (805.0 ± 517.23 IU/L) in the serum of patients with colon cancer (stage pT3) compared with control (114.6 ± 49.77 IU/L). The enzyme was purified by the precipitation of the serum protein using 40% $(NH4)_2SO4$ and then removing the remaining salts by dialysis. The column of gel (Sephadex G.100) was used to separate the enzyme from another protein, in this step a single peak was obtained. The effective part of lipoxygenase is at yield 71.42% and folds 11.033. The ion exchange chromatography (DEAE–CeA50) was used to isolate LOX isoenzyme, and two bands (LOX1 and LOX2) were acquired with different degree of purity 16.372 and 12.16 folds, respectively. The result displayed a noteworthy increase in the GGT activity in patients (58.69 ± 16.94 IU/L) compared with control (12.79 ± 5.68 IU/L) $p \leq 0.0001$. The increase in the activity of LOX can be potentially used as a tumor marker for colorectal cancer.

Keywords: colon cancer, lipoxygenase (LOX), gamma-glutamyl transferase (GGT), LOX isoenzyme, linoleic acid

1. Introduction

Tumors usually arise as a result of mutations in the cellular DNA [1–7]. The mutations occur in two types of genes, oncogenes and tumor suppressor genes. Oncogenes stimulate cell division, and increasing the activity of these genes encourages cancer cells to grow abnormally and work on Protect cells from apoptosis. Tumor suppressor genes or apoptosis genes work to stop cell division and help the immune system protect tissue [8]. In the case of a tumor, these genes stop, because they oppose its formation by correcting errors in DNA transcription.

It should be noted that cancer occurs in all cases due to mutation, but not all mutations cause cancer. Cancer results from the abnormal activation of cellular genes that regulate cell growth and divisions. Determining the stage of the tumor expresses the extent of the tumor's progress and exacerbation and is necessary before starting the treatment. Thus we conclude that cancer is a disorder that results from the failure of cells to die, rather than the process of cell proliferation, as the proliferation is not matched by a sufficient number of cells that die, which leads to their accumulation [9–12].

The metabolism of fats in the human body, especially the arachidonic acid metabolism pathway, plays a major role in chronic inflammation and colon carcinogenesis [13], as phospholipase A2 (PLA2) enzymes stimulate the formation of free fatty acids such as arachidonic acid from phospholipids associated with the cell membrane, which have been shown to participate in the formation of cancer in laboratory mouse models [14].

LOX has an important role to stimulate inflammatory reactions. Reactive oxygen free radicals can cause inflammation that activates the release of cytokines and the activation of LOX. Inflammation is associated with many diseases, such as cancer, cardiovascular and neurodegenerative diseases. LOX contributes to the synthesis of leukotrienes and prostaglandins. These are associated with disease development [15]. The most important enzymes in the pathway of arachidonic acid metabolism [16] are LOX and COX, which are found in high concentrations in many tumors, including lung cancer [17], prostate cancer [18], brain cancer [19], rectal cancer [20], skin cancer [21], and breast cancer [22] where the GGT enzyme enters in the metabolic pathway of leukotrienes C4 [23].

2. Materials and methods

2.1 Collection of samples

Blood samples of 80 colon cancer patients (aged 40–80 years) who attend the Teaching Oncology Hospital at the City of Medicine and the National Center for Oncology, Baghdad for the period (18-2-2018 to 28-2-2019), were obtained.

A total of 50 blood samples were collected from apparently healthy individuals as a control group (aged 40–80 years). The samples were collected by drawing blood from the vein (5 mL) using a syringe and placing the blood in a gel tube.

The tubes were placed in the centrifuge at 1252 g for 10 minutes to obtain serum. The serum was kept by Eppendorf tube in deep-freeze at −20°C until testing.

2.2 Measuring the LOX activity in blood serum

The method of measuring the activity of the LOX enzyme [24] is based on stimulating the oxygen reaction with the unsaturated fatty acids containing (cis, cis −1.4-pentadiene). It consists of a sequential system of double bonds that increase absorption at a wavelength of 234 nm where the absorption intensity is directly proportional to the concentration of the enzyme [25]. The unit of enzyme is defined as the amount of enzyme that changes in absorbance by 0.001 / sec at wavelength 234 nm under ideal conditions.

2.3 Estimation protein concentration

The biuret method was used to estimate the concentration of the protein in the samples [26].

2.4 Separation and purification of LOX from serum patients of colon cancer

LOX is purified using the following steps:

2.4.1 Precipitation by ammonium sulfate

The serum proteins were deposed by adding 0.9 gm of ammonium sulfate (0.40%) to 4 ml of serum for patients with colon cancer, which was gradually added in ice bath with magnetic stirrer (15 minutes) until all the ammonium sulfate has been dissolved. Then the solution was placed in the centrifuge for 15 minutes and at a speed of 17,608 g to separate the precipitation from the leachate, the precipitate was dissolved with the least amount of the buffer solution (Buffer phosphate pH 7(0.001 M)). Then, the enzyme activity and protein concentration were measured.

2.4.2 Dialysis

The process of dialysis for the dissolved protein was done to remove the ammonium sulfate residues that were used to precipitate the proteins, using a dialysis bag. The dissolved protein was added into the bag and immersed in the buffer solution (Buffer phosphate (0.001 M) pH 7). This process was carried out for 24 hours, with the solution being changed periodically. This step of purification was done at 4° C to maintain the activity of the enzyme. The activity and protein concentration of the enzyme were measured after the end of the process.

2.4.3 Gel filtration

The gel filtration technique is based on the difference in molecular weights. This step was used to purify the LOX enzyme from proteins and associated salts. The filter column of the Sephadex G.100 was used.

- A column separating diameter of 2 cm and length of 70 cm with a filter at the end of which prevents the granulation of the resin outside was used, the process of casting the column was performed by using resin solution and pouring the resin solution on the walls slowly and homogeneously so as not to form air bubbles that impede the separation process, the column was then washed with a quantity of buffer solution (Buffer phosphate (0.001 M) pH 7), and the flow velocity was set at 1 mL/min.

- 4 mL of product in dialysis step were added slowly and gradually over the resin surface and on the column walls and left for 5 minutes to soak into the resin.

- The gel filtration process was initiated using 250 mL of the buffer solution (Buffer phosphate (0.001 M) pH 7). The extracts were extracted from the gel filtration column at a size of 5 mL per part.

- The activity and the protein concentration of the LOX enzyme were evaluated.

2.4.4 Ion exchange chromatography

This technique was used to purify the isoenzyme of the LOX.

- DEAE-Cellulose (A50) was prepared by dissolving 20 gm of DAEA-Cellulose A50 in 250 mL of Buffer phosphate pH 7, leaving the solution suspended for 24 hours and at 4° C. The solution was switched several times from time to time to remove the soft minutes from the suspended solution until the pH reaches 7.

- NaCl solution (1 M) was prepared by dissolving 5.85gm of sodium chloride in 100 mL of (Buffer phosphate (0.001 M) pH 7) solution. Other solution was obtained with graduated concentrations of NaCl (0.1, 0.25, 0.5, 0.75 M).

- A glass column diameter of 3 cm and length of 30 cm contains a filter at the end, which prevents the resin granules from leaking out of it was used, the process of casting the column was performed by using resin solution with pouring the resin solution on the walls slowly and homogeneously so as not to form air bubbles that impede the process of ion exchange, then the column was washed with 250 mL of the buffer solution (Buffer phosphate (0.001 M) pH 7) and the flow time and velocity were set at 1 mL/min.

- 3 ml of protein from the gel filtration step were added slowly on the column walls and left to soak into the column. The separation process was initiated using (500 mL) of the buffer solution containing NaCl (25, 50, 75, 100 mM) progressive concentrations and the elute parts (3 mL) were collected for each part. Then the activity of the LOX and the protein concentration was evaluated.

2.4.5 Measuring GGT activity in blood serum

The Szasz method [27] was used to measure the effectiveness of the GGT enzyme, and the reaction equation is shown in Eq. (1):

$$\mathrm{L-\gamma-Glutamul-3-carboxy-4-nitroanilid+Glycylglycin} \overset{\gamma-\mathrm{GT}}{\Rightarrow} \mathrm{L-\gamma-Glutamul-Glycylglycin+5-Amino-2-nitro-benzoat} \tag{1}$$

In Eq. (1) the reaction of measured the effectiveness of the GGT.

The activity of the enzyme is directly proportional to the formation of 5-amino-2-nitro-benzoate at a wavelength of 405 nm.

2.5 Statistical analysis

Statistical analysis was carried out using SPSS (version 16). Graphs were drawn using Excel (2010), where ANOVA, arithmetic mean and standard deviation were used. The minimum probability factor ($p \le 0.05$) was statistically significant.

3. Results and discussion

The study included 80 males with colon cancer. The study also included 38 samples of healthy (control) males. The age range for both groups was between 40 and 80 years.

3.1 Measurement of LOX activity in blood serum

The activity of LOX was estimate in patients with stage pT3 colon cancer.

The results of the study included the statistical values of colon cancer patients and the biochemical variables measured in patients and control group.

The results showed that there was an increase in the activity of LOX in the blood serum of patients with colon cancer. A statistical comparison between the effectiveness of LOX in patients' and control showed a significant excess in enzyme effectiveness in patients with probability $P \leq 0.0001$ compared with control, as shown in **Figure 1**.

Overall, the results indicated an increase in the activity of LOX in the serum of colon cancer patients, previous scientific literature did not indicate that the enzyme's activity was measured from the serum of colon cancer patients, but indicated an increase in the activity of the enzyme in human colon cancer cell lines [28–30], this high effectiveness was reported to be highly correlated with reproduction of cancer cells, angiogenesis and resistance to apoptosis [31, 32].

Also the increase in enzyme activity is due to the increase in the digestion of unsaturated fatty acids and the release of Eicosanoid compounds that promote the growth of cancerous tumors [33].

Separation and Purification of LOX from Serum Patients of Colon Cancer: LOX was separated and purified in several steps as shown in the **Table 1**.

The first step was precipitating and separating the enzyme from blood serum by using ammonium sulfate salt at a concentration 0.40%. In the second step, the dialysis was performed to obtain a degree of purity and desalting. In the third step size-exclusion chromatography technique was used to purify the LOX from the proteins and other salts associated with the enzyme. The filtration column of the Sephadex G-100 resin was used in this step, a single peak was obtained at yield 71.42% and 11.033 times of purification as shown in **Figure 2**.

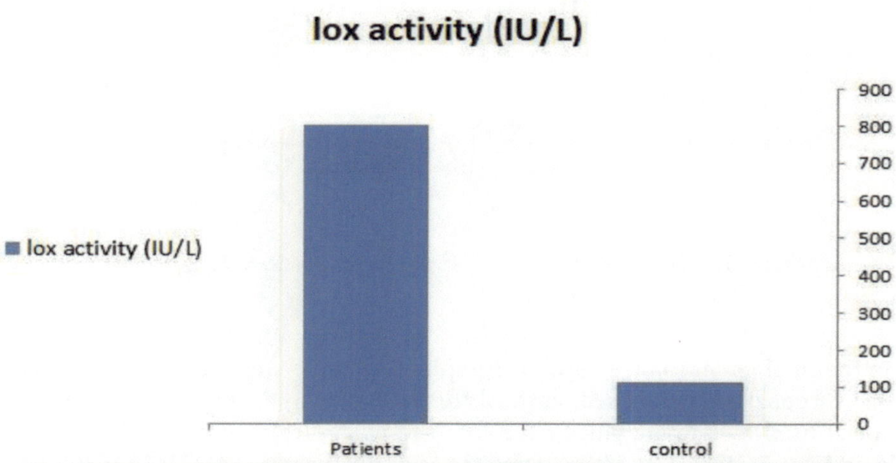

Parameter	Control Mean±S.D N=50	Patients Mean±S.D N=80	T test	P value
LOX (IU/L)	114.6± 49.77	805± 517.23	5.94	0.000

Figure 1.
The effectiveness of LOX in sera of control and patient.

Step	Elute (ml)	Activity (IU/L)	Total activity (IU)	Protein con. (g/L)	Total protein (g)	Specific activity (IU/g)	Purification (fold)	Yield %
Crude	6	420	2.52	78.3	0.4698	5.363	1	100
Ammonium sulfate (0–40)	5	480	2.4	24	0.12	20	3.729	95.23
Dialysis	4	540	2.16	13.6	0.0544	39.705	7.403	85.71
Gel filtration sephadex G100	5	360	1.8	6.093	0.0365	59.17	11.033	71.42
Ion exchange DEAE-C A50 Isoenzyme-II	3	180	0.54	2.05	0.00615	87.804	16.372	28.57
Isoenzyme-I	3	120	0.36	1.84	0.00552	65.217	12.16	21.42

Table 1.
Separation and purification of the lox enzyme from serum patients of colon cancer yield.

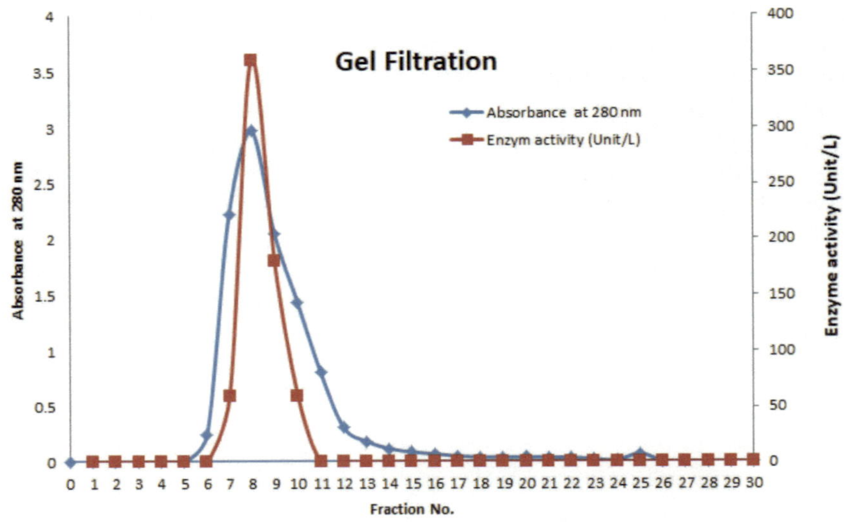

Figure 2.
Activity and absorbance at 280 nm for the fraction of gel filtration step of Sephadex G-100 resin.

In the final ion exchange chromatography technique step was used to separate the LOX isoenzyme that based on the difference in charge. DEAE-Cellulose A50 resin was used, two isoenzymes were obtained with varying degrees of purity at a yield 28.57%, 21.42%, respectively and times of purification 16.372, 12.16 as shown in **Figure 3**.

It has been noted in previous scientific literature that LOX was purified from various sources such as the serum of patients with cardiovascular disease [34], with asthma [35] and with breast cancer [36].

Previous scientific literature has also indicated that the enzyme was purified from the colon cancer cell line [37] but did not indicate that the enzyme was purified from the serum of colon cancer patients. Also the scientific literature indicated that the enzyme was purified from various other sources, including

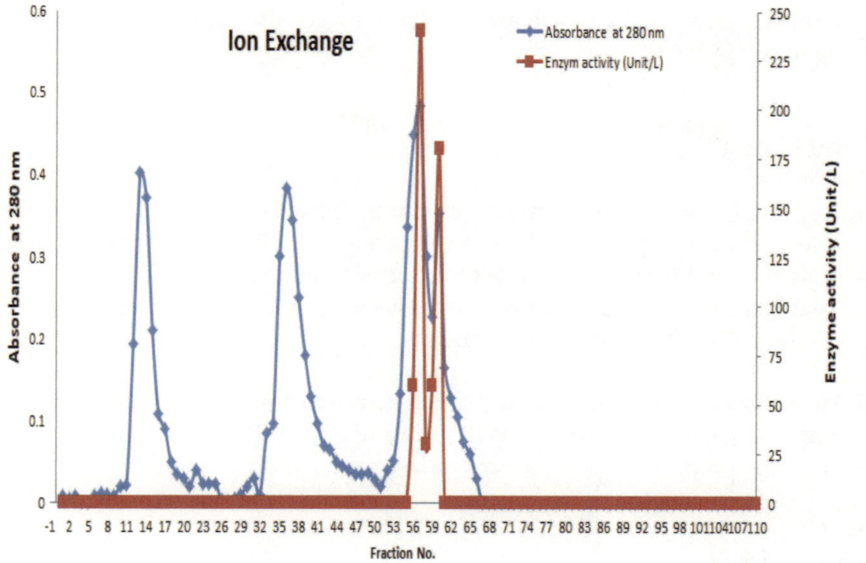

Figure 3.
Activity and absorbance at 280 nm for the fraction of ion exchange step by using DEAE cellulose A-50 resin.

soybeans, where the number of times of purification was 7.7 times at yield of 41% [38]. The enzyme was also purified from Human Placenta with a yield of 21.84% [39].

3.2 Measurement of GGT activity in blood serum

The results of the statistical analysis also showed a higher activity of GGT in colon cancer patients compared to control as shown in **Figure 4**.

Previous scientific literature has indicated a high GGT activity in the serum of colon cancer patients [40, 41]. The reason for the high activity of GGT is due to that the GGT is involved in generating free radicals and peroxidation

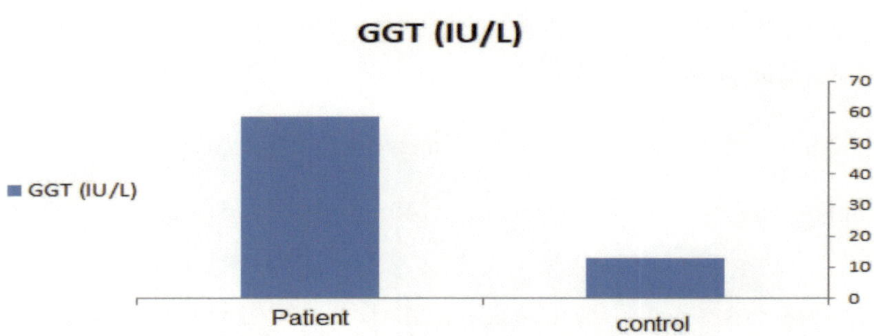

Parameter	Control Mean±S.D N=50	Patients Mean±S.D N=40	T test	P value
GGT (IU/L)	12.79± 5.68	58.69 ± 16.94	11.48	0.000

Figure 4.
The activity of GGT in sera of patients and control groups.

of unsaturated fatty acids, which are involved in various stages of tumorigenesis [42, 43].

4. Conclusion

1. This and other studies show an increase in the activity of LOX in patients with colon cancer compared to the healthy group. This increase in enzyme activity in patients can potentially be used as a tumor marker to detect the presence of colon cancer and also measure disease activity, before and after treatment, in conjunction with other tumor markers.

2. There was a significant increase in the activity of the enzyme GGT in patients with colon cancer compared to the healthy group. This may have clinical and prognostic significance. Further work is progressing in this field.

Authors' declaration

We hereby confirm that all the Figures and Tables in the manuscript are mine ours. Besides, the Figures and images, which are not mine ours, have been given the permission for re-publication attached with the manuscript. The author has signed an animal welfare statement.

Ethical clearance

The project was approved by the local ethical committee in Tikrit University.

Author details

Muslim Abas Abed AlAdlee[1*] and Sahar Ghazi Imran[2]

1 General Directorate of Diyala Education, Ministry of Education, Baqubah, Republic of Iraq

2 General Directorate of Diyala Education, Ministry of Science and Technology, Baqubah, Republic of Iraq

*Address all correspondence to: mu_mh_2006@yahoo.com

References

[1] Murphy K, Weaver C. Janeway's Immunobiology. New York: Garland Science; 2016

[2] Pazdur R, Wagman LD, Camphausen KA, Hoskins WJ. Cancer Management. A Multidisciplinary Approach. 11th ed. New York: CMP Healthcare Media; 2009

[3] Cooper GM, Hausman RE. The development and causes of cancer. The Cell: A Molecular Approach. 2000;**2**: 725-766

[4] Jones PA, De Clerck YA. Extracellular matrix destruction by invasive tumor cells. Cancer and Metastasis Reviews. 1982;**1**(4):289-317

[5] Seyfried TN, Huysentruyt LC. On the origin of cancer metastasis. Critical Reviews in Oncogenesis. 2013;**18**(1-2):43

[6] Huether SE, McCance KL. Understanding Pathophysiology. 3rd ed. U.S.A.; 2004. pp. 301-311

[7] Kilian M, Mautsch I, Gregor JI, Heinichen D, Jacobi CA, Schimke I, et al. Influence of conjugated and conventional linoleic acid on tumor growth and lipid peroxidation in pancreatic adenocarcinoma in hamster. Prostaglandins, Leukotrienes and Essential Fatty Acids. 2003;**69**(1): 67-72

[8] Kandiah M, Tan PCJ. Inverse relationship between body mass index and premenopausal breast cancer risk in Malaysian women. Asia Pacific Journal of Clinical Nutrition. 2004;**13**

[9] Seyfried TN, Shelton LM. Cancer as a metabolic disease. Nutrition & Metabolism. 2010;**7**(1):7

[10] Macrae FA, Bendell J, Tanabe KK. Clinical Presentation, Diagnosis, and Staging of Colorectal Cancer. 2016

[11] Heer PD. *Molecular and Biological Interactions in Colorectal Cancer*. Department of Surgery, Faculty of Medicine, Leiden University Medical Center (LUMC), Leiden University; 2007

[12] Øines M, Helsingen LM, Bretthauer M, Emilsson L. Epidemiology and risk factors of colorectal polyps. Best Practice & Research Clinical Gastroenterology. 2017;**31**(4):419-424

[13] Gomes RN, Felipe da Costa S, Colquhoun A. Eicosanoids and cancer. Clinics. 2018;**73**

[14] Murakami M. Lipoquality control by phospholipase A2 enzymes. Proceedings of the Japan Academy, Series B. 2017; **93**(9):677-702

[15] Srivastava P, Vyas VK, Variya B, Patel P, Qureshi G, Ghate M. Synthesis, anti-inflammatory, analgesic, 5-lipoxygenase (5-LOX) inhibition activities, and molecular docking study of 7-substituted coumarin derivatives. Bioorganic Chemistry. 2016;**67**:130-138

[16] Reddy KK, Rajan VKV, Gupta A, Aparoy P, Reddanna P. Exploration of binding site pattern in arachidonic acid metabolizing enzymes. Cyclooxygenases and Lipoxygenases. BMC Research Notes. 2015;**8**(1):152

[17] Hall Z, Ament Z, Wilson CH, Burkhart DL, Ashmore T, Koulman A, et al. Myc expression drives aberrant lipid metabolism in lung cancer. Cancer Research. 2016;**76**(16):4608-4618

[18] Garg R, Blando JM, Perez CJ, Lal P, Feldman MD, Smyth EM, et al. COX-2 mediates pro-tumorigenic effects of PKCε in prostate cancer. Oncogene. 2018;**37**(34):4735

[19] Qiu J, Shi Z, Jiang J. Cyclooxygenase-2 in glioblastoma

multiforme. Drug Discovery Today. 2017;**22**(1):148-156

[20] Tuncer S, Banerjee S. Eicosanoid pathway in colorectal cancer: Recent updates. World Journal of Gastroenterology. 2015;**21**(41):11748

[21] Rundhaug JE, Mikulec C, Pavone A, Fischer SM. A role for cyclooxygenase-2 in ultraviolet light-induced skin carcinogenesis. Molecular Carcinogenesis: Published in cooperation with the University of Texas MD Anderson Cancer Center. 2007;**46**(8):692-698

[22] Kennedy BM, Harris RE. Cyclooxygenase and lipoxygenase gene expression in the inflammogenesis of breast cancer. Inflammopharmacology. 2018;**26**(4):909-923

[23] Han B, Luo G, Shi ZZ, Barrios R, Atwood D, Liu W, et al. γ-Glutamyl leukotrienase, a novel endothelial membrane protein, is specifically responsible for leukotriene D4 formation in vivo. The American Journal of Pathology. 2002;**161**(2): 481-490

[24] Liu K. Soybean Chemistry Technology and Utilization. Vol. 12. Tokyo: ITP International Thomson publishing, Chapman & Hall Book; 1998. pp. 415-420

[25] Holkova I, Bilka F, Rauova D, Bezakova L. Purification and properties of lipoxygenase from opium poppy seedlings (*Papaver somniferum* L.). Turkish Journal of Biology. 2016;**40**(4): 772-780

[26] Gornall AG, Bardawill CJ, David MM. Determination of serum proteins by means of the biuret reaction. Journal of Biological Chemistry. 1949; **177**(2):751-766

[27] Szasz G. A kinetic photometric method for serum γ-glutamyl transpeptidase. Clinical Chemistry. 1969;**15**(2):124-136

[28] Tunçer S, Keşküş AG, Çolakoğlu M, Çimen I, Yener C, Konu Ö, et al. 15-Lipoxygenase-1 re-expression in colorectal cancer alters endothelial cell features through enhanced expression of TSP-1 and ICAM-1. Cellular Signalling. 2017;**39**:44-54

[29] Che XH, Chen CL, Ye XL, Weng GB, Guo XZ, Yu WY, et al. Dual inhibition of COX-2/5-LOX blocks colon cancer proliferation, migration and invasion in vitro. Oncology Reports. 2016;**35**(3):1680-1688

[30] Lee SI, Zuo X, Shureiqi I. 15-Lipoxygenase-1 as a tumor suppressor gene in colon cancer: Is the verdict in? Cancer and Metastasis Reviews. 2011;**30**(3):481-491

[31] Moore GY, Pidgeon GP. Cross-talk between cancer cells and the tumour microenvironment: The role of the 5-lipoxygenase pathway. International Journal of Molecular Sciences. 2017; **18**(2):236

[32] Hoque A, Lippman SM, Wu TT, Xu Y, Liang ZD, Swisher S, et al. Increased 5- lipoxygenase expression and induction of apoptosis by its inhibitors in esophageal cancer: A potential target for prevention. Carcinogenesis. 2005;**26**(4): 785-791

[33] Wächtershäuser A, Steinhilber D, Loitsch SM, Stein J. Expression of 5-lipoxygenase by human colorectal carcinoma Caco-2 cells during butyrate-induced cell differentiation. Biochemical and Biophysical Research Communications. 2000;**268**(3):778-783

[34] Mahmood AA, Rashed RN. Separation of lipoxygenase and estimation of its level in blood of males with cardiovascular disease. Rafidain Journal of Science. 2013;**24**(2E):65-81

[35] Al-Barqawi A. Separation of the Lipoxygenase Enzyme from the Serum of Healthy Men and External Treatment of Enzyme in Asthma Patients, PhD [Dissertation]. Iraq Babylon: College of Science, University of Babylon; 2017

[36] Knosh J. Purification of Lipoxygenase Enzyme and Estimation of some Biochemical Variables in Serums Women with Breast Cancer, PhD [Dissertation]. Iraq tikrit: College of Education for Pure Sciences, University of Tikrit; 2017

[37] Kamitani H, Geller M, Eling T. Expression of 15-lipoxygenase by human colorectal carcinoma Caco-2 cells during apoptosis and cell differentiation. Journal of Biological Chemistry. 1998;**273**(34): 21569-21577

[38] Robinson DS, Wu Z, Domoney C, Casey R. Lipoxygenases and the quality of foods. Food Chemistry. 1995;**54**(1): 33-43

[39] Kheirullah A, Aberumand M, Nikkzmir A, Malekaskar AM, Alimuhamadi M. The inhibitory effect of potassium cyanide, sodium azide & some divalent ions on lipoxygenase activity of the purified human placental. Iran Journal of Pharmacy Science. 2013; **9**(1):39-45

[40] Ojo O, Asaolu M, Akinlua OA, Atiba A. Serum marker enzymes activities in cancer patients. Journal of Chemistry. 2016;**4**(2):15-21

[41] Yardim-Akaydin S, Deviren C, Miser-Salihoglu E, Caliskan-Can E, Atalay MC. mRNA expressions of gamma-glutamyl transferase genes in different types of cancer. FABAD Journal of Pharmaceutical Sciences. 2017;**42**(1):21

[42] Negre-Salvayre A, Auge N, Ayala V, Basaga H, Boada J, Brenke R, et al. Pathological aspects of lipid peroxidation. Free Radical Research. 2010;**44**(10):1125-1171

[43] Hann HW, Wan S, Myers RE, Hann RS, Xing J, Chen B, et al. Comprehensive analysis of common serum liver enzymes as prospective predictors of hepatocellular carcinoma in HBV patients. PLoS One. 2012;**7**(10): e47687

Section 5

Colorectal Cancer – Preoperative and Intraoperative Imaging Techniques

Chapter 9

The Utility of Magnetic Resonance Imaging in the Multidisciplinary Treatment of Patients with Rectal Cancer

Ioana Hălmaciu, Andrei Suciu Bogdan, Cristian Russu, Vlad Olimpiu Butiurcă, Nicolae Bacalbașa, Simu Patricia Maria Luminița, Nicolescu Cosmin and Călin Molnar

Abstract

Rectal cancer is one of the most common types of cancer in both men and women. In recent years, the importance of magnetic resonance imaging (MRI) has greatly increased in the multidisciplinary treatment of patients with rectal cancer. MRI has a particularly important role in the most accurate preoperative staging of these patients, both in terms of assessing the local invasion of the tumor and in terms of assessing the status of pelvic lymph nodes. Many patients with rectal cancer, especially those in the advanced stage of the disease, in the preoperative period undergo neoadjuvant radio chemotherapy. The evaluation of the clinical response of these patients to neoadjuvant therapy is of crucial importance both in terms of personalized treatment and in terms of their prognosis. In this regard, MRI has its clearly defined role at present in evaluating the efficacy of neoadjuvant therapy, as well as in postoperative follow-up.

Keywords: MRI, rectal cancer, staging, lymph nodes, multidisciplinary treatment

1. Introduction

Rectal cancer is currently a real public health problem, being the second most common type of cancer in women and the third most common type of cancer in men. Surgical treatment with curative intent (rectal resection with total mesorectal excision - TME) is the only therapeutic possibility that can ensure the healing of these patients [1].

In recent decades, the prognosis of these patients has significantly improved following the introduction in clinical practice of neoadjuvant radio chemotherapy, both to improve the life expectancy and to reduce the incidence of local recurrence. In this regard, studies show that in 15–27% of patients with rectal cancer, neoadjuvant radio-chemotherapy has caused a significant decrease in the size of tumors [2]. Therefore, a particularly important role in clinical practice is the

IntechOpen

response identification to neoadjuvant therapy in these patients. At the same time, a particularly important role in the prognosis of patients, in addition to the response to neoadjuvant radio chemotherapy, is the surgery itself and especially the achievement of a total mesorectal excision (TME) as accurate as possible and obtaining negative surgical resection margins [3, 4].

2. The utility of magnetic resonance imaging in patients with rectal cancer

In recent years, abdominal and pelvic magnetic resonance imaging (MRI) has established itself as a gold standard method in the evaluation of patients with rectal cancer because of its crucial role in identifying non-responsive patients to neodjuvant radio chemotherapy [5, 6]. However, a particularly important role in the preoperative and postoperative clinical evaluation of these patients is played by accurate images of the anatomical structures of the pelvis, rectal tumor and their relationship with the surrounding anatomical structures [7].

In this sense, the most used MRI sequence in the preoperative evaluation of these patients for visualization of the rectum, tumor, and its relationship with surrounding tissues is High-spatial-resolution T2-weighted imaging [7]. On the other hand, one of the major advantages of rectal MRI scanning in T2 sequences is that 3 layers of the rectal wall can be differentiated. The inner layer is represented by the mucosa and submucosa, the middle layer is represented by the muscularis propria, and the outer layer is represented by the mesorectal fat. This allows for a much more accurate understanding of tumor invasion of the rectal wall and surrounding structures compared to other imaging studies [8, 9].

One of the disadvantages of MRI is the rather long time required to perform this investigation and therefore it is recommended that patients be positioned in a supine position for maximum comfort. But despite this inconvenience the benefit of this imaging method is major [10]. Current studies debate the optimal MRI resolution in the evaluation of patients with rectal cancer (1.5 T or 3 T). While 3 T cameras provide much better spatial resolution, they also have a higher susceptibility to artifacts during diffusion-weighted imaging (DWI) [10–12].

2.1 Local staging in rectal cancer using MRI

Newer studies have shown that MRI can identify patients who are at increased risk of local recurrence. In this sense, it has been shown that patients with tumors that invade only the rectal mucosa have a good long-term prognosis, while patients with invasion of the mesorectal fascia and pelvic organs in the vicinity of the rectum have a particularly high risk of recurrence [13–15]. In this respect MRI has a special utility for the detection of extramural tumor invasion as well as mucin deposits at this level [16]. On the other hand, more and more studies have shown that, in the case of superficial rectal tumors, EUS (endorectal ultrasound) has a special value in the identification of tumors and invasion of surrounding structures, while EUS is less useful in the case of tumors that penetrate the mesorectal fascia, respectively the anatomical structures in the vicinity of the rectum [17, 18].

Regarding the technique of performing MRI in these patients, in order to obtain good quality anatomical images, most authors recommend that the scan plane be perpendicular to the rectal wall at the level of the tumor with a slice thickness of maximum 3 mm. The sections are made in coronal, sagittal and axial plane [19]. On the other hand, there are debates in the literature regarding the use of intravenous contrast in these patients. Most authors do not recommend the routine use of intravenous contrast [16]. However, there are authors who consider that the use of gadolinum contrast increases the accuracy of detecting transmural tumor invasion as well as vascular invasion [9, 20, 21].

There is further controversy in regards to patient preparation for MRI. Some authors recommend the administration of spasmolytic drugs prior to imaging studies especially in patients with upper rectal tumors and if 3 T devices are used. Other authors recommend that the use of diffusion-weighted MRI be preceded by endorectal filling. But in these cases, dilation of the rectum can affect the measurement of the distance between the mesorectal fascia and the tumor [22, 23]. To eliminate this inconvenience, some authors recommend that a maximum of 60 ml of gel be used for endorectal filling [24].

One of the major advantages of performing MRI in patients with rectal cancer is that it is possible to accurately identify both the circumferential invasion of the tumor in the rectal mucosa and its transmural invasion. This fact is especially important because newer studies have shown that one of the main factors that can lead to local recurrence is incomplete resection, especially in the lateral aspect of the resection specimen [25]. At the same time, pelvic MRI has the ability to accurately detect the macroscopic type of rectal tumor (polypoid, ulcerative) and the presence or absence of mucin at this level [9].

When performing rectal MRI in T2 sequences, the rectal mucosa appears hypointense, the submucosa hyperintense, and the muscularis propria appears as a circumferential hypersignal. Precise identification of the layers of the rectal wall thus allows a precise location of the tumor at the level of the rectal wall [26]. According to the TNM classification of rectal cancer, in stage T1, the tumor is limited to the mucosa and submucosa, in stage T2, the tumor does not extend beyond the muscularis propria, in stage T3, the tumor exceeds muscularis propria and in stage T4, the tumor extends beyond the rectal wall [19] (**Figure 1**).

If the tumor invades the mesorectal fat it is considered to be stage T3 and if it invades the peritoneum of the pelvic cavity, it is interpreted as stage T4. The invasion of intersphincter space is considered a T3 stage. and the invasion of the external anal sphincter is considered a T4 stage [27–29] (**Figure 2**).

A limiting factor in these cases is the existence of fibrous tissue in the rectal wall or in the tissues around the tumor. The existence of fibrosis at this level can make it difficult properly stage the patient, especially by over staging [30]. In this respect, there are studies in the literature which have shown that it is sometimes difficult to differentiate by MRI, peritumoral fibrosis from residual tumor deposits, especially in patients who have undergone neoadjuvant radiochemotherapy. Therefore, most

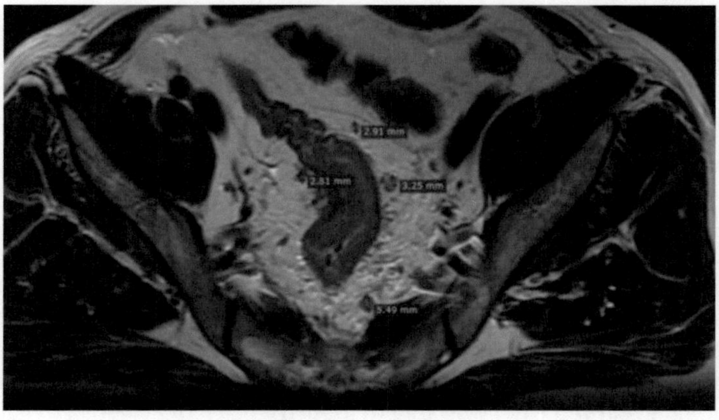

Figure 1.
MRI image, axial view, the tumor invades the mesorectal fascia.

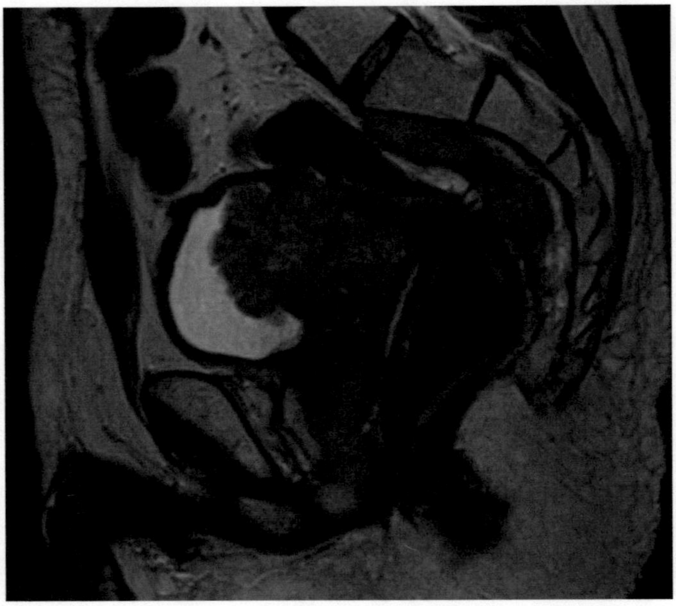

Figure 2.
MRI image, sagital view – tumor recurrence invasive in the bladder and prostate.

authors in the literature recommend that, in patients who have undergone neo-adjuvant radio-chemotherapy, MRI examination should be performed by physicians experienced in this type of pathology [31].

Further MRI findings regard the relationship of the tumor with the anal sphincter as well as the distance between the tumor and the anocutaneous line. Tumors located less than 6 cm are considered low rectal tumors, tumors whose lower edge is located 7–11 cm from the ano-cutaneous line are considered medium rectal tumors, and tumors whose lower limit is located more than 11 cm from the ano-cutaneous line are considered superior rectal tumors [29]. The precise location of the tumor and its relationship to the anal sphincters are particularly important in determining the type of surgery to be performed in these patients (abdomino-perianal resection, abdominal resection) and the extent of the surgery to be performed.

Given the importance of precise localization of the rectal tumor relative to the anocutaneous line in determining the subsequent therapeutic decision in these patients, there are many studies that have investigated the specificity and sensitivity of MRI compared to colonoscopy in establishing the exact distance between the lower edge of the tumor and ano-cutaneous line.

In this regard, there are studies that have shown that MRI cannot rule out performing colonoscopy in these patients, especially because of the fact that colonoscopy offers the possibility of collecting biopsies for histopathological examination. But in many cases the assessment of the distance between the lower edge of the rectal tumor and the anocutaneous line during colonoscopy is subjective, both due to local anatomical details and the experience of the person performing colonoscopy, so many authors conclude that pelvic MRI it is much more useful in establishing the distance between the lower edge of the tumor and the ano-cutaneous line [32–35].

In patients with rectal cancer, a particularly important factor that determines their long-term prognosis, both in terms of the occurrence of local recurrence and survival is represented by extramural vascular invasion (EMT). Recent studies have shown that, T2-weighted MRI was able to identify EMT in 80–90% of cases. EMT is manifested by the existence of morphological changes in the blood vessels adjacent to the tumor [29, 36–38].

Another particularly important prognostic factor that can be identified in these patients using MRI and is represented by the distance between the tumor margin and the mesorectal fascia. Thus, it has been shown that in patients in whom the distance between the rectal tumor and the mesorectal fascia is less than 1 mm, the risk of local recurrence is approximately 22%; if the distance is greater than 1 mm, the risk of local recurrence is only 5% [39, 40]. Regarding the assessment of the distance between the tumor edge and the mesorectal fascia, a factor that may limit the effectiveness of MRI is the existence of a low layer of mesorectal fat between the anterior wall of the rectum and the seminal vesicles in men, respectively the posterior wall of the vagina in women. In these cases, it has been shown that MRI sensitivity and specificity may be affected [41].

Regarding the accuracy of MRI, in the correct evaluation of the T descriptor of the TNM classification of rectal cancer, a very important role is played by the experience of the radiologist performing the investigation [42, 43]. Thus, population studies have shown that the sensitivity of MRI in the correct evaluation of the T descriptor varies between 29 and 57% and the specificity varies between 50 and 83% [43–47]. These results are due, in part, to the experience of the examining physician and, on the other hand, to the difficulty of differentiating in some cases a stage T1 tumor from a stage T2 tumor. In some cases, the desmoplastic reaction of the tumor makes a tumor look like T3 stage on MRI when in fact, following surgical specimen examining the surgical resection piece is actually a T2 stage [48].

Last but not least, the knowledge of local anatomical details, of the relations of the rectal tumor formation with the surrounding structures, allows the surgical team an adequate programming of the resection surgery, thus diminishing the possible intraoperative surprises regarding local invasion of the rectal tumor. In this way, the morbidity and postoperative mortality of these patients can be significantly reduced.

2.2 Detection of lymph node metastases using MRI in patients with rectal cancer

The existence of loco-regional lymph node metastases at the time of diagnosis is a poor prognostic factor in patients with rectal cancer, the first lymph nodes affected being those located in the mesorectum. In the case of rectal cancer, loco-regional lymph nodes are considered to be the obturator lymph nodes, internal iliac lymph nodes and the ones located in the mesorectum [49–51]. Therefore, the correct assessment of the existence of lymph node metastases in patients with rectal cancer is of particular importance in the preoperative assessment of these patients, the experience of the examining physician having a particularly important role in these cases [52, 53] (**Figure 3**).

It is often difficult to assess the status of loco-regional lymph nodes using MRI and it has been found that in about 25% of cases loco-regional lymphadenopathy which were considered as lymph node metastases were not confirmed positive on the histology report [54, 55]. However, some studies have shown that the use of high-resolution T2-weighted sequences can improve the sensitivity and specificity of MRI in the detection of lymph node metastases. These results are due to the fact that, especially in the case of patients undergoing neo-adjuvant radiochemotherapy, local fibrosis makes it difficult to correctly assess the status of loco-regional lymph nodes [56–58].

A much debated topic in the literature is the diagnostic criteria for lymph node metastases based on MRI examination. Thus, there are authors who consider that lymph node adenopathy with a diameter larger than 5 mm represents malignant lymphadenopathy, and those with a diameter below 5 mm are benign [59]. On the other hand, other authors consider that the most faithful sign of suspicion for malignancy is represented by the fact that the diameter of the loco-regional lymph

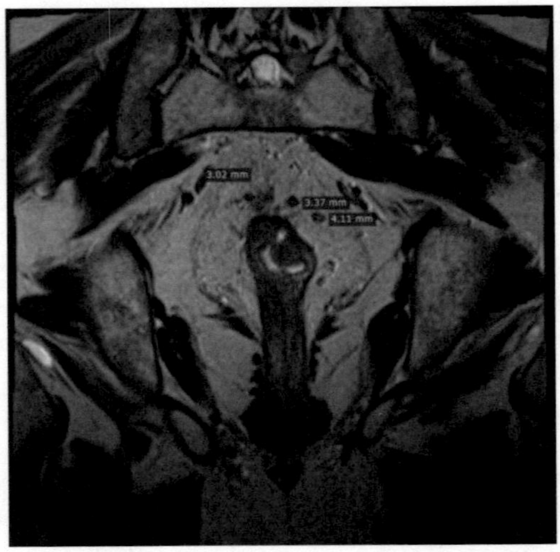

Figure 3.
Adjacent lymph nodes in mesorectal fat up to 4 mm in size. 4 mm extramesorectal lymph node.

nodes decreases in size or increases in size after the practice of neo-adjuvant radio-chemotherapy [60, 61]. On the other hand, other authors consider as criteria for malignancy of the lymph nodes, based on MRI examination, the existence of extracapsular invasion or enlargement of the lymph nodes located on the walls of the pelvic cavity (extramesorectal), or changes in their morphology (presence or absence of heterogeneity) [62, 63].

However, the specificity of the diagnosis of malignant lymphadenopathy with MRI is around 70%, mainly due to fibrotic changes or mucinous degeneration of these lymph nodes, these results being due also to the fact that there are studies that have shown the existence of fibrotic changes also in case of benign lymphatic nodules [64]. There are also studies in the literature that recommend the practice of MRI with dynamic contrast-enhanced, in patients with rectal cancer, in order to increase the accuracy of MRI diagnosis of lymph node involvement. In the case of the administration of dynamic contrast, it is considered that, usually, the malignant lymph nodes, when examined in T2 sequences, have edges in hypersignal, and their center presents hyposignal [65].

2.3 Detection of distant metastases using MRI in patients with rectal cancer

Recently, the importance of MRI in the preoperative evaluation of rectal cancer patients has increased greatly despite the abdominal CT examination, especially due to the fact that diffusion-weighted MRI is much more effective in detecting small liver metastases compared to abdominal CT imaging [66]. There are also studies in the literature that have shown that the sensitivity and specificity of MRI in the detection of liver metastases is superior even to PET-CT [67, 68]. Therefore, there are authors who recommend performing a whole body MRI, in patients with rectal cancer [69]. On the other hand, the sensitivity and specificity of the detection of pulmonary metastases, in patients with rectal cancer, is lower in the case of MRI compared with chest CT scan [70].

Recently, in order to detect the existence of distant metastases, in patients with rectal cancer, PET-MRI is increasingly used. This method eliminates the lower sensitivity and specificity of MRI in the detection of lung metastases and brings in addition the increased sensitivity and specificity of MRI for the detection of liver metastases, compared to abdominal CT scan [71].

2.4 Evaluation of the response to neo-adjuvant radiochemotherapy

The prognosis of patients with rectal cancer has significantly improved, in recent years, on the one hand by introducing the neo-adjuvant radiochemotherapy in their treatment, as well as by improving imaging methods that allow a more accurate preoperative staging of these patients [72, 73]. Thus, it has been shown that the introduction of neo-adjuvant radiochemotherapy in patients with advanced loco-regional forms of rectal cancer has led to an improvement in their survival, decreased the risk of local recurrence and, in some cases, has even been recorded a complete pathological response, improving as well the postoperative morbidity and mortality of these patients. Also, for these patients it was found a better compliance to postoperative radio-chemotherapy [74–76].

With the initiation of neo-adjuvant radio-chemotherapy of particular clinical importance is the identification of patients with no response to this therapy, with incomplete clinical response or with a complete clinical response (the absence of residual tumor, the absence of neoplastic lymph nodes in the mesorectum). The identification of these groups of patients is very important given the principles of personalized medicine. It is also of crucial importance to identify patients who do not respond to radiochemotherapy, in which case it is beneficial for them to initiate the surgical treatment as soon as possible [77–80].

In this regard, in recent years there are authors who, in rectal cancer patients with neo-adjuvant radiochemotherapy to whom a complete clinical response is recorded, recommend either the practice of a resection surgery with preservation of the rectum or only the clinical follow-up of these patients, without the indication of a surgical treatment. In these situations, a complete clinical response is recorded in approximately 24% of cases [80, 81]. Some authors have shown that the usual MRI techniques (T2 weighted) cannot always correctly assess the clinical response to neo-adjuvant radiochemotherapy, recommending in these cases the use of functional MRI techniques (dynamic contrast-enhanced MRI - DCE-MRI and diffusion-weighted imaging - DWI). These techniques have the advantage of providing much more accurate information about the existence of the residual tumor.

In this sense, in the case of the use of DWI-MRI, the so-called diffusion coefficient that evaluates the diffusion capacity of water at the tissue level is particularly important in evaluating the tumor response to neo-adjuvant radiochemotherapy. This coefficient is inversely proportional to tissue cellularity. Usually, viable tumor cells prevent the diffusion of water to the tissues, while necrotic tumor cells allow the diffusion of water at this level [82, 83]. The diffusion coefficient is also particularly useful in differentiating viable tumor tissue from inflamed areas, respectively necrosis areas. Thus, some authors consider that the value of this coefficient has predictive value in terms of response to neo-adjuvant radiochemotherapy of these patients [84].

DCE-MRI can provide important information about the vascularization of the tumor, the permeability of these vessels, as well as about the structure of the extracellular space. Also, this method has the possibility to identify the areas of hypoxia as well as the intensity of the microvascularization at the level of the tumor formation, both from a quantitative and a qualitative point of view. In this regard, there are studies in the literature that have shown that the existence of increased vascular permeability in the tumor before initiating neo-adjuvant radiochemotherapy is associated with a good therapeutic response, in these cases. Other authors have also shown that the existence of mucin at the level of the tumor formation is associated with a poor therapeutic response in these cases [84–87].

The major advantages of using MRI in evaluating the clinical response to neo-adjuvant radiochemotherapy are represented on the one hand by highlighting the morphological changes that occur at the level of the rectal tumor (size, vascularity, structure) as well as the changes that occur in the pelvic lymph nodes. The limiting factor that may influence the accuracy of the method in these cases is the occurrence of local fibrosis after radiotherapy or post irradiation proctitis [88].

2.5 The utility of MRI in the postoperative follow up of the patients with rectal cancer

Local recurrence occurs in approximately 30% of patients operated for rectal cancer. Early identification of local recurrence in these patients is of particular importance both for the therapeutic management of these patients as well as for their long-term prognosis [89]. Local recurrence is characterized by the appearance of a tumor formation at the level of the anastomosis, at the level of the operating bed or at the level of the pelvic lymph nodes. At the time of local recurrence, only about 20% of these patients are still suitable for surgical treatment [90].

Although currently the most used imaging method in postoperative follow-up of patients with operated rectal cancer is abdomino-pelvic CT scan, recently there are more and more studies in the literature that recommend performing abdominal-pelvic MRI in these patients. Those who promote this method are based on the fact that in the detection of pelvic neoplasms, the specificity and sensitivity of pelvic MRI in differentiating areas of fibrosis from tumor recurrence is much higher than pelvic CT scan [91, 92]. At the same time, it has been shown that, in the case of small liver metastases, abdominal MRI has a better detection rate compared to abdominal CT. Also, another argument for the utility of pelvic MRI in these cases is given by the fact that, compared to the pelvic CT, MRI offers a much better spatial resolution, and can also provide functional information (tissue diffusion, local vascularization) [93]. Recent studies have shown that when using diffusion-weighted MRI (DWI-MRI) there is the possibility of identifying tumor recurrence, in these cases, faster than when using conventional MRI techniques or when using abdominal CT [94, 95].

3. Conclusions

The pelvic MRI examination has a special utility both in the preoperative evaluation of the patients with rectal cancer and in the postoperative follow-up of these patients. Nowadays, this method represent the "gold standard" imagistic method in the evaluation of these patients.

Author details

Ioana Hălmaciu[1], Andrei Suciu Bogdan[1*], Cristian Russu[2], Vlad Olimpiu Butiurcă[2], Nicolae Bacalbașa[3], Simu Patricia Maria Luminița[4], Nicolescu Cosmin[1] and Călin Molnar[2]

1 Anatomy and Embryology Department, "George Emil Palade" University of Medicine, Pharmacy, Science, and Technology of Targu Mures, Romania

2 General Surgery Department, "George Emil Palade" University of Medicine, Pharmacy, Science, and Technology of Targu Mures, Romania

3 University of Medicine and Pharmacy "Carol Davila" Bucharest, Center for Excellence in Translational Medicine, Fundeni Clinical Institute, Bucharest, Romania

4 Radiology Department, University County Hospital, Targu Mure, Romania

*Address all correspondence to: suciubogdanandrei@yahoo.com

References

[1] Gürses B, Böge M, Altınmakas E, Balık E. Multiparametric MRI in rectal cancer, Diagn Interv Radiol. 2019 May;25(3):175-182. doi: 10.5152/dir.2019.18189.

[2] Maas M, Nelemans PJ, Valentini V, et al. Longterm outcome in patients with a pathological complete response after chemoradiation for rectal cancer: a pooled analysis of individual patient data. Lancet Oncol 2010; 11:835-844

[3] Heald RJ, Ryall RD. Recurrence and survival after total mesorectal excision for rectal cancer. Lancet 1986;1(8496):1479-1482.

[4] Krook JE, Moertel CG, Gunderson LL, et al. Effective surgical adjuvant therapy for high-risk rectal carcinoma. N Engl J Med 1991;324(11):709-715.

[5] Hötker AM, Garcia-Aguilar J, Gollub MJ. Multiparametric MRI of rectal cancer in the assessment of response to therapy: a systematic review. Dis Colon Rectum 2014; 57:790-799

[6] Attenberger UI, Pilz LR, Morelli JN, et al. Multi-parametric MRI of rectal cancer - do quantitative functional MR measurements correlate with radiologic and pathologic tumor stages? Eur J Radiol 2014; 83:1036-1043.

[7] Horvat N, Carlos Tavares Rocha C, Clemente Oliveira B, Petkovska I, Gollub MJ. MRI of Rectal Cancer: Tumor Staging, Imaging Techniques, and Management. Radiographics. 2019 Mar-Apr;39(2):367-387. doi: 10.1148/rg.2019180114. Epub 2019 Feb 15.

[8] F. Iafrate, A. Laghi, P. Paolantonio., Preoperative staging of rectal cancer with MR imaging:correlation with surgical and histopathologic findings. Radiographics, 26 (2006), pp. 701-714

[9] Srisajjakul S, Prapaisilp P, Bangchokdee S., Pitfalls in MRI of rectal cancer: What radiologists need to know and avoid., Clin Imaging. Jul-Aug 2018; 50:130-140. doi: 10.1016/j.clinimag.2017.11.012.

[10] Taylor FG, Swift RI, Blomqvist L, Brown G. A systematic approach to the interpretation of preoperative staging MRI for rectal cancer. AJR Am J Roentgenol 2008;191(6):1827-1835.

[11] Gollub MJ, Arya S, Beets-Tan RG, et al. Use of magnetic resonance imaging in rectal cancer patients: Society of Abdominal Radiology (SAR) rectal cancer disease-focused panel (DFP) recommendations 2017. Abdom Radiol (NY) 2018 May 21

[12] Kim H, Lim JS, Choi JY, et al. Rectal cancer: comparison of accuracy of local-regional staging with two- and three-dimensional preoperative 3T MRI. Radiology 2010;254(2):485-492.

[13] Gowdra Halappa V, Corona Villalobos CP, Bonekamp S, et al. Rectal imaging: part 1—high-resolution MRI of carcinoma of the rectum at 3 T. AJR Am J Roentgenol 2012;199(1): W35–W42

[14] Beets-Tan RGH et al (2018) Magnetic resonance imaging for clinical management of rectal cancer: Updated recommendations from the 2016 European Society of Gastrointestinal and Abdominal Radiology (ESGAR) consensus meeting. Eur Radiol 28(4):1465-1475

[15] Engelen SME, Maas M, Lahaye MJ, Leijtens JWA, Berlo CLH van, Jansen RLH et al (2013) Modern multidisciplinary treatment of rectal cancer based on staging with magnetic resonance imaging leads to excellent local control, but distant control remains a challenge. Eur J Canc 49(10):2311-2320

[16] Balyasnikova S, Brown G. Optimal Imaging Strategies for Rectal Cancer Staging and Ongoing Management. Curr Treat Options Oncol. 2016 Jun;17(6):32. doi: 10.1007/s11864-016-0403-7.

[17] Marusch F et al (2002) Routine use of transrectal ultrasound in rectal carcinoma: results of a prospective multicenter study. Endoscopy 34(5):385-390

[18] Boot J, Gomez-Munoz F, Beets Tan RGH. Imaging of rectal cancer, Radiologe 2019 Dec;59(Suppl 1):46-50. doi: 10.1007/s00117-019-0579-5.

[19] Moreno CC, Sullivan PS, Mittal PK., MRI Evaluation of Rectal Cancer: Staging and Restaging, Curr Probl Diagn Radiol. 2017 May-Jun;46(3):234-241. doi: 10.1067/j.cpradiol.2016.11.011. Epub 2016 Nov 21

[20] H. Okizuka, K. Sugimura, T. Yoshizako, Y. Kaji, A. Wada., Rectal carcinoma: prospective comparison of conventional and gadopentetate dimeglumine enhanced fat suppressed MR imaging. J Magn Reson Imaging, 6 (3) (1996), pp. 465-471

[21] R.F. Vliegen, G.L. Beets, M.F. von Meyenfeldt, A.G. Kessels, E.E. Lemaire, J.M. van Engelshoven, et al. Rectal cancer: MR imaging in local staging—is gadolinium-based contrast material helpful? Radiology, 234 (1) (2005), pp. 179-188

[22] Beets-Tan RGH, Lambregts DMJ, Maas M, Bipat S, Barbaro B, Curvo-Semedo L, Fenlon HM, Gollub MJ, Gourtsoyianni S, Halligan S, Hoeffel C, Kim SH, Laghi A, Maier A, Rafaelsen SR, Stoker J, Taylor SA, Torkzad MR, Blomqvist L., Magnetic resonance imaging for clinical management of rectal cancer: Updated recommendations from the 2016 European Society of Gastrointestinal and Abdominal Radiology (ESGAR) consensus meeting. Eur Radiol. 2018 Apr;28(4):1465-1475. doi: 10.1007/s00330-017-5026-2. Epub 2017 Oct 17.

[23] Slater A, Halligan S, Taylor SA, Marshall M (2006) Distance between the rectal wall and mesorectal fascia measured by MRI: Effect of rectal distension and implications for preoperative prediction of a tumour-free circumferential resection margin. Clin Radiol 61:65-70

[24] Dal Lago A, Minetti AE, Biondetti P, Corsetti M, Basilisco G (2005) Magnetic resonance imaging of the rectum during distension. Dis *Colon Rectum* 48:1220-1227

[25] P. Quirke, P. Durdey, M.F. Dixon, N.S. Williams., Local recurrence of rectal adenocarcinoma due to inadequate surgical resection. Histopathological study of lateral tumor spread and surgical excision., Lancet, 2 ((8514) (1986), pp. 996-999

[26] E. Iannicelli, S. Di Renzo, M. Ferri, et al. Accuracy of high-resolution MRI with lumen distention in rectal cancer staging and circumferential margin involvement prediction. Korean J Radiol, 15 (2014), pp. 37-44

[27] U. Tapan, M. Ozbayrak, S. Tatl. MRI in local staging of rectal cancer: An update. Diagn Interv Radiol, 20 (2014), pp. 390-398

[28] H. Kaur, H. Choi, Y.N. You, et al. MRI for preoperative evaluation of primary rectal cancer: Practical considerations. RadioGraphics, 32 (2012), pp. 389-409

[29] J.S. Park, Y.-J. Jang, G.-S. Choi, et al. Accuracy of preoperative MRI in predicting pathology stage in rectal cancers: Node-for-node matched histopathology validation of MRI features. Dis Col Rectum, 57 (2014), pp. 32-38

[30] Tapan U., Ozbayrak M., Tatli S., MRI in local staging of rectal cancer: an update. Diagn Interv Radiol . Sep-Oct 2014;20(5):390-398. doi: 10.5152/dir.2014.13265.

[31] Van der Paardt M., Zagers MB., Beets-Tan RGH., Stoker J., Bipat S., Patients Who Undergo Preoperative Chemoradiotherapy for Locally Advanced Rectal Cancer Restaged by Using Diagnostic MR Imaging: A Systematic Review and Meta-Analysis. Radiology. 2013 Oct;269(1):101-112. doi: 10.1148/radiol.13122833. Epub 2013 Jun 25

[32] G. Baatrup, M. Bolstad, J.H. Mortensen., Rigid sigmoidoscopy and MRI are not interchangeable in determining the position of rectal cancers. Eur J Surg Oncol, 35 (11) (2009), pp. 1169-1173

[33] D.S. Keller, R. Paspulati, A. Kjellmo, et al. MRI-defined height of rectal tumours. Br J Surg, 101 (2) (2014), pp. 127-132

[34] D. Meylemans, F. Penninckx, D. Vanbeckevoort, A.M. Wolthuis, S. Fieuws, A. D'Hoore., Endoscopic versus radiology-based location of rectal cancer. Acta Chir Belg, 114 (6) (2014), pp. 364-369

[35] Chung E, Kang D, Lee HS, Cho ES, Kim JH, Park EJ, Baik SH, Lee KY, Kang J., Accuracy of pelvic MRI in measuring tumor height in rectal cancer patients with or without preoperative chemoradiotherapy., Eur J Surg Oncol . 2019 Mar;45(3):324-330. doi: 10.1016/j.ejso.2018.08.029. Epub 2018 Oct 9.

[36] Shirozu K, Isomoto H, Kakegawa T, Morimatsu M. A prospective clinicopathologic study of venous invasion in colorectal cancer. Am J Surg 1991; 162:216-222.

[37] Freedman LS, Macaskill P, Smith AN. Multivariate analysis of prognostic factors for operable rectal cancer. Lancet 1984; 2:733-736.

[38] Smith NJ, Barbachano Y, Norman AR, Swift RI, Abulafi AM, Brown G. Prognostic significance of magnetic resonance imaging-detected extramural vascular invasion in rectal cancer. Br J Surg 2008; 95:229-236

[39] Wibe A, Rendedal PR, Svensson E, et al. Prognostic significance of the circumferential resection margin following total mesorectal excision for rectal cancer. Br J Surg 2002; 89:327-334.

[40] Karatag O, Karatag GY, Ozkurt H, et al. The ability of phased-array MRI in preoperative staging of primary rectal cancer: correlation with histopathological results. Diagn Interv Radiol 2012; 18:20-26.

[41] Peschaud F, Cuenod CA, Benoist S, et al. Accuracy of magnetic resonance imaging in rectal cancer depends on location of the tumor. Dis Colon Rectum 2005; 48:1603-1609

[42] Klessen C, Rogalla P, Taupitz M. Local staging of rectal cancer: The current role of MRI. Eur Radiol. 2007; 17: 379– 389.

[43] Xu L, Zhang C, Zhang Z, Qin Q, Sun X., Value of 3Tesla MRI in the preoperative staging of mid-low rectal cancer and its impact on clinical strategies., Asia Pac J Clin Oncol. 2020 Oct;16(5): e216-e222. doi: 10.1111/ajco.13368. Epub 2020 Aug 6

[44] Rovera F, Dionigi G, Boni L, Cutaia S, Diurni M, Dionigi R. The role of EUS and MRI in rectal cancer staging. Surg Oncol. 2007; 16(Suppl 1): S51– S52

[45] Suzuki C, Torkzad MR, Tanaka S, et al. The importance of rectal cancer MRI protocols on interpretation accuracy. World J Surg Oncol. 2008; 6: 89.

[46] Torkzad MR, Hansson KA, Lindholm J, Martling A, Blomqvist L. Significance of mesorectal volume in staging of rectal cancer with magnetic resonance imaging and the assessment of involvement of the mesorectal fascia. Eur Radiol. 2007; 17: 1694-1619.

[47] Videhult P, Smedh K, Lundin P, Kraaz W. Magnetic resonance imaging for preoperative staging of rectal cancer in clinical practice: High accuracy in predicting circumferential margin with clinical benefit. Colorectal Dis. 2007; 9: 412– 419.

[48] Sethi R, Lee SH. Imaging in colorectal cancer. In: SR Brown, JE Hartley, J Hill, N Scott, G Williams, eds. Contemporary coloproctology. London: Springer; 2012: 123-138.

[49] Taylor, F. G., Quirke, P., Heald, R. J., Moran, B., Blomqvist, L., Swift, I. et al & MERCURY study group (2011). Preoperative high-resolution magnetic resonance imaging can identify good prognosis stage I, II, and III rectal cancer best managed by surgery alone: a prospective, multicenter, European study. Ann Surg, 253(4), 711-719.

[50] Edge SB, Byrd DR, Compton CC (2010). AJCC cancer staging handbook: from the AJCC cancer staging manual, 7th ed. New York, NY: Springer, 2010:718

[51] Koh, D. M., Brown, G., Temple, L., Blake, H., Raja, A., Toomey, et al (2005) Distribution of mesorectal lymph nodes in rectal cancer: in vivo MR imaging compared with histopathological examination. Initial observations. European radiology, 15(8), 1650-1657.

[52] C.C. Moreno, P.S. Sullivan, B.T. Kalb, et al. Magnetic resonance imaging of rectal cancer: staging and restaging evaluation., Abdom Imaging, 40 (7) (2015), pp. 2613-2629

[53] Fornell-Perez R, Perez-Alonso E, Aleman-Flores P, Lozano-Rodriguez A, Loro-Ferrer JF. Nodal staging in the rectal cancer follow-up MRI after chemoradiotherapy: use of morphology, size, and diffusion criteria., Clin Radiol. 2020 Feb;75(2):100-107. doi: 10.1016/j.crad.2019.08.003. Epub 2019 Sep 9.

[54] S. Bipat, A.S. Glas, F.J.M. Slors, et al. Rectal cancer: local staging and assessment of lymph node involvement with endoluminal US, CT, and MR imaging—a meta-analysis. Radiology, 232 (3) (2004), pp. 773-783

[55] J.J. Van Den Broek, F.S.W. Van Der Wolf, M.J. Lahaye, et al. Accuracy of MRI in restaging locally advanced rectal cancer after preoperative chemoradiation. Dis *Colon Rectum*, 60 (3) (2017), pp. 274-283

[56] G. Brown, C.J. Richards, M.W. Bourne, et al. Morphologic predictors of lymph node status in rectal cancer with use of high-spatial-resolution MR imaging with histopathologic comparison. Radiology, 227 (2) (2003), pp. 371-377

[57] D.M. Koh, G. Brown, J.E. Husband. Nodal staging in rectal cancer Abdom Imaging, 31 (6) (2006), pp. 652-659

[58] Bud V., Suciu BA., Butiurca V, Brinzaniuc K., Copotoiu R., Copotoiu C., Sin A., New ways of bronchial stump closure after lung resection: experimental study, Rom J Morphol Embryo 2013;54(11):115-119

[59] L.A. Heijnen, M. Maas, R.G. Beets-Tan, et al. Nodal staging in rectal cancer: why is restaging after chemoradiation more accurate than primary nodal staging? Int J Colorectal Dis, 31 (6) (2016), pp. 1157-1162

[60] J.S. Park, Y.J. Jang, G.S. Choi, et al. Accuracy of preoperative MRI in predicting pathology stage in rectal cancers: node-for-node matched histopathology validation of MRI features Dis *Colon Rectum*, 57 (1) (2014), pp. 32-38

[61] L.A. Heijnen, D.M.J. Lambregts, M.J. Lahaye, et al. Good and complete responding locally advanced rectal tumors after chemoradiotherapy: where are the residual positive nodes located on restaging MRI? Abdom Radiol, 41 (7) (2016), pp. 1245-1252

[62] Zhang, M. R., Xie, T. H., Chi, J. L., Li, Y., Yang, L., Yu, Y. Y., Sun, X. F., & Zhou, Z. G. (2016). Prognostic role of the lymph node ratio in node positive colorectal cancer: a meta-analysis. Oncotarget, 7(45), 72898-72907

[63] Madbouly, K. M., Abbas, K. S., & Hussein, A. M. (2014). Metastatic lymph node ratio in stage III rectal carcinoma is a valuable prognostic factor even with less than 12 lymph nodes retrieved: a prospective study. American journal of surgery, 207(6), 824-831.

[64] Pangarkar S, Mistry K, Choudhari A, Smriti V, Ahuja A, Katdare A, Engineer R, Ostwal V, Ramadwar M, Saklani A, Baheti AD., Accuracy of MRI for nodal restaging in rectal cancer: a retrospective study of 166 cases., Abdom Radiol (NY). 2021 Feb;46(2):498-505. doi: 10.1007/s00261-020-02708-y. Epub 2020 Aug 19.

[65] Alberda WJ, Dassen HP, Dwarkasing RS, Willemssen FE, van der Pool AE, de Wilt JH, Burger JW, Verhoef C., Prediction of tumor stage and lymph node involvement with dynamic contrast-enhanced MRI after chemoradiotherapy for locally advanced rectal cancer. Int J Colorectal Dis. 2013 Apr;28(4):573-580. doi: 10.1007/s00384-012-1576-6. Epub 2012 Sep 22.

[66] Marion-Audibert AM, Vullierme MP, Ronot M et al (2018) Routine MRI with DWI sequences to detect liver metastases in patients with potentially resectable pancreatic ductal carcinoma and normal liver CT: a prospective multicenter study. AJR Am J Roentgenol 211: W217–W225

[67] Suciu BA., Halmaciu I., Vunvulea V., Brinzaniuc K., Is there any correlation between the occurrence of spontaneous pneumothorax and changes in the weather conditions worldwide? Eur J Cardio-Thorac Surg. 2018;53(4):895-896

[68] Sivesgaard K, Larsen LP, Sørensen M, Kramer S, Schlander S, Amanavicius N, et al. Diagnostic accuracy of CE-CT, MRI and FDG PET/CT for detecting colorectal cancer liver metastases in patients considered eligible for hepatic resection and/or local ablation. Eur Radiol. 2018; 28:4735-4747

[69] Queiroz MA, Ortega CD, Ferreira FR, Nahas SC, Cerri GG, Buchpiguel CA., Diagnostic accuracy of FDG-PET/MRI versus pelvic MRI and thoracic and abdominal CT for detecting synchronous distant metastases in rectal cancer patients., Eur J Nucl Med Mol Imaging. 2021 Jan;48(1):186-195. doi: 10.1007/s00259-020-04911-x. Epub 2020 Jun 20.

[70] Heye T, Ley S, Heussel CP, Dienemann H, Kauczor HU, Hosch W, et al. Detection and size of pulmonary lesions: how accurate is MRI? A prospective comparison of CT and MRI. Acta Radiol. 2012; 53:153-160.

[71] Yoon JH, Lee JM, Chang W, Kang HJ, Bandos A, Lim HJ, Kang SY, Kang KW, Ryoo SB, Jeong SY, Park KJ., Initial M Staging of Rectal Cancer: FDG PET/MRI with a Hepatocyte-specific Contrast Agent versus Contrast-enhanced CT, Radiology. 2020 Feb;294(2):310-319. doi: 10.1148/radiol.2019190794. Epub 2019 Dec 3.

[72] Horvat N, Veeraraghavan H, Khan M, Blazic I, Zheng J, Capanu M, Sala E, Garcia-Aguilar J, Gollub MJ, Petkovska I., MR Imaging of Rectal Cancer: Radiomics Analysis to Assess Treatment Response after Neoadjuvant Therapy., Radiology. 2018 Jun;287(3):833-843. doi: 10.1148/radiol.2018172300. Epub 2018 Mar 7.

[73] Heald RJ, Ryall RD. Recurrence and survival after total mesorectal excision for rectal cancer. Lancet 1986;1(8496):1479-1482.

[74] National Comprehensive Cancer Network. NCCN Clinical Practice Guidelines in Oncology (NCCN Guidelines) Rectal Cancer version 2.2017. https://www.nccn.org/professionals/physician_gls/pdf/rectal.pdf.

[75] Halmaciu I., Suciu BA., Trambitas C., Vunvulea V., Ivanescu A., Clipa A., Adascalitei P., Brinzaniuc K., Fodor D., It is Useful to Use Plastic Anatomical Models in Teaching Human Anatomy? Mater Plast. 2018;55(3):414-418

[76] Habr-Gama A, Perez RO, Nadalin W, et al. Operative versus nonoperative treatment for stage 0 distal rectal cancer following chemoradiation therapy: long-term results. Ann Surg 2004;240(4):711-717

[77] Capirci C, Valentini V, Cionini L, De Paoli A, Rodel C, Glynne-Jones R, Coco C, Romano M, Mantello G, Palazzi S. Prognostic value of pathologic complete response after neoadjuvant therapy in locally advanced rectal cancer: long-term analysis of 566 ypCR patients. Int J Radiat Oncol Biol Phys. 2008; 72:99-107

[78] Maas M, Nelemans PJ, Valentini V, Das P, Rödel C, Kuo LJ, Calvo FA, García-Aguilar J, Glynne-Jones R, Haustermans K. Long-term outcome in patients with a pathological complete response after chemoradiation for rectal cancer: a pooled analysis of individual patient data. Lancet Oncol. 2010; 11:835-844

[79] García-Albéniz X, Gallego R, Hofheinz RD, Fernández-Esparrach G, Ayuso-Colella JR, Bombí JA, Conill C, Cuatrecasas M, Delgado S, Ginés A, Miquel R, Pagés M, Pineda E, Pereira V, Sosa A, Reig O, Victoria I, Feliz L, María de Lacy A, Castells A, Burkholder I, Hochhaus A, Maurel J. Adjuvant therapy sparing in rectal cancer achieving complete response after chemoradiation. World J Gastroenterol 2014; 20(42): 15820-15829

[80] Kim, HJ, Song, JH, Ahn, HS. Wait and see approach for rectal cancer with a clinically complete response after neoadjuvant concurrent chemoradiotherapy. Colorectal Dis 2017; 32: 723-727.

[81] Janjan, NA, Crane, C, Feig, BW. Improved overall survival among responders to preoperative chemoradiation for locally advanced rectal cancer. Am J Clin Oncol 2001; 24: 107-112.

[82] Petrillo, A, Fusco, R, Granata, V. MR imaging perfusion and diffusion analysis to assess preoperative short course radiotherapy response in locally advanced rectal cancer: standardized index of shape by DCE-MRI and intravoxel incoherent motion-derived parameters by DW-MRI. Med Oncol 2017; 34: 198.

[83] Gibbs P, Liney GP, Pickles MD, Zelhof B, Rodrigues G, Turnbull LW. Correlation of ADC and T2 measurements with cell density in prostate cancer at 3.0 Tesla. Invest Radiol 2009; 44: 572-76. doi: https://doi.org/10.1097/RLI.0b013e3181b4c10e

[84] Pham TT, Liney GP, Wong K, Barton MB., Functional MRI for quantitative treatment response prediction in locally advanced rectal cancer., Br J Radiol. 2017 Apr;90(1072):20151078. doi: 10.1259/bjr.20151078. Epub 2017 Mar 7

[85] Suciu BA., Halmaciu I., Fodor D., Trambitas C., Godja D., Clipa A., Nicolescu C., Brinzaniuc K., Vunvulea V., Comparative Study on the Need for Postoperative Analgesic Medication

After Surgical Treatment of Inguinal Hernia with Surgical Mesh through Laparoscopic or Classic Approach., Mater Plast. 2018;55(3):380-384

[86] Zahra MA, , Hollingsworth KG, , Sala E, , Lomas DJ, , Tan LT. Dynamic contrast-enhanced MRI as a predictor of tumour response to radiotherapy. Lancet Oncol 2007; 8: 63-74. doi: https://doi.org/10.1016/S1470-2045(06)71012-9

[87] Tofts PS, Brix G, Buckley DL, Evelhoch JL, Henderson E, Knopp MV, et al. Estimating kinetic parameters from dynamic contrast-enhanced T (1)-weighted MRI of a diffusable tracer: standardized quantities and symbols. J Magn Reson Imaging 1999; 10: 223-32. doi: https://doi.org/10.1002/(SICI)1522-2586(199909)10:3<223:AID-JMRI2>3.0.CO;2-S

[88] Memom S., Lynch AC., Bressel M., Wise AG., Heriot AG., Systematic review and meta-analysis of the accuracy of MRI and endorectal ultrasound in the restaging and response assessment of rectal cancer following neoadjuvant therapy. Colorectal Dis. 2015 Sep;17(9):748-761. doi: 10.1111/codi.12976.

[89] Lee SL., Shin YR., Kim K., The added value of pelvic surveillance by MRI during postoperative follow-up of rectal cancer, with a focus on abbreviated MRI., Eur Radiol. 2020 Jun;30(6):3113-3124. doi: 10.1007/s00330-020-06711-1. Epub 2020 Feb 18

[90] Goldberg RM, Fleming TR, Tangen CM et al (1998) Surgery for recurrent colon cancer: strategies for identifying resectable recurrence and success rates after resection. Eastern Cooperative Oncology Group, the North Central Cancer Treatment Group, and the Southwest Oncology Group. Ann Intern Med 129:27-35

[91] Dresen RC, Kusters M, Daniels-Gooszen AW et al (2010) Absence of tumor invasion into pelvic structures in locally recurrent rectal cancer: prediction with preoperative MR imaging. Radiology 256:143-150

[92] Titu LV, Nicholson AA, Hartley JE, Breen DJ, Monson JR (2006) Routine follow-up by magnetic resonance imaging does not improve detection of resectable local recurrences from colorectal cancer. Ann Surg 243:348-352

[93] Torricelli P, Pecchi A, Luppi G, Romagnoli R (2003) Gadolinium-enhanced MRI with dynamic evaluation in diagnosing the local recurrence of rectal cancer. Abdom Imaging 28:19-27

[94] Lambregts DM, Lahaye MJ, Heijnen LA et al (2016) MRI and diffusion-weighted MRI to diagnose a local tumour regrowth during long-term follow-up of rectal cancer patients treated with organ preservation after chemoradiotherapy. Eur Radiol 26:2118-2125

[95] Lambregts DMJ, Maas M, Boellaard TN et al (2020) Long-term imaging characteristics of clinical complete responders during watch-and-wait for rectal cancer-an evaluation of over 1500 MRIs. Eur Radiol 30:272-280

Chapter 10

Intraoperative Ultrasound in Colorectal Surgery

Sinziana Ionescu

Abstract

Intraoperative ultrasound (IOUS) in colorectal surgery can be used both in benign and in malignant lesions. In benign cases, such as Crohn's disease and diverticulitis, it can orient toward the extension of the surgical intervention. In malignant cases, such as colorectal cancer with liver metastases, IOUS/CE-IOUS (contrast-enhanced) improved the intraoperative management of liver metastases by dictating the resection margins in relation to the tumor extension. The IOUS method allows for exact tumor location, intestinal wall visualization, and malignant tumor penetration. The IOUS revealed the tumor and its margin in rectal lesions, making the sphincter-sparing operation easier to perform. In patients with small polyps and early colon and rectum cancers, IOUS works well as a one-of-a-kind intraoperative localization technique. In comparison with IOUS, CE-IOUS offered better detection and resection guidance. Intraoperative ultrasound enables surgeons to easily localize small, non-palpable lesions of the large bowel. Furthermore, it can determine even the aggressive potential of these lesions with high precision.

Keywords: colorectal, intraoperative ultrasound, laparoscopic ultrasound, colorectal surgery, robotic ultrasound

1. Introduction

Intraoperative ultrasound is a complex and highly interactive imaging study field that is one of the ultrasonography's fastest growing fields. Intraoperative ultrasound has a wide spectrum of uses, which are expanding all the time.

Intraoperative ultrasound is used effectively in neurosurgery to operate on the brain and spinal cord, and it is mostly used in intra-abdominal surgery to operate on the liver, biliary tract, and pancreas.

Intraoperative vascular surgical disease assessment and intraoperative ultrasound imaging can also guide endarterectomy interventions. In patients with colorectal liver metastases, liver resections with negative margins increase survival (CRLM).

Intraoperative ultrasound (IOUS) is a useful tool that provides information about liver lesions, allowing surgeons to adjust their surgical technique to ensure total removal and, as a result, increase disease-free survival (DFS). Another important use of intraoperative ultrasound in colorectal surgery is to localize lesions at the level of the colon and of the rectum in order to properly adjust the extension of the resection (**Figure 1**).

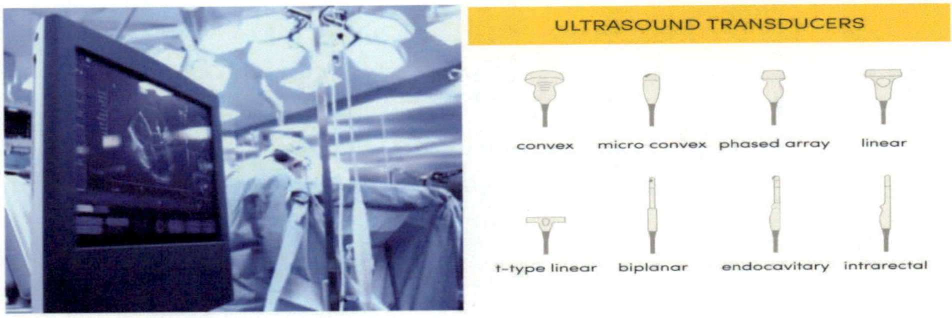

Figure 1.
Intraoperative monitor of ultrasound and various types of ultrasound probes.

2. General characteristics of intraoperative ultrasound

2.1 Intraoperative ultrasound in open surgery

Intraoperative ultrasonography (IOUS), according to Machi and coauthors [1] can provide a wide range of diagnostic information that would otherwise be unavailable or unavailable, as well as a guide or help with various surgical procedures in real time. With the technical development of the proper equipment, IOUS is currently used in a wide variety of surgical interventions, such as hepato-biliary, pancreatic, endocrine, cardiovascular, and neurologic surgeries. Among its numerous advantages, we underline safety, quickness, accuracy, and versatility. Therefore, IOUS is a valuable technique that surgeons are recommended to master to improve intraoperative decision-making. Furthermore increasing the attention for details, ultrasound Doppler allows the user to visualize blood flow and can assess the blood supply in and near the area of interest, thus avoiding injury to important vessels during dissection, as found by Vapenstad and collab [2]. Various intraoperative transducers are available for use, as mentioned by Marcal and team [3] in abdominal surgery: Linear array, curvilinear array, and phased array IOUS transducers are made available by different vendors. One of the most important criteria is that the probe fits snugly into the surgical incision and can be easily maneuvered in a narrow operative space. Higher-frequency transducers, in comparison with lower frequency transducers, can produce higher-resolution images.

Due to the faster attenuation, as the wave passes through the tissue, high-frequency echography waves have a mild tissue penetration. Moreover, from a didactic perspective, the operating room is a place in which the surgeon (more than in the case of other specialties) has a favorable environment to learn operative ultrasound use and interpretation, since the surgeon is already familiar with the anatomical structures that have to be examined during the procedure.

2.2 Laparoscopic ultrasound

Laparoscopic ultrasound is a relatively new method in point of surgical sonography, whose arrival can be attributed to the need for the development of specialized transducers that could fit through conventional laparoscopic trocars. The quality, reliability, and ease of use of such units have evolved quickly, so that laparoscopic ultrasonography became routine. One of the advantages of this procedure is that it helps the surgeon to peer into the tissues being operated on, compensating for the inability to palpate those tissues physically.

As a result, not only did it help to replicate open surgery, but it also helped to improve existing laparoscopic surgical techniques. The monitoring of the tips of ultrasound (US) laparoscopes presents several particular challenges.

Instead of a camera, an ultrasound laparoscope's tip has an ultrasound array.

As a result, computer vision tracking methods cannot be used to detect the tip using the image from the laparoscope. The control levers on the laparoscope handle can be used to adjust the tip of the probe.

In contrast to endoscopes, which are rigid throughout, and the tip's pose can be calculated solely by tracking the handle, ultrasound laparoscopes require an additional sensor installed on the tip to obtain the pose, as defined in Chinmay's work [4].

An ultrasound array is located at the tip of the considered ultrasound laparoscope.

The probe's tip is movable, and the surgeon operating the laparoscope may use the control levers to adjust the tip's trajectory even further.

These levers are attached to the laparoscope's tip.

The movement of the laparoscope tip is usually regulated by two levers.

The laparoscope tip may be relocated in a hemispheric space inside the patient's body using them (**Figure 2**).

Alecu and coauthors [5] came to the following conclusions in a report on the efficiency of visualization and the general benefits of laparoscopic ultrasonography in abdominal surgery:

1. Diagnostic laparoscopy and intraoperative contact ultrasonography are combined in laparoscopic ultrasonography;

2. laparoscopic ultrasound is a simple and effective examination procedure;

3. laparoscopic ultrasonography is the technique of choice for intraoperative CBD exploration;

4. laparoscopic ultrasonography may improve abdominal malignancy exploration, resulting in a more accurate diagnosis.

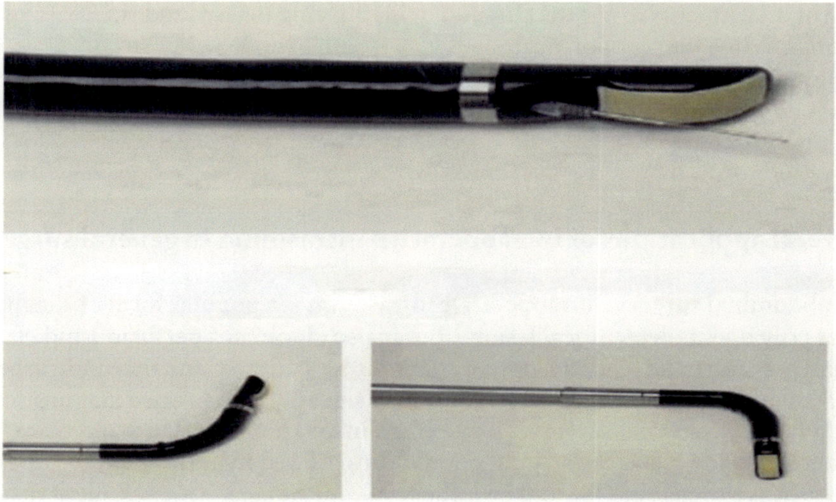

Figure 2.
(a-c) A laparoscopic probe has a needle biopsy enhancement (a, above) and two lower images (b, c) showing the flexibility of the tip of the probe.

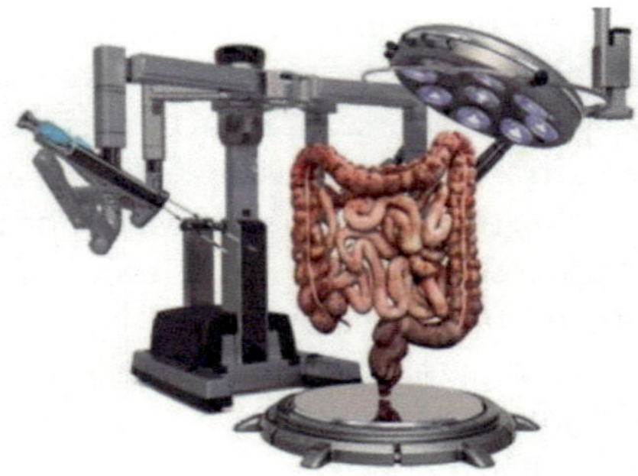

Figure 3.
A surgical robot and the schematic approach to the colorectal area.

2.3 Robotic ultrasound

The combination of an ultrasound imaging technique with a robotic device in medical procedures is known as the Robots' ultrasound process (RUS).

Robots are often suitable for ultrasound integration because of their unquestionable capacity for high precision, dexterity, and repeatability.

Despite the fact that the field is still relatively new, it has already developed a slew of robotic systems for use in dozens of medical procedures, such as the one by Priester and collab [6].

Consider the following example: the use of robotic ultrasound in partial nephrectomy with a robot.

According to Di Cosmo and coauthors [7], using a robotic ultrasound probe during partial nephrectomy enables the surgeon to optimize tumor detection with maximum autonomy while also benefiting from the robot's precision and articulation during this crucial phase of the procedure.

Furthermore, ultrasound can help to reduce the time spent in ischemia (IT).

The benefits of nephron-sparing surgery over radical nephrectomy are identified using a pool of data that shows oncological and survival equivalence.

As robot-assisted partial nephrectomy (RAPN) techniques evolved, the use of different instruments to aid the surgeon in identifying masses and their vascular network became more sophisticated.

The authors of this study [7] investigated the current use of intraoperative ultrasound as an operative tool to enhance the localization of small renal masses during RAPN (**Figure 3**).

3. Several applications of intraoperative ultrasound in general surgery

In abdominal surgery, intraoperative ultrasound is a popular form of diagnosis.

Not only does it detect focal lesions, but it also eliminates perfusion and elasticity analyses with color-coded Doppler sonography, contrast-enhanced ultrasound, and elastography, all of which allow for highly sensitive and precise diagnostics, especially in oncological surgery, as described in an article by Hackl and team [8]. Another study looked at the staging possibilities offered by intraoperative ultrasound as was the case of Oba and coauthors [9]. Intraoperative assessment needed to appreciate the extent and location of Crohn's disease has not been standardized and currently involves a mixture of surgeons' experience, tactile feedback, and macroscopic appearance. In a study titled "Assessing the Feasibility and Safety of Using Intraoperative Ultrasound in Ileocolic Crohn's Disease—The IUSS CROHN

Study," Celentano and team [10] devised a strategy for a thorough intraoperative ultrasound scan of the small bowel to overcome this variability. This feasibility study mentioned above demonstrated the safety of intraoperative ultrasound and allowed the development of a standardized protocol for the intraoperative ultrasound.

4. Intraoperative ultrasound in colorectal surgery

4.1 Early and precise detection of liver metastases with consecutive treatment: Resection, RFA, cryosurgery

According to Walker and collab [11], up to two-thirds of colorectal cancer (CRC) patients develop colorectal liver metastases (CRLMs), with one-quarter of patients having synchronous metastases.

Surgical resection for CRLM provides the best chance of a successful outcome.

Computerized tomography and magnetic resonance imaging are often used to stage CRC prior to surgery.

Intraoperative ultrasound (IOUS) and contrast-enhanced IOUS (CE-IOUS) scans have been shown to detect additional metastases not visible on preoperative imaging.

Colorectal surgeons do not commonly use IOUS during primary resection for CRC.

The confident use of IOUS/CE-IOUS after primary resection of CRC can aid decision-making by giving the most sensitive type of liver staging, even when compared to magnetic resonance imaging. This is especially significant in the age of laparoscopic procedures, as the colorectal surgeon loses the ability to palpate the liver and its lesions.

The use of IOUS/CE-IOUS by colorectal surgeons has been hampered by a number of factors.

Time constraints, familiarity with procedures, a perceived learning curve, cost effects, and numerous limitations of the modality due to operator variations are just a few of them.

Incorporating IOUS into colorectal surgeons' basic training and subsequent research into the potential benefits of IOUS/CE-IOUS could theoretically lower these barriers, allowing for more widespread use of IOUS during primary resection for CRC. In a research performed by Desolneux and coauthors [12], the central idea was to determine the clinical utility (CU) of contrast-enhanced intraoperative ultrasound (CE-IOUS) using sulfur hexafluoride microbubbles during CRLM surgery. The conclusion was that although the primary endpoint was not met for one protocol violation, secondary endpoints indicate that CE-IOUS has an intermediate added value for surgeons treating CRLMs (**Figure 4**).

4.2 Localization of colorectal tumors

In a study published by Greif and collab [13] with the goal of determining the accuracy of intraoperative ultrasound (IOUS) as a localizing technique for colorectal resections and its impact on surgical management, it was discovered that IOUS can be used as a sole method of intraoperative localization and provide additional information in patients with small polyps and early cancers of the colon and rectum.

Furthermore, a study by Luck and team [14] discovered that in an *in vitro* setting, a direct ultrasound of the colon utilizing a high-frequency surgical probe gave accurate pictures of neoplastic tumors. This method may play a part in the

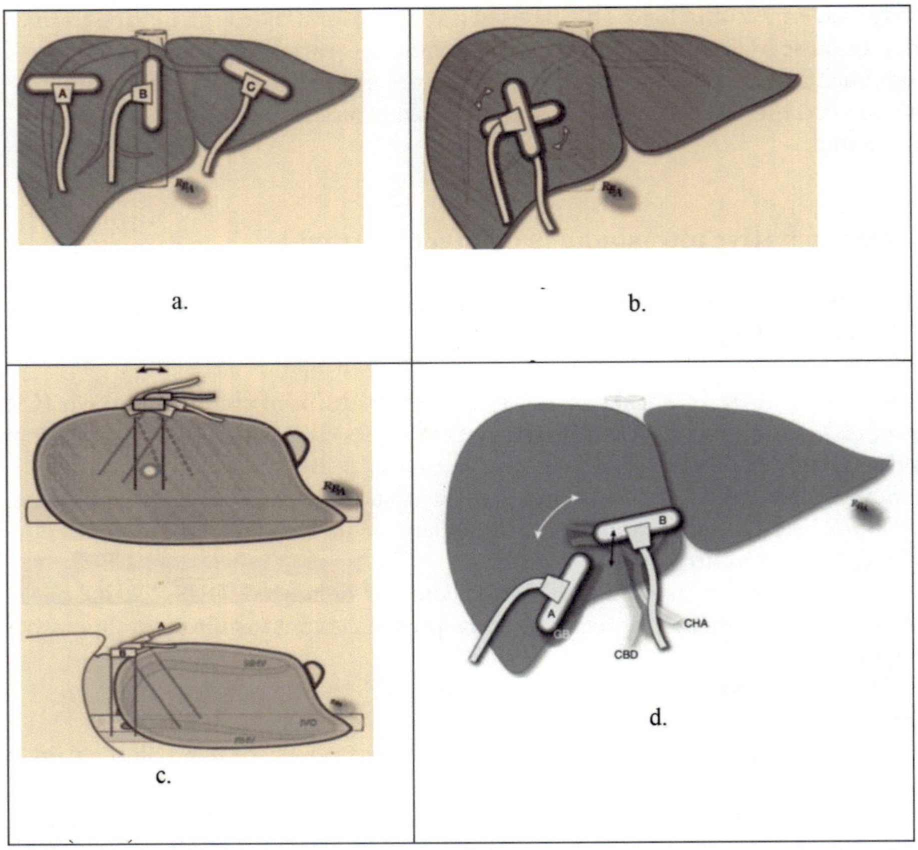

Figure 4.
(a) Standard intraoperative transducer position for liver scanning. (b) Rotational transducer movement, the probe is rotated clockwise or counterclockwise on a fixed point, in order to see in two planes. (c) Rocking/tilting the transducer without (above) or with (down) saline immersion. (d) Positions of the probe in order to look at the biliary tree—Main divisions.

intraoperative location of lesions and assessment of colorectal cancer. Furthermore, the same research adds to the overall picture by stating that excellent ultrasound images were obtained, particularly when the colonic lumen was filled with saline.

This technique found and correctly located all lesions, as well as several impalpable synchronous polyps.

The remains of a malignant polyp not evident with intraoperative colonoscopy were discovered by specimen ultrasound in two specimens.

The image's clarity allowed for cancer staging.

The benefit of using laparoscopic high-resolution ultrasonography in conjunction with color power Doppler to locate colonic polyp lesions during a laparoscopic colon resection, as stated by Panaro and coauthors [15], is that intraoperative colonoscopy is avoided.

Intraoperative colon ultrasonography can pinpoint colonic polyp lesions that are not visible during laparoscopy, and it is a quick and painless alternative to other imaging techniques.

4.3 Guidance of the technique of quadratus lumborum block for postoperative pain management in colorectal surgery

In an article authored by Deng [16], it was underlined that laparoscopic ultrasound can be used for guiding the injection site in quadratus lumborum block

(QLB) for pain management. The study looked at 74 patients who were scheduled for laparoscopic colorectal surgery and were divided into two classes at random.

Following surgery, patients were given a single dose of QLB or TAPB administered bilaterally using ultrasound guidance.

Twenty-microliter of 0.375% ropivacaine was injected into each hand.

All patients were given sufentanil as a patient-controlled intravenous analgesia (PCIA), and the results showed that the QLB is a more powerful postoperative analgesia than the TAPB in patients undergoing laparoscopic colorectal surgery because it decreases sufentanil intake.

4.4 Doppler assessment of flow and vessel division

AS early as 1980, studies evaluating colonic blood flow through intraoperative Doppler ultrasound showed that laser Doppler flowmetry represents a potentially very interesting non-invasive, continuous method for the quantitative study of human intestinal blood flow, such as the one performed by Ahn and team [17]. In parallel to the study on humans and completing the general picture with valuable information regarding blood flow, a study by Kashiwagi and collab [18] will be further described. In order to determine the minimal threshold of tissue blood flow (TBF) for safe colonic anastomosis, an experiment was performed in dogs: The wound healing process of anastomotic sites was correlated with varying degrees of TBF, measured by laser Doppler velocimetry (LDV). The conclusion of the above-mentioned study was in terms of TBF, if the LDV value at the anastomotic site is at least 1.0, equivalent to about 30% of the TBF of the intact colonic wall, then the anastomosis is considered healthy and dehiscence is unlikely.

In a study presented by Seike and coauthors [19], colonic blood flow at the proximal site of the anastomosis was measured by laser Doppler flowmetry in 96 patients with the rectum and sigmoid colon cancer while clamping IMA or LCA, and the conclusion of the research that looked at which point of ligature would be optimal was that colonic blood flow at the proximal site of the anastomosis was crucial. Patients who undergo ultralow anterior resection and have a high reduction by IMA clamping need various intraoperative efforts to avoid ischemia at the stage of the anastomosis.

According to another study reported by Hallbook [20], laser Doppler flowmetry was used to measure transmural colonic blood flow before the formation of a plain (n = 16) or pouch (n = 14) anastomosis during the surgery. Before dissecting the bowel, the vascular supply was recorded at two locations: one near to the intended bowel end and another 8 cm away.

After dissection and, where possible, pouch creation, but before the anastomosis was completed, a second recording was made at the same sites.

Following bowel dissection, blood flow levels at the site intended for the anastomosis were substantially reduced in the end-to-end anastomosis community.

Following bowel dissection and pouch building, blood supply levels at the site of the anastomosis were comparable in the pouch community (side-to-end anastomosis).

Unaffected blood supply at the pouch anastomosis site can be a beneficial factor for anastomotic healing, according to the findings.

Furthermore, when it comes to the small bowel partner of an anastomosis, such as the ileocolic anastomosis after right hemicolectomy or the confection of a small bowel J pouch, blood flow supply must be assessed.

This can now be done more accurately with the aid of an ICG quantitative flow technique, but laser Doppler can still be used for orientation, as demonstrated in a study published by Johansson and coauthors [21]. The precision of the blood flow evaluation by Doppler is such that one can look at the sutureline blood flow in colonic anastomoses, to compare the impact of a mechanical versus a manual anastomosis on the blood supply to the anastomosed area, as was emphasized by Chung and team [22].

4.5 Ultrasound elastography to detect fibrotic bowel strictures in Crohn's disease

Another study conducted by Chen [23] looked at the distinction of intestinal fibrosis from inflammation in Crohn's disease (CD)-associated strictures, as presented by Vestito [24] in a systematic review with meta-analysis to assess whether ultrasound elastography can have a diagnostic role in detecting fibrotic bowel strictures in patients with Crohn's disease. The study included consecutive CD patients with ileal/ileocolonic strictures who had shear wave elastography (SWE) within 1 week of surgical resection.

The grade and severity of both fibrosis and inflammation in the resected bowel specimen were compared to the SWE of the stenotic bowel wall.

One of the key points of this study was that SWE is a viable and effective method for detecting intestinal fibrosis in CD patients.

Combining SWE and bowel vascularization on traditional ultrasound after validation could be used to direct a management strategy in CD patients by identifying the form of intestinal stricture.

5. Conclusion

This chapter explores the general advantages of intraoperative ultrasound in improving the outcome of the surgical diagnosis, staging, and patient outcome. Specifically, intraoperative colorectal ultrasound can be used both at the level of the primary tumor, as at the level of the lymph nodes, and at the level of the secondary determinations, especially liver metastases.

Conflict of interest

The author declares no conflict of interest.

Author details

Sinziana Ionescu[1,2]

1 Bucharest Oncology Institute, Bucharest, Romania

2 "Carol Davila" University of Medicine and Pharmacy, Bucharest, Romania

*Address all correspondence to: sinzianaionescu30@gmail.com

References

[1] Machi J, Oishi AJ, Furumoto NL, Oishi RH. Intraoperative ultrasound. The Surgical Clinics of North America. 2004;**84**(4):1085-1111. DOI: 10.1016/j.suc.2004.04.001

[2] Våpenstad C, Rethy A, Langø T, et al. Laparoscopic ultrasound: A survey of its current and future use, requirements, and integration with navigation technology. Surgical Endoscopy. 2010;**24**:2944-2953. DOI: 10.1007/s00464-010-1135-6

[3] Marcal LP, Patnana M, Bhosale P, Bedi DG. Intraoperative abdominal ultrasound in oncologic imaging. World Journal of Radiology. 2013;**5**(3):51-60. DOI: 10.4329/wjr.v5.i3.51

[4] file:///Users/ionescusinziana/Downloads/SAMANT_Chinmay_2019_ED269.pdf

[5] Alecu L, Lungu C, Pascu A, Costan I, Corodeanu G, Deacu A, et al. Ecografia intraoperatorie în chirurgia laparoscopică [Intraoperative ultrasonography during laparoscopic surgery]. Chirurgia. 2000;**95**(6):557-564

[6] Priester AM, Natarajan S, Culjat MO. Robotic ultrasound systems in medicine. IEEE Transactions on Ultrasonics, Ferroelectrics, and Frequency Control. 2013;**60**(3):507-523. DOI: 10.1109/TUFFC.2013.2593

[7] Di Cosmo G, Verzotti E, Silvestri T, Lissiani A, Knez R, Pavan N, et al. Intraoperative ultrasound in robot-assisted partial nephrectomy: State of the art. Archivio Italiano di Urologia, Andrologia. 2018;**90**(3):195-198. DOI: 10.4081/aiua.2018.3.195

[8] Hackl C, Bitterer F, Platz Batista da Silva N, Jung EM, Schlitt HJ. Intraoperative ultrasound in visceral surgery. Chirurg. 2020;**91**(6):474-480. DOI: 10.1007/s00104-020-01142-6

[9] Oba A, Inoue Y, Ono Y, Ishizuka N, Arakaki M, Sato T, et al. Staging laparoscopy for pancreatic cancer using intraoperative ultrasonography and fluorescence imaging: The SLING trial. The British Journal of Surgery. 2021;**108**(2):115-118. DOI: 10.1093/bjs/znaa111

[10] Celentano V, Beable R, Ball C, Flashman KG, Reeve R, Fogg C, et al. Feasibility of intraoperative ultrasound of the small bowel during Crohn's disease surgery. Techniques in Coloproctology. 2020;**24**(9):965-969. DOI: 10.1007/s10151-020-02268-9

[11] Walker TLJ, Bamford R, Finch-Jones M. Intraoperative ultrasound for the colorectal surgeon: Current trends and barriers. ANZ Journal of Surgery. 2017;**87**(9):671-676. DOI: 10.1111/ans.14124

[12] Desolneux G, Isambert M, Mathoulin-Pelissier S, Dupré A, Rivoire M, Cattena V, et al. Contrast-enhanced intra-operative ultrasound as a clinical decision making tool during surgery for colorectal liver metastases: The ULIIS study. European Journal of Surgical Oncology. 2019;**45**(7):1212-1218. DOI: 10.1016/j.ejso.2019.03.002

[13] Greif F, Aranovich D, Hananel N, Knizhnik M, Belenky A. Intraoperative ultrasound in colorectal surgery. Journal of Clinical Ultrasound. 2009;**37**(7):375-379. DOI: 10.1002/jcu.20600

[14] Luck A, Copley J, Hewett P. Ultrasound of colonic neoplasia. Surgical Endoscopy. 2000;**14**:185-188. DOI: 10.1007/s004649900097

[15] Panaro F, Casaccia M, Cavaliere D, Torelli P. Laparoscopic colon resection with intraoperative polyp localisation with high resolution ultrasonography coupled with colour power Doppler. Postgraduate Medical Journal.

2003;**79**(935):533-534. DOI: 10.1136/pmj.79.935.533

[16] Deng W, Long X, Li M, Li C, Guo L, Xu G, et al. Quadratus lumborum block versus transversus abdominis plane block for postoperative pain management after laparoscopic colorectal surgery: A randomized controlled trial. Medicine. 2019;**98**(52):e18448. DOI: 10.1097/MD.0000000000018448

[17] Ahn H, Lindhagen J, Lundgren O. Measurement of colonic blood flow with laser Doppler flowmetry. Scandinavian Journal of Gastroenterology. 1986;**21**(7):871-880. DOI: 10.3109/00365528609011132

[18] Kashiwagi H. The lower limit of tissue blood flow for safe colonic anastomosis: An experimental study using laser Doppler velocimetry. Surgery Today. 1993;**23**(5):430-438. DOI: 10.1007/BF00309502

[19] Seike K, Koda K, Saito N, et al. Laser Doppler assessment of the influence of division at the root of the inferior mesenteric artery on anastomotic blood flow in rectosigmoid cancer surgery. International Journal of Colorectal Disease. 2007;**22**:689-697. DOI: 10.1007/s00384-006-0221-7

[20] Hallböök O, Johansson K, Sjödahl R. Laser Doppler blood flow measurement in rectal resection for carcinoma—Comparison between the straight and colonic J pouch reconstruction. British Journal of Surgery. 1996;**83**(3):389-392. DOI: 10.1002/bjs.1800830330

[21] Johansson K, Ahn H, Lindhagen J. Intraoperative assessment of blood flow and tissue viability in small-bowel ischemia by laser Doppler flowmetry. Acta Chirurgica Scandinavica. 1989;**155**(6-7):341-346

[22] Chung RS. Blood flow in colonic anastomoses. Effect of stapling and suturing. Annals of Surgery. 1987;**206**(3):335-339. DOI: 10.1097/00000658-198709000-00011

[23] Chen YJ, Mao R, Li XH, Cao QH, Chen ZH, Liu BX, et al. Real-time shear wave ultrasound elastography differentiates fibrotic from inflammatory strictures in patients with Crohn's disease. Inflammatory Bowel Diseases. 2018;**24**(10):2183-2190. DOI: 10.1093/ibd/izy115

[24] Vestito A, Marasco G, Maconi G, Festi D, Bazzoli F, Zagari RM. Role of ultrasound elastography in the detection of fibrotic bowel strictures in patients with Crohn's disease: Systematic review and meta-analysis. Ultraschall in der Medizin. 2019;**40**(5):646-654. DOI: 10.1055/a-0865-1842

Chapter 11

The Use of Indocyanine Green in Colorectal Surgery

Sinziana Ionescu

Abstract

This chapter looks at the use of indocyanine green (ICG) in colorectal surgery, by exploring at first the definition of vital dyes generally used in the surgical field, afterward the benefits of fluorescence-guided surgery, and furthermore, it enumerates several uses of ICG in the broad surgical field. The identification of tumor nodules in the peritoneum can help with proper cancer staging, and the same advantage is brought by the accurate detection of the sentinel lymph node, which concerns the use of ICG specifically in colorectal surgery, and this can be summed up through the following assets brought by the technique: (a) intraoperative fluorescence angiography as an adjuvant in the process of anastomosis, (b) fluorescence-guided detection of lymph node metastases in colorectal cancer and the sentinel lymph node technique, which was proved better than formal methods in some studies, (c) the positive fluorescence of a liver nodule as small as "only" 200 tumor cells, (d) the help in diagnosing a fistula, (e) the possibility to be used for tumor tattooing also, and (f) the help in maintaining a clean surgical field and preventing wound infection in abdominoperineal resection.

Keywords: colorectal, fluorescence, ICG, ICG-NIR, colorectal surgery, intraoperative staining

1. Introduction

As the general surgical techniques have polished with more and more precise gestures, which in time lead to the appearance and development of even robotic surgery, the same phenomenon happened when it comes to adjuvant methods to better identify, visualize, and resect a specific structure/tissue during the intervention. Fluorescence can bring important assets when it comes to seeing better—the vessels, the lymph nodes, and the tumor itself. Some organs, such as the case of the ureter, are also much better underlined with the technique of NIR-ICG (near-infrared light and indocyanine green [ICG]), and therefore, the risk of producing a lesion secondary to incomplete visualization is smaller. This chapter closely looks at the literature on the theme of ICG in colorectal surgery, offering also a general frame made out of significant research, mainly systematic reviews and randomized controlled trials about the use of ICG in visceral surgery.

IntechOpen

2. Types of dyes used in surgery

2.1 Classical dyes

According to the definition given by the Merriam-Webster dictionary, a dye or a stain is able to penetrate living cells or tissues without inducing immediate obvious degenerative changes and thus, it is also called a vital stain. Supravital staining implies the removal of living cells from an organism, whereas intravital staining involves injecting (or otherwise administering) the dye into the organism. The term "vital stain" is sometimes used to refer to an intravital stain, and in some other situations, it is interchangeable with a supravital stain, the main idea being that the cell being looked at is still alive. In a more strict way of speaking, the term "vital staining" has a meaning which is opposite to "supravital staining." If living cells take up the stain during supravital staining, living cells exclude the dye during "vital staining"; for example, they color negatively and only dead cells color positively, and hence, viability can be measured by counting in percentage the amount of total cells that stain negatively. Because the nature of the dye defines if the staining is either supravital or intravital, a mix of supravital and vital dyes can be employed to better categorize cells into various groups (e.g., viable, dead, dying) (**Figures 1** and **2**).

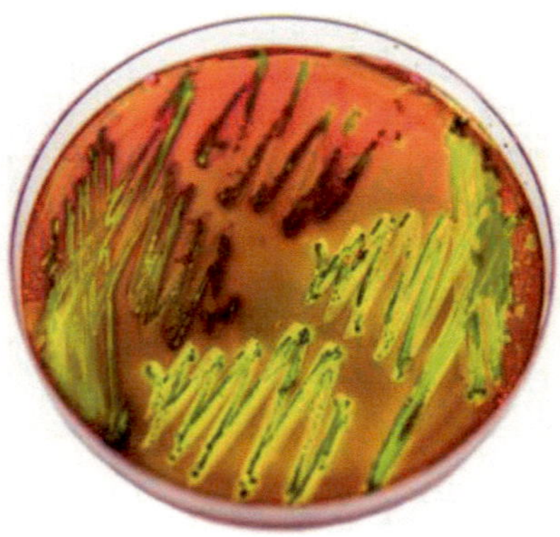

Figure 1.
Metallic green sheen characteristic colonies of Escherichia coli on eosin methylene blue agar (EMB) in close-up.

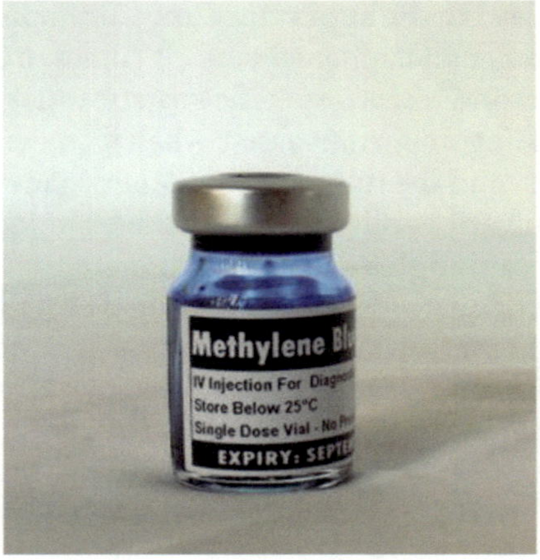

Figure 2.
A vial of methylene blue.

Tissue staining, also known as chromoscopy, can be used as an adjuvant technique in gastrointestinal endoscopy to help with the recognition of subtle lesions, such as is the case with polyps or, more so, allows to directly target biopsies, which may happen in the case of Barrett's esophagus, in order to increase the precision of the diagnosis. Four endoscopic staining techniques have been described—vital staining (the use of an agent that is absorbed by the intestinal epithelium), contrast staining (the use of a substance to accentuate the aspect of the surface), reactive staining (the use of an agent that can fire chemical reactions), and tattooing (a technique using agents such as India ink to underline a special lesion on the mucosa).

Tissue stains used in gastrointestinal surgery, as mentioned by Fennerty [1], can be classified as follows:

a. tattooing agents

1. India ink is used for permanent marking of the mucosal site for relocalization at the time of surgery or endoscopy, also used in the esophagus, stomach, and colon, which is safe without side effects.

2. Indocyanine green is a shorter-duration tattooing agent with more information offered in the following section.

b. absorptive stains

1. Lugol's iodine (stains normal glycogen containing squamous mucosa of the esophagus, allowing recognition of abnormal squamous epithelium—dysplasia—or metaplastic epithelium—Barrett s esophagus),

2. methylene blue and toluidine blue (stains the absorptive epithelium small bowel and colon), allowing the identification of metaplastic epithelium in the esophagus (Barrett s esophagus) and stomach (gastric intestinal metaplasia), can also find a negative stain in gastric metaplasia at the level of the duodenal bulb.

c. contrast stains

1. indigo carmine and cresyl violet (accentuates mucosal topography, allowing recognition of abnormal small bowel sprue and colonic mucosa inflammatory bowel disease, polyps).

d. reactive stains

1. Congo red (identifies acid-secreting portions of the stomach postoperatively and documents achlorhydria) and

2. phenol red (identifies alkaline areas of the stomach).

2.2 Fluorescent dyes

According to the definition offered by www.britannica.com, fluorescence is the emission of electromagnetic radiation, usually visible light, caused by the excitation of atoms in a material, which then reemit almost immediately (within about 10 s). The initial excitation is frequently determined by the absorption of energy from

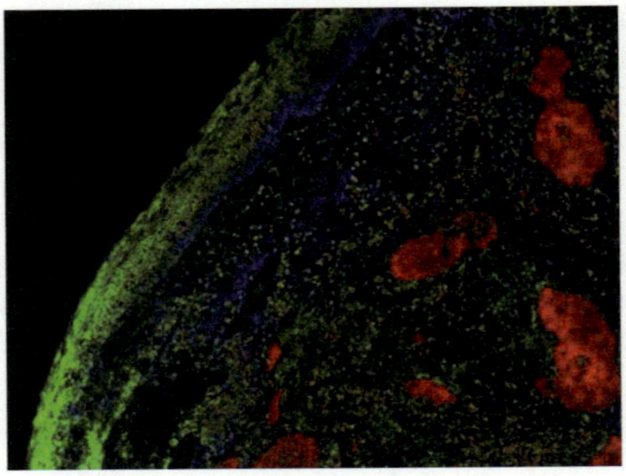

Figure 3.
High-resolution fluorescent microscope image of clusters of tumor cells in red surrounded by normal cells and normal skin in green. Photo source: www.shutterstock.com.

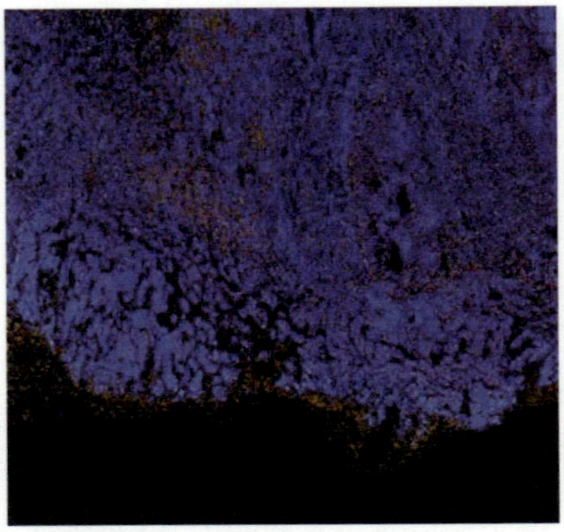

Figure 4.
Research sample slide of tumor tissue where cells have been stained for different proteins using a fluorescently tagged antibody. Presented as false-color image on white background.

incident radiation of particles, as is the case with X-rays or electrons (**Figure 3**). Due to the fact that reemission happens so quickly, the fluorescence stops when the exciting source is removed, unlike the phenomenon of phosphorescence (**Figure 4**), which later persists as an afterglow.

3. The use of ICG in surgery

3.1 General aspects

Fluorescence imaging techniques have become increasingly common in recent years. ICG-based fluorescence, in particular, is now widely used in a variety of diagnostic and treatment procedures, according to the research made by Nowaka and co [2]. ICG is currently the most commonly used fluorescent agent due to its gradual degradation and the rarity of the severe adverse effects described. ICG is a water-soluble, amphiphilic tricarbocyanine probe with a molecular weight of 776 Da, relatively nontoxic, unstable compound, a dye in clinic use bound by albumin in the intravascular space until rapid clearance by the liver. Severe allergic reactions associated with the use of ICG are very rare (1:10,000) with an incidence of 0.05% and mostly occur in patients allergic to iodine. It has various applications in different fields, such as cardiology, ophthalmology, and neurosurgery, but its fluorescent properties have only recently been applied to the intraoperative estimation of tissue blood supply. Apart from ICG, other substances can act as fluorophores (fluorescent chemical compounds that are able to reemit light upon light excitation), such as methylene blue, five-aminolevulinic acid, fluorescein sodium.

What is fluorescence-guided surgery (FSG)? FSG is employed because white visible light makes various tissues appear either identical or highly similar, and proper tumor identification can be difficult, according to www.isfgs.org [3]. Moreover, the surgeon just sees the tissues from the superficial layers under natural light. Nonetheless, structures that were previously invisible can be seen now and recognized by using ICG in a different light length. By combining visual abilities with special dyes, it is now possible to avoid such organs or structures during the surgical process in order to avoid harming them. Other benefits of the FSG include the ability to minimize operative time and the need for second-look procedures by facilitating the rapid detection of structures and lesions while avoiding excessive harm.

3.2 The use of ICG in general surgery interventions, outside the colorectal area

ICG has found application in several fields of general surgery, especially colorectal surgery (seen in the next section of the present article), esophageal surgery, and emergency evaluation of intestinal perfusion in cases of mesenteric ischemia, kidney transplantation, hepatobiliary, and endocrine surgery.

3.2.1 ICG in peritoneal carcinomatosis

ICG can improve the harvesting of tumors during surgery and can properly adjust both the indications, as the extent of the intervention. In a systematic review performed in 2020 by Baiocchi [4], which took into account 192 screened papers with six series meeting the eligibility criteria, there were analyzed in total 353 peritoneal nodules, the neoplasms in question being—colorectal, hepatocellular, ovarian, endometrial. The above-mentioned study had as a purpose to look at the available clinical data regarding the value of ICG fluorescence imaging for intraoperative detection of peritoneal carcinomatosis during open surgery and the main aspects studied settled to the conclusion that sensitivity varied from 72.4 to 100%, while the specificity ranged from 54.2 to 100%.

3.2.2 ICG in liver surgery

The ICG fluorescence method is being used more and more in liver surgery due to the fact that it permits the real-time display of the segmental anatomy of the organ, depending on the tumor's characteristics, and, more so, it is possible to perform direct or indirect identification of hepatic lesions and metastases. Additionally, ICG imaging allows more sensitive detection of tumor foci and, therefore, also a higher R0 resection rate. However, in a systematic review of the literature on the application of ICG imaging in open and laparoscopic liver surgery performed by Sucher et al. [5], the conclusion was drawn toward the aspect that the application resulted mainly useful for superficial lesions, as the depth of penetration of NIR is only 8–10 mm. In liver resections, post-hepatectomy liver failure (PHLF) can occur although an adequate liver volume is kept in place. Diverse dynamic functional tests, such as the indocyanine green test (ICG), could only appreciate globally the liver function, with no definition toward the functional ability of the hepatic remnant. Magnetic resonance imaging (MRI) with liver-specific contrast agents makes the evaluation of both liver function and volume possible. A preoperative combination between dynamic quantitative tests, such as ICG, with MRI or HBS (hepato-bilio-scintigraphy), should provide a more complete functional evaluation. One should opt for various functional tests to predict PHLF that should be selected according to patient's characteristics, disease, and center experience, as shown by Tomassini and the team [6].

3.2.3 ICG-NIR to assess skin flap perfusion

The incidence of skin flap necrosis after mastectomies can reach 11–24%. Laser-assisted ICG angiography appears as a promising technique to assess skin flap perfusion. In a systematic review performed by Driessen et al. [7], it was found that all studies looking at the current ICG methodology and ability to predict outcome showed a substantial decrease in skin necrosis when the ICG was used.

3.2.4 ICG-NIR to assess peritoneal endometriosis

Endometriosis is a very commonly encountered disease that is found in up to 10% of the female population. The use of (ICG) has been advocated for the proper location of endometriotic lesions intraoperatively. NIR-ICG is useful in appreciating the blood supply of bowel anastomoses after segmental resection, according to a systematic review done by Ianieri et al. [8] that looked at 53 studies.

3.2.5 ICG to identify the ureter

Iatrogenic ureteral injury in abdominal surgery is rare at the moment, although it can still result in significant morbidity and mortality. Inspection and palpation are two traditional methods of measuring iatrogenic ureteral damage, which can be difficult during laparoscopic procedures. The use of NIRF imaging to aid in better visualization of the ureters is currently being investigated. The report's goal performed by Slooter et al. [9] was to picture the currently available and experimental dyes in ureter visualization and to further evaluate their feasibility of using them and, more so, to look at their effectiveness.

3.2.6 ICG to identify a bleeding site in the GI area

Several studies, among which the one performed by Copaescu [10], aimed to look at the reliability of a novel fluorescence-guided laparoscopic technique to correctly find the site of unknown gastrointestinal bleeding, with the help of the vascular washout properties of indocyanine green (ICG). The bleeding site was correctly identified and the patient benefited from a minimally invasive technique, and it was, therefore, possible to avoid an open surgical exploration.

3.2.7 ICG in sentinel lymph node in different neoplasms

This represents another important topic in different surgical fields, for instance, urology, gynecology, and general surgery.

3.2.7.1 Breast cancer

In the early stage of breast cancer, ICG-fluorescence-based sentinel lymph node (SLN) detection is being considered. A systematic review looking at 2301 patients from 19 studies found that ICG-fluorescence could complement the radioisotope method or provide an alternative. Another study regarding the ICG lymph node technique in breast cancer was a literature review presented by Benson [11] in which a significantly better sentinel node detection rate was found with ICG than with the standard radioisotope method (**Figure 5**).

3.2.7.2 Cervical cancer

Techniques that combine the ability to identify technetium-99 and a blue dye have been widely used for sentinel lymph node biopsy (SLNB), but there has recently been a surge of interest in the use of fluorescent staining, such as indocyanine green (ICG), to improve the rate of SLN detection. Even though recent guidelines recommend sentinel lymph node biopsy in addition to PLND, SLN biopsy alone is not yet the gold standard because there is insufficient prospective evidence, especially in terms of long-term oncological protection. The prospective randomized clinical trial SENTICOL III will answer to these signaled issues, as a study by Balaya et al. [12] mentions. In addition to the facts mentioned above, the prospectively randomized FILM trial evaluated ICG to be superior in lymph node detection compared to isosulfan blue dye in patients with stage I endometrial or cervical cancer, an evaluation performed by Frumovitz and team [13]. Meanwhile, the study's conclusions created a context for the FDA's approval of ICG for lymph node mapping. NCCN guidelines mention sentinel lymph node mapping by ICG in cervical cancer patients, according to Koh et al. [14].

3.3 The use of ICG in colorectal surgery

3.3.1 Intraoperative fluorescence angiography in colorectal surgery used for the evaluation of the anastomosis

Anastomotic leakage remains among the most feared and challenging complications after colorectal resection. The etiology of leaks includes patient factors, technical factors, and anastomotic perfusion. The known etiology of leaks includes the following: different patient factors, technical factors, and anastomotic blood supply. An intact anastomotic irrigation pattern is particularly vital in the process of anastomotic healing. The air leak testing and intraoperative colonoscopy are

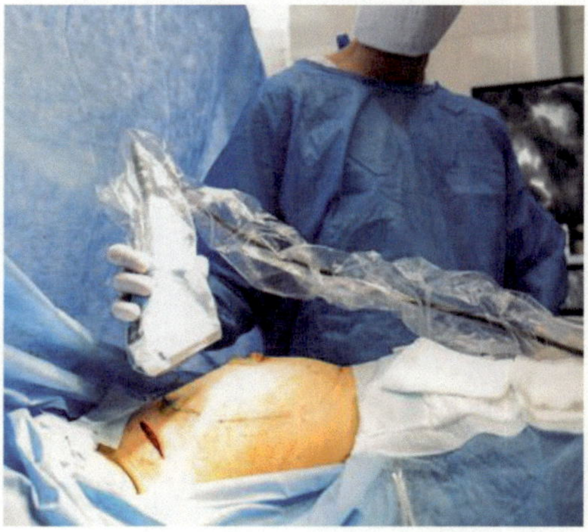

Figure 5.
The surgeon uses a portable fluorescence imaging device during breast removal. Photo source: www.shutterstock.com.

methods that can be done to establish the anastomotic integrity intraoperatively. Among the major causes of anastomotic leakage is impaired vascularization and a minimal deficit in blood supply, both aspects being difficult to detect under white light. Fluorescence angiography with indocyanine green (ICG-FA) is employed in colorectal surgery in order to evaluate the blood supply in the area of an anastomosis. Studies with ICG-FA in open and laparoscopic interventions indicated a lower rate of anastomotic leakage; for example, the PILLAR II study reported a leakage rate of 1.4%. There were researches in this field, such as is the case of Carus and Pick [15] that reported impressive results in clinical outcome and patient prognosis. Likewise, the use of ICG-FA in the group of patients studied potentially led to a reduction of the leakage rate by 48%. Another systematic review from Blanco-Colino and Espin-Basany [16] looks at 1302 patients from five nonrandomized studies in which fluorescence imaging significantly decreased the anastomotic leak in cases operated on for colorectal cancer. Lower leak rates were found in rectal cancer surgery, as well (ICG 1.1% vs. non-ICG 6.1%; $p = 0.02$) (**Figure 6**).

3.3.2 Fluorescence-guided detection of lymph node metastases in colorectal cancer and the sentinel lymph node technique

Indocyanine green fluorescence imaging can also be used as a potential tool for enhancing the accuracy of the staging of patients with primary colorectal cancer through the detection of sentinel lymph nodes. The search in electronic databases was performed and eligible data were taken from 248 patients in a review published by Emile et al. [17], which looked at the overall sensitivity and specificity of (ICG) (NIR) fluorescence in sentinel lymph node detection in colorectal cancer. The median values for the sensitivity, specificity, and accuracy rates were 73.7, 100, and 75.7, respectively. Other several studies, even though none was a prospective one, considered the ICG method feasible in colorectal cancer and also for lower rectal tumors, especially in order to detect the lymphatic drainage across the lateral lymph nodes, as studied by the teams of Nagata et al. [18], Kawahara et al. [19], Cahill et al. [20], and Liberale et al. [21]. Another method used in correctly and precisely identifying the lymph node involvement is one-step nucleic acid (OSNA), as it can offer a quick method of characterization of the lymph nodes. On the other hand, near-infrared (NIR) laparoscopy, together with indocyanine green (ICG), can identify relevant nodal tissue *in situ* during surgery. The association between the OSNA, laparoscopy, and NIR-ICG was studied in an RCT by Yeung et al. [22],

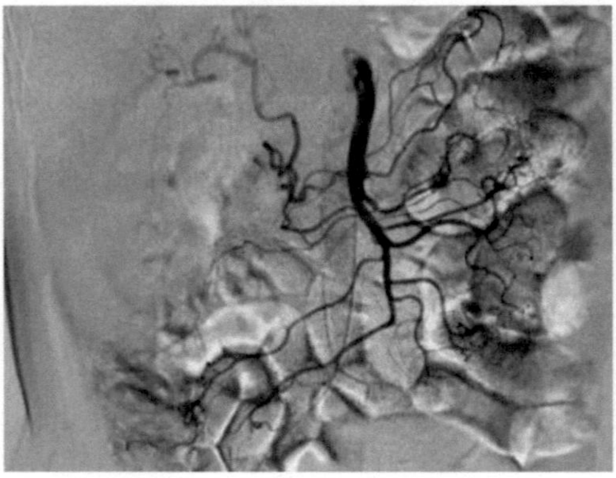

Figure 6.
X-ray angiography of the inferior mesenteric artery (IMA) with contrast media. Its supplies arterial blood to organs of hindgut-distal 1/3 of the transverse, splenic flexure, descending colon, sigmoid, rectum.

a research during which ICG was administered around the tumor, while endoscopy was conducted at a moment previous to the operation. NIR-identified fluorescent lymph nodes were first labeled and then sent for whole-node OSNA review. Both traditional histology and OSNA were used to examine and analyze "fresh" lymph nodes dissected from the typical resection specimen. Furthermore, the fluorescent lymph node status was compared to that of non-ICG nodes in order to determine their predictive value. OSNA is concordant with normal histology, but only a minority of nodes detectable by complete pathological examination was identified for OSNA on fresh dissection, according to the study's findings. To provide an intraoperative evaluation of nodal tissue in patients with colorectal cancer, OSNA can be performed at the same time as NIR and ICG lymphatic mapping. Patients with colorectal cancer can benefit from this treatment.

A study performed by Vuijk et al. [23] looking at the lymph node involvement in gastrointestinal tumors assessed the sentinel lymph node technique with Nanocoll, and ICG- and CEA-targeted fluorescent imaging, and settled to the following conclusions: sentinel lymph node interventions in gastric cancer resections using indocyanine green (ICG) linked to Nanocoll outperformed normal ICG, but could not offer details on possible lymph node metastasis. Besides that aspect, the carcinoembryonic antigen (CEA)-targeted fluorescent imaging technique by using SGM-101 was successful in both pancreatic and colorectal cancers. A large phase III multicenter trial with the corresponding results would be able to complete the missing data.

Simultaneously, in which concerns lymph node invasion, the concept of ultrastaging appeared recently in the specific literature. Furthermore, studies were compiled, such as the one by Hirche et al. [24], in which regards ultrastaging of colon cancer by sentinel node biopsy using fluorescence navigation with ICG Overall, the ICG fluorescence technique found a mean of 1.7 sentinel lymph node (SLN) in 25 out of 26 patients (with a detection rate of 96%). Metastatic involvement of the SLN was detected in 9 out of 11 nodal positive patients by conventional histopathology. The sensitivity of the method was 82% in the case of colon carcinoma. The drawn conclusion of the abovementioned study was that the ICG fluorescence technique is a new but feasible method for SLNB of colon carcinoma and permits ultrastaging with improved accuracy, but with limited validity (so far) due to the small number of cases (**Figures** 7 and **8**).

3.3.3 ICG in metastatic colorectal cancer

ICG is metabolized by the liver and accumulates in areas of slower bile metabolism, a situation that can be encountered in primary liver cancers and colorectal secondary determinations (metastases), as found by the teams of Peloso et al. [25] and van der Vorst [26]. A tumor cluster of cells as small as 200 tumor cells can be identified by ICG, allowing surgeons to find foci of a minimum of 1 mm,

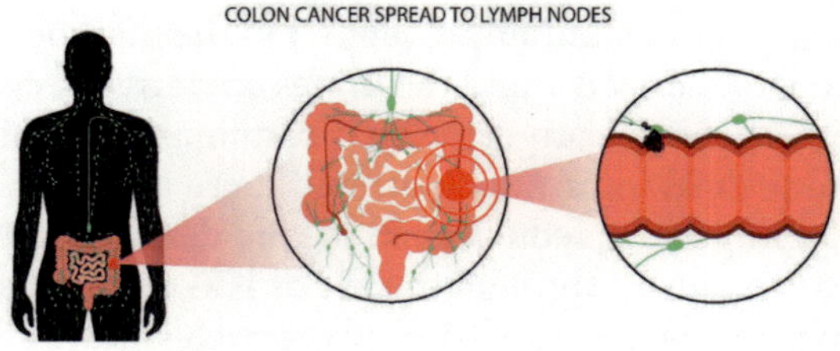

Figure 7.
Colorectal cancer concept. Development of cancer from the colon or rectum to the whole large intestine. Stages of spreading tumor to the lymph nodes and vector flat illustration of other internal organs.

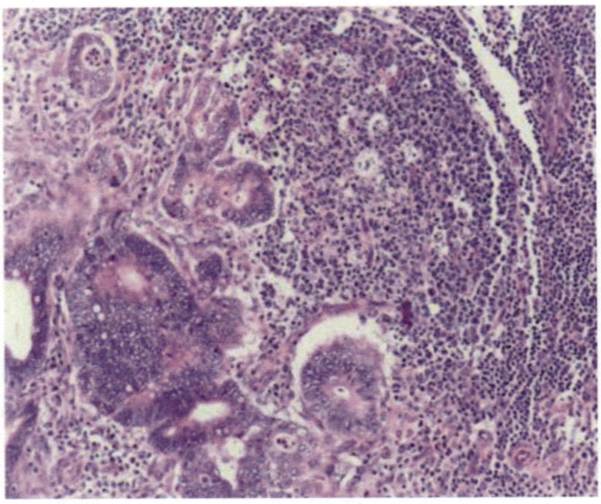

Figure 8.
Metastatic colon carcinoma, in lymph node. Tumor component is on the left and lymphoid component is on the right, magnification 200×.

as it was shown by Ishizawa et al. [27]. The practical aspect of finding liver masses is that they have to be superficial, and the fluorescence methods can look at the maximum depth of infiltration of up to 10 mm. A combination of the application of intraoperative ultrasound and fluorescence techniques was shown to increase the identification rate of colorectal metastatic lesions, as it was researched by Kaibori et al. [28]. In patients suffering from liver fibrosis, nevertheless, areas that have a slow bile metabolism might give false-positive fluorescence. ICG fluorescence can be employed to qualitatively and quantitatively depict changes at a molecular and cellular level in the living organism, and to objectively display liver tumor information, to define hepatic tumor boundaries, and to detect residual tumors, achieving an intraoperative real time coloration and the successful navigation of the liver parenchyma in the targeted zone, as mentioned by Shizawa et al. [29]. A recent meta-analysis included studies on 587 patients showing that ICG fluorescence in the field of liver surgery does decrease operative time, blood loss, hospital stay, and postoperative complications if we are to mention a study done by Qi et al. [30]. As mentioned in subchapter 3.2.2 (ICG in liver surgery), the ICG fluorescence technique is for sure viewed as an intraoperative method that allows the detection of additional superficial hepatic metastases of colorectal cancer, a fact underlined by Liberale and team [31] in an article in which PubMed and Medline literature databases were searched for articles on the use of ICG in the setting of clinical studies on CRC (**Figures 9** and **10**).

3.3.4 Evidence of ICG usefulness in robotically assisted colorectal surgery

As previously shown in the previous subsections of the chapter, ICG fluorescence imaging is increasingly being used, tested, and documented in different areas of abdominal surgery. The constant improvement in the method and in the technological possibilities enables easy use and facilitates operative decision-making, also in robotically assisted colorectal surgery, as it is communicated in a study published by Vilz et al. [32]. Additional information offered there was that the first individual studies underlined an important reduction in the incidence of anastomotic leakage after colorectal anastomosis through the use of ICG fluorescence angiography (FA, 9.1% vs. 16.3%; p = 0.04). First feasibility research studies also emphasized lymph node detection or navigation, as well as the possibility to visualize the ureter (**Figure 11**).

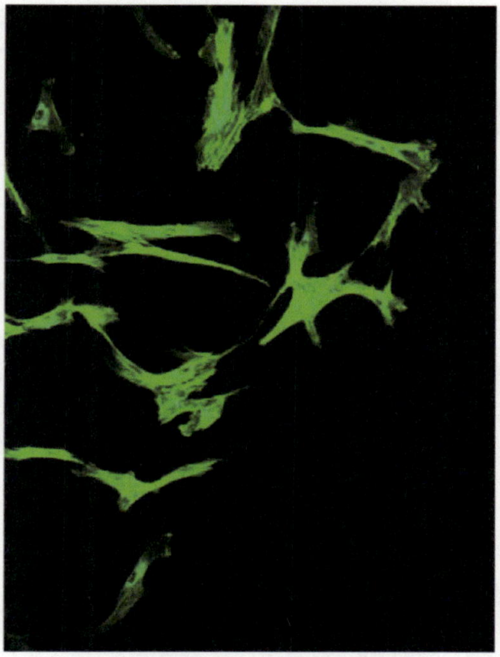

Figure 9.
Immunofluorescence of multiple human tumor metastatic cells growing in tissue culture for research purposes.

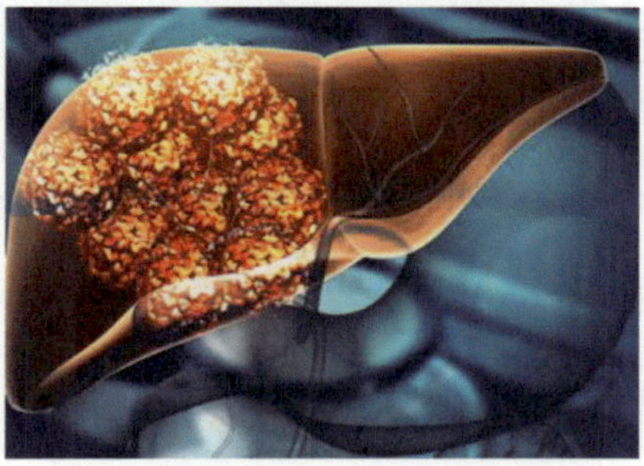

Figure 10.
Human liver cancer cell growth. 3D illustration.

3.3.5 Evidence of ICG usefulness in laparoscopic colorectal resection

In regard to tumor localization, ICG-coated endoscopic clips can bring a promising new technique, as seen in a study by Lee et al. [33]. The precise localization of a tumor before surgery is vital, more so in the early stages of cancer, and the amplitude of the surgical intervention must be established. The accurate localization of a colorectal lesion ensures proper margins for resection and prevents surgical removal of healthy segments of the colon; furthermore, it can reduce the duration of surgery and prevent unnecessary colon traction and tumor handling, which could result in dissemination of tumor cells. The method abovementioned involves placing endoscopic clips coated or mounted with near-infrared fluorescent material, such as ICG, at the lesion site and determining the location of the tumor by consequently detecting the fluorescent signal through the intestinal wall (through the use of a near-infrared laparoscope).

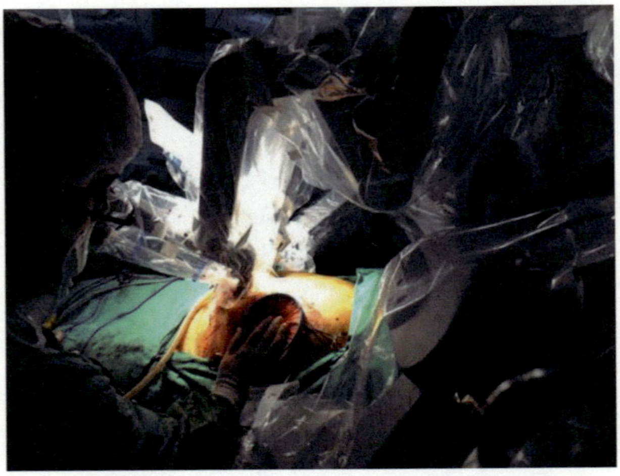

Figure 11.
Robotic surgery in the operation room.

In a research by de Nardi and team [34], a randomized trial was formulated, involving 252 cases in which laparoscopic left-sided colon and rectal resection were performed. The algorithm randomized 1:1 to intraoperative ICG or to subjective visual evaluation of the bowel blood supply without ICG. The main results were the following: ICG angiography documented insufficient blood supply of the colic stump, which implied extended bowel resection in 13 cases (11%). In the control group, 11 patients (9%) had a fistula; meanwhile, in the study group, six patients (5%) developed one anastomotic leak (p = n.s.).

Based on the general elements reviewed, it was summed up that intraoperative ICG fluorescence angiography can efficiently find correctly the vasculature of the colic stump and anastomosis in situations when colorectal resection is performed.

Despite the fact that this method guided proximal bowel resection in 13 instances, the ICG arm did not find a statistically meaningful decrease in anastomotic bowel leak rate. Transanal ICG angiography has been shown to be both feasible and effective in imaging the mucosal and anastomotic blood supply in research conducted by Sherwinter [35]. Future research in a larger community of patients is needed to fully understand the technique's potential to detect flaws in tissue perfusion that could lead to an anastomotic breakdown. Twenty patients with benign and malignant lesions underwent low anterior resection for the analysis. Indocyanine green (ICG) was injected through a peripheral iv catheter after the anastomosis was completed. Transanally, an endoscopic near-infrared imaging device (NIR) was used to test the blood supply at the level of the colon mucosa, the rectum, and the anastomotic staple axis (**Figure 12**).

3.3.6 ICG monitoring for perineal wound contamination in abdominoperineal resection

The incidence of the incisional surgical site infections in colorectal surgery was reported between 5 and 26%. Surgical site infections (SSI) in an abdominoperineal resection (APR) appear more than in other types of interventions in the case of patients with colorectal cancer. Toshiyuki et al. [36] found that perineal wounds are the most vulnerable sites, and they may be triggered by stool contamination. Indocyanine green (ICG) fluorescence testing was employed as a marker of perineal wound contamination. The study had as a method to inject indocyanine green into the rectum transanally before the operation, and fluorescence images were obtained

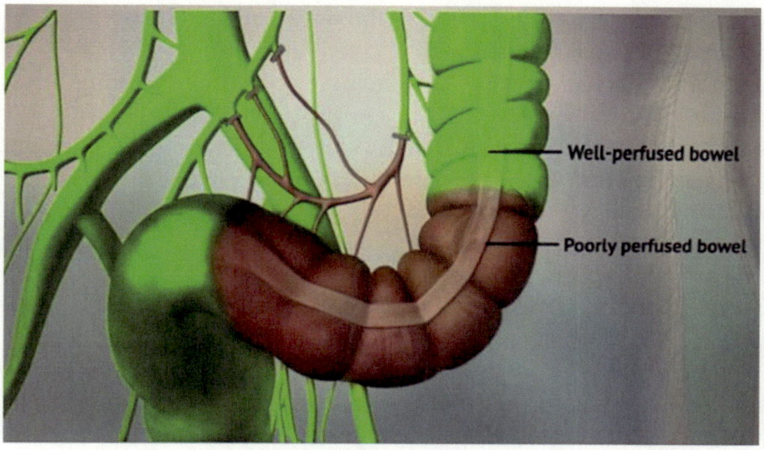

Figure 12.
Schematics of fluorescence angiography in the colorectal area.

during the operation in patients who underwent APR. The findings, though sparse, are promising: one subject had an SSI after having no clear gross contamination, and a trace of ICG fluorescence was found in the perianal skin.

The other two cases were free of SSI, and skin treatment was carried out thoroughly before ICG contamination was removed in those cases.

Even after the normal antiseptic skin preparation, a trace of stool contamination can remain in the perineal skin area, according to the study's findings.

Furthermore, careful skin preparation is needed and it is compulsory if we are to minimize stool contamination in APR subjects (**Figure 13**).

3.3.7 Surgical usefulness of ICG as an alternative to India ink for endoscopic marking

India ink has been largely used for preoperative colonic tattooing, but different complications have been reported. A study performed by Miyoshi et al. [37] looked at the surgical usefulness of ICG as an alternative to India ink for endoscopic marking and evaluated 40 patients between the time of ICG marking and the intervention, the median time period was 4 days (range, 1–73 days).

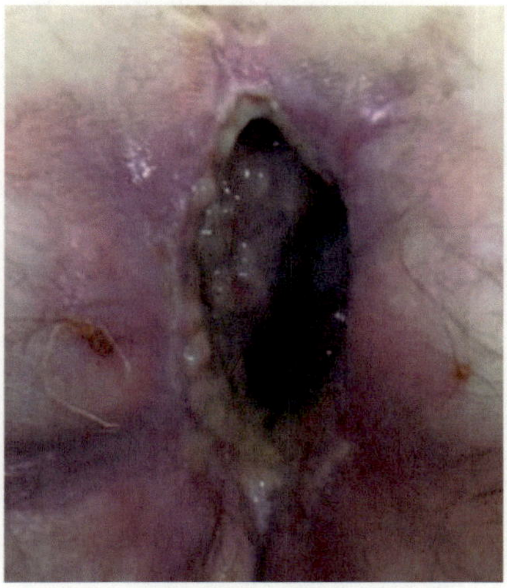

Figure 13.
A perineal wound with infection and inflammation after colorectal surgery.

At the time of surgery, all 29 patients who were operated on within 8 days of tattooing stained positive in green with ICG dye.

Positive staining was clearly obviated in just two of the remaining 10 cases after 9 days or more.

The staining faded over time and finally vanished.

There was no mention of the dye's perioperative side effects.

The authors concluded that this study supports the use of ICG as a safe approach that may be consistently detected within 8 days of endoscopic injection (**Figure 14**).

3.3.8 Preoperative detection of occult enterovesical fistulas in patients with Crohn's disease

Efficacy of oral or rectal administration of indocyanine green solution. In a study realized by Sou et al. [38] whose objectives were to detect enterovesical occult microfistulas in patients with Crohn's disease before the fistulas had become readily apparent, nonhazardous enteral administration of indocyanine green solution was performed. The methods that were used collected a total of 12 patients with Crohn's disease who were suspected from their clinical manifestations of having enterovesical fistulas. Urine was collected and tested for contamination with indocyanine green by using a colorimeter to detect fistulas following oral or rectal administration of the indocyanine green solution. In addition, the efficacy of the indocyanine green test was compared to that of the "classical" X-ray sample.

The ICG test was positive in 11 of the 12 cases after either oral or rectal administration, resulting in a 92% correct diagnosis rate (11/12 patients).

The percentage of right diagnoses using an X-ray analysis, on the other hand, was just 17% (2/12 patients).

Furthermore, none of the eight patients with secret fistulas could be accurately diagnosed using an X-ray analysis, but all showed promising results when the indocyanine green approach was used.

The researchers concluded that the indocyanine green test had a 92% accuracy rate in diagnosing obscure fistulas and was highly diagnostic, while traditional examinations are often complicated and inaccurate (**Figure 15**).

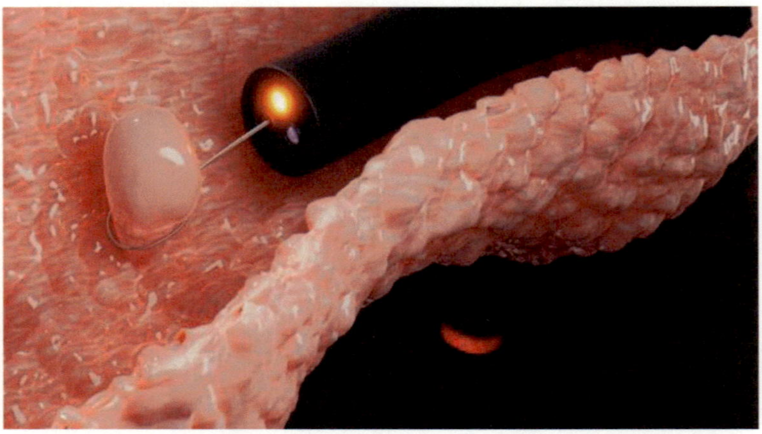

Figure 14.
Colon polyp removal. Endoscope inside colonoscopy for colon polyps.

3.3.9 The affinity of ICG in the detection of colorectal peritoneal carcinomatosis

Peritoneal metastases can appear in 30–40% of patients with colorectal cancer and in a quarter of the patients might be the cause of death. ICG-guided surgery was able to detect additional lesions, and some studies reported up to 21.4% with a direct impact on modifying the surgical resection technique (**Figure 16**).

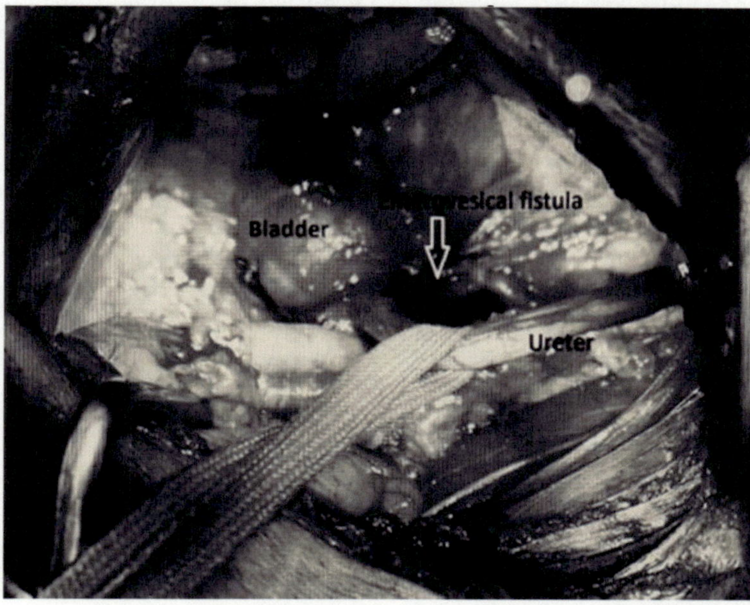

Figure 15.
Intraoperative macroscopic enterovesical fistula.

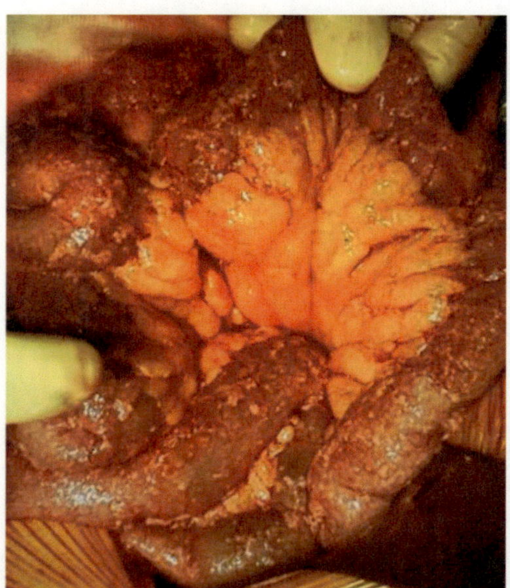

Figure 16.
Extensive lesions of peritoneal carcinomatosis.

4. Conclusions

Fluorescence-assisted surgery using near-infrared (NIR) light is a relatively new technique.

To improve the visible spectrum, this technique uses a combination of dyes and NIR imaging equipment.

As a result, it may provide more detailed anatomic and functional details, allowing for a more complete resection of a neoplasm or the protection of essential normal structures. Indocyanine green fluorescence technique is a surgical tool with increasing perioperative and intraoperative applications in colorectal surgical interventions. In colorectal surgery, in particular, several studies have shown that intraoperative fluorescence imaging is a safe and feasible method to evaluate anastomotic perfusion, and its use might positively affect the patient's clinical outcome by decreasing the incidence of anastomotic leaks. The number of virtual uses for indocyanine green is enhancing and developing, including new ways to detect and control colorectal metastases to the liver. All these advances expanded by the further evolution in time with more prospective trials could offer great information and value for both surgeons and patients, by improving the accuracy and outcomes of general surgery and surgical oncology.

Conflict of interest

The author declares no conflict of interest.

Author details

Sinziana Ionescu[1,2]

1 Bucharest Oncology Institute, Bucharest, Romania

2 "Carol Davila" University of Medicine and Pharmacy, Bucharest, Romania

*Address all correspondence to: sinzianaionescu@gmail.com

References

[1] Fennerty MB. Tissue staining (chromoscopy) of the gastrointestinal tract. Canadian Journal of Gastroenterology. 1999;**13**(5):423-429

[2] Nowak K, Karampinis I, Gerken ALH. Application of fluorescent dyes in visceral surgery: State of the art and future perspectives. Visceral Medicine. 2020;**36**:80-87

[3] www.ifsg.org

[4] Baiocchi GL, Gheza F, Molfino S, Arru L, Vaira M, Giacopuzzi S. Indocyanine green fluorescence-guided intraoperative detection of peritoneal carcinomatosis: Systematic review. BMC Surgery. 2020;**20**(1):158. DOI: 10.1186/s12893-020-00821-9

[5] Sucher R, Brunotte M, Seehofer D. Indocyanine green fluorescence staining in liver surgery. Chirurg. 2020;**91**(6):466-473. DOI: 10.1007/s00104-020-01203-w

[6] Tomassini F, Giglio MC, De Simone G, Montalti R, Troisi RI. Hepatic function assessment to predict post-hepatectomy liver failure: What can we trust? A systematic review. Updates in Surgery. 2020;**72**(4):925-938. DOI: 10.1007/s13304-020-00859-7. Epub 2020 Aug 4

[7] Driessen C, Arnardottir TH, Lorenzo AR, Mani MR. How should indocyanine green dye angiography be assessed to best predict mastectomy skin flap necrosis? A systematic review. Journal of Plastic, Reconstructive & Aesthetic Surgery. 2020;**73**(6):1031-1042. DOI: 10.1016/j.bjps.2020.02.025. Epub 2020 Feb 18

[8] Ianieri MM, Corte LD, Campolo F, Cosentino F, Catena U, Bifulco G, et al. Indocyanine green in the surgical management of endometriosis: A systematic review. Acta Obstetricia et Gynecologica Scandinavica. 2021;**100**(2):189-199. DOI: 10.1111/aogs.13971. Epub 2020 Sep 7

[9] Slooter MD, Janssen A, Bemelman WA, Tanis PJ, Hompes R. Currently available and experimental dyes for intraoperative near-infrared fluorescence imaging of the ureters: A systematic review. Techniques in Coloproctology. 2019;**23**(4):305-313. DOI: 10.1007/s10151-019-01973-4. Epub 2019 Apr 27

[10] Copăescu C, Bîrlog C, Turcu F, Săftoiu A. A novel indocyanine green fluorescence-guided laparoscopic technique to map the site of obscure. Chirurgia (Bucur). 2021;**116**(1):89-101. DOI: 10.21614/chirurgia.116.1.89

[11] Benson J. Indocyanine green fluorescence for sentinel lymph node detection in early breast cancer. Annals of Surgical Oncology. 2016;**23**(1):6-8

[12] Balaya V, Guani B, Bonsang-Kitzis H, Deloménie M, Ngô C, Macias RM, et al. Sentinel lymph node biopsy in early-stage cervical cancer: Current state of art. Bulletin du Cancer. 2020;**107**(6):696-706. DOI: 10.1016/j.bulcan.2019.06.011. Epub 2019 Oct 15

[13] Frumovitz M, Plante M, Lee PS, Sandadi S, Lilja JF, Escobar PF, et al. Near-infrared fluorescence for detection of sentinel lymph nodes in women with cervical and uterine cancers (FILM): A randomised, phase 3, multicentre, non-inferiority trial. The Lancet Oncology. 2018;**19**(10):1394-1403

[14] Koh WJ, Abu-Rustum NR, Bean S, Bradley K, Campos SM, Cho KR, et al. Cervical Cancer, Version 3.2019, NCCN Clinical Practice Guidelines in Oncology. Journal of the National Comprehensive Cancer Network. 2019;**17**(1):64-84

[15] Carus T, Pick P. Intraoperative fluorescence angiography in colorectal surgery. Chirurg. 2019;**90**(11):887-890. DOI: 10.1007/s00104-019-01042-4

[16] Blanco-Colino R, Espin-Basany E. Intraoperative use of ICG fluorescence imaging to reduce the risk of anastomotic leakage in colorectal surgery: A systematic review and meta-analysis. Techniques in Coloproctology. 2018;**22**(1):15-23. DOI: 10.1007/s10151-017-1731-8. Epub 2017 Dec 11

[17] Emile SH, Elfeki H, Shalaby M, Sakr A, Sileri P, Laurberg S, et al. Sensitivity and specificity of indocyanine green near-infrared fluorescence imaging in detection of metastatic lymph nodes in colorectal cancer: Systematic review and meta-analysis. Journal of Surgical Oncology. 2017;**116**(6):730-740. DOI: 10.1002/jso.24701. Epub 2017 Jun 1

[18] Nagata K, Endo S, Hidaka E, Tanaka J, Kudo SE, Shiokawa A. Laparoscopic sentinel node mapping for colorectal cancer using infrared ray laparoscopy. Anticancer Research. 2006;**26**(3B):2307-11.55

[19] Kawahara H, Nimura H, Watanabe K, Ko-bayashi T, Kashiwagi H, Yanaga K. Where does the first lateral pelvic lymph node receive drainage from? Digestive Surgery. 2007;**24**(6):413-7.56

[20] Cahill RA, Anderson M, Wang LM, Lindsey I, Cunningham C, Mortensen NJ. Near-infra-red (NIR) laparoscopy for intraoperative lymphatic road-mapping and sentinel node identification during definitive surgical resection of early-stage colorectal neoplasia. Surgical Endoscopy. 2012;**26**(1):197-204

[21] Liberale G, Galdon MG, Moreau M, Vankerckhove S, El Nakadi I, Larsimont D, et al. Ex vivo detection of tumoral lymph nodes of colorectal origin with fluorescence imaging after intraoperative intravenous injection of indocyanine green. Journal of Surgical Oncology. 2016;**114**(3):348-353

[22] Yeung TM, Wang LM, Colling R, Kraus R, Cahill R, Hompes R, et al. Intraoperative identification and analysis of lymph nodes at laparoscopic colorectal cancer surgery using fluorescence imaging combined with rapid OSNA pathological assessment. Surgical Endoscopy. 2018;**32**(2):1073-1076. DOI: 10.1007/s00464-017-5644-4. Epub 2017 Jun 22

[23] Vuijk FA, Hilling DE, Mieog JSD, Vahrmeijer AL. Fluorescent-guided surgery for sentinel lymph node detection in gastric cancer and carcinoembryonic antigen targeted fluorescent-guided surgery in colorectal and pancreatic cancer. Journal of Surgical Oncology. 2018;**118**(2):315-323. DOI: 10.1002/jso.25139. Epub 2018 Sep 14

[24] Hirche C, Mohr Z, Kneif S, Doniga S, Murawa D, Strik M, et al. Ultrastaging of colon cancer by sentinel node biopsy using fluorescence navigation with indocyanine green. International Journal of Colorectal Disease. 2012;**27**(3):319-324. DOI: 10.1007/s00384-011-1306-5. Epub 2011 Sep 13

[25] Peloso A, Franchi E, Canepa MC, Barbieri L, Briani L, Ferrario J, et al. Combined use of intraoperative ultrasound and indocyanine green fluorescence imaging to detect liver metastases from colorectal cancer. HPB (Oxford). 2013;**15**(12):928-934

[26] van der Vorst JR, Schaafsma BE, Hutteman M, Verbeek FP, Liefers GJ, Hartgrink HH, et al. Near-infrared fluorescence-guided resection of colorectal liver metastases. Cancer. 2013;**119**(18):3411-3418

[27] Ishizawa T, Masuda K, Urano Y, Kawaguchi Y, Satou S, Kaneko J, et al. Mechanistic background and clinical applications of indocyanine green fluorescence imaging of hepatocellular carcinoma. Annals of Surgical Oncology. 2014;**21**(2):440-448

[28] Kaibori M, Matsui K, Ishizaki M, Iida H, Oku-mura T, Sakaguchi T, et al. Intraoperative detection of superficial liver tumors by fluorescence imaging using indocyanine green and 5-aminolevulinic acid. Anticancer Research. 2016;**36**(4):1841-1849

[29] Shizawa T, Fukushima N, Shibahara J, Ma-suda K, Tamura S, Aoki T, et al. Real-time identification of liver cancers by using indocyanine green fluorescent imaging. Cancer. 2009;**115**(11):2491-2504

[30] Qi C, Zhang H, Chen Y, Su S, Wang X, Huang X, et al. Effectiveness and safety of indocyanine green fluorescence imaging-guided hepatectomy for liver tumors: A systematic review and first meta-analysis. Photodiagnosis and Photodynamic Therapy. 2019;**28**: 346-353

[31] Liberale G, Bourgeois P, Larsimont D, Moreau M, Donckier V, Ishizawa T. Indocyanine green fluorescence-guided surgery after IV injection in metastatic colorectal cancer: A systematic review. European Journal of Surgical Oncology. 2017;**43**(9):1656-1667. DOI: 10.1016/j.ejso.2017.04.015. Epub 2017 May 8

[32] Vilz TO, Kalff JC, Stoffels B. Evidence of indocyanine green fluorescence in robotically assisted colorectal surgery : What is the status? Der Chirurg. 2021;**92**(2):115-121. DOI: 10.1007/s00104-020-01340-2. Epub 2021 Jan 11

[33] Lee DW, Sohn DK, Han KS, Hong CW, Park HC, Oh JH. Promising novel technique for tumor localization in laparoscopic colorectal surgery using indocyanine green-coated endoscopic clips. Diseases of the Colon & Rectum. 2021;**64**(1):e9-e13. DOI: 10.1097/DCR.0000000000001876

[34] De Nardi P, Elmore U, Maggi G, Maggiore R, Boni L, Cassinotti E, et al. Intraoperative angiography with indocyanine green to assess anastomosis perfusion in patients undergoing laparoscopic colorectal resection: Results of a multicenter randomized controlled trial. Surgical Endoscopy. 2020;**34**(1):53-60. DOI: 10.1007/s00464-019-06730-0. Epub 2019 Mar 21

[35] Sherwinter DA. Transanal near-infrared imaging of colorectal anastomotic perfusion. Surgical Laparoscopy, Endoscopy & Percutaneous Techniques. 2012;**22**(5):433-436. DOI: 10.1097/SLE.0b013e3182601eb8

[36] Kitai T, Kawashima M, Fujii H, Mashima S, Shimahara Y. Indocyanine green fluorescence monitoring of perineal wound contamination in abdominoperineal resection: A preliminary report. Surgery Today. 2011;**41**(8):1037-1040. DOI: 10.1007/s00595-010-4417-7. Epub 2011 Jul 20

[37] Miyoshi N, Ohue M, Noura S, Yano M, Sasaki Y, Kishi K, et al. Surgical usefulness of indocyanine green as an alternative to India ink for endoscopic marking. Surgical Endoscopy. 2009;**23**(2):347-351. DOI: 10.1007/s00464-008-9938-4. Epub 2008 Apr 29

[38] Sou S, Yao T, Matsui T, Takemura S, Sakurai T, Takenaka K, et al. Preoperative detection of occult enterovesical fistulas in patients with Crohn's disease: Efficacy of oral or rectal administration of indocyanine green solution. Diseases of the Colon & Rectum. 1999;**42**(2):266-270. DOI: 10.1007/BF02237140

Section 6

Colorectal Cancer – Surgical Techniques and Outcomes

Chapter 12

Emergency Treatment of Transverse Colon Cancer

Nicolescu Cosmin, Andrei Suciu Bogdan, Adrian Tudor, Cristian Russu, Mircea Gherghinescu, Vlad Olimpiu Butiurca, Marian Botoncea, Catalin-Dumitru Cosma and Călin Molnar

Abstract

This chapter deals with the emergency treatment of transverse colon cancer. The main complications that classify transverse colon cancer in an emergency setting are obstruction, perforation accompanied by localized or generalized peritonitis, and hemorrhage which may be occult or cataclysmic with hemorrhagic shock. We present the technical principles of radical surgical resection using embryological, anatomical, and oncological concepts. In this chapter we also discuss the principles of lymphadenectomy associated with complete excision of the mesocolon with high vascular ligation, in particular with T3 or T4 cancers requiring D2/D3 lymphadenectomy. The use of infrapyloric, gastro-epiploic, and prepancreatic lymphadenectomy is recommended due to the frequent metastases in these regional lymph nodes.

Keywords: transverse colon cancer, emergency, transverse cancer, colon cancer, large bowel obstruction

1. Introduction

The incidence of transverse colon cancer in an emergency setting is approximately 77–80%. Five percent of all colon cancer are located at the level of transverse colon, hepatic flexure cancer represents 3% whilst splenic flexure represents 2% [1, 2]. The complications associated with transverse colon cancer are represented by large bowel obstruction, tumor perforation, or more commonly diastatic perforation and hemorrhagic syndrome [3].

Based on embryological and anatomical considerations, the colonic frame can be divided into the proximal ("right") colon represented by the cecum, the ascending colon and the proximal or right 2/3 of the transverse colon, and the distal ("left") colon represented by the distal 1/3 of the transverse colon, the descending colon, the sigmoid colon, the rectum and the proximal 2/3 of the anal canal [4–7].

Since the proximal colon is derived from the midgut the incidence of transverse colon cancer is higher in females. Thus, mucinous tumors are more common, which present an increased risk of genetic mutations ↑ CIMP, ↑ BRAF, ↑ MSI, ↑ CMS1, ↑ CMS3, ↑ KRAS, and where survival has a limited prognosis compared to distal colon cancers [8–10].

The recommended surgical technical principles for proximal colon cancer complications are simple and are represented by resection and anastomosis in the first intent in most scenarios, while in the case of distal colon cancer complications, surgeons perform resections and colostomies (terminal or loop colostomy) or in rare cases of hemodynamically stable patients, per-primam anastomoses.

The majority of transverse colon tumors and their complications follow the general characteristics of colorectal cancers. Thus, in an emergency setting, patients have already developed complications the disease is generally found in advanced stages (T3-T4) [11]. Due to the presence of complications at the time of diagnostic, radical intent surgery is most of the time impossible; surgeons cannot perform a radical D2 or D3 lymphadenectomy, due to local cancer spread and the technical impossibility to remove the tumor together with the anterior and posterior sheets of the visceral peritoneum. To follow Hohenberger principles introduced in 2009 [12] to completely resect the mesocolon and perform high vascular ligature, in the case of complicated transverse colon cancer becomes impossible in most cases [12, 13].

Embryologically, the small intestine starting from D3, the cecum, the ascending colon, and the proximal or right 2/3 of the transverse colon derive from the midgut. The vascular supply is represented by ileocolic vessels, right colic artery, and middle colic artery, all derivative from superior mesenteric vessels. The parasympathetic innervation of these segments of the intestine is represented by the vagus nerve.

For the distal third (or left third), the descending colon, sigmoid, rectum, and the proximal 2/3 of the anal canal the embryological origin are represented by the hindgut and the vascular supply by the left colic branches of the inferior mesenteric vessels. The parasympathetic innervation is represented by the pelvic splanchnic nerves S2-S4. The transition zone from the parasympathetic vagal to the sacred is called the Cannon-Bohm point [14]. This corresponds to Griffith's point where Drummond's marginal arch anastomoses with the ascending branch of the middle colic artery [15].

2. Anatomical particularities

The proximal colon is anatomically the most dilated segment in the colonic frame, having the largest diameter at the level of the cecum (8 cm), while the ascending colon being is 6 cm in diameter and the transverse colon 5 cm. The transverse colon is the longest segment of the colic frame, having a length of about 50 cm as well as being the most mobile segment of the colon [16].

The arterial sources of the ascending colon are represented by the branches of the superior mesenteric artery. They are the ileocolic artery, the right colic artery which may be inconsistent, the middle colic artery with the right and left branches, the left colic artery with the ascending branch which has its origin in the inferior mesenteric artery. In addition to these arterial sources for each segment, some anastomoses from the marginal artery of Drummond (MA) – the marginalis colic artery (arteria marginalis coli), the anastomotic source between the superior and inferior mesenteric artery [14, 17]. Another important anastomotic arterial source, also the anastomosis between the two important arterial sources, is represented by Riolan's arch, also called Moskowitz's arch or meandering mesenteric artery. An important aspect of this marginal arch is present in the splenic flexion, the so-called Griffith area in which there is the possibility to interrupt this arterial anastomosis, thus having direct implications in resections of the transverse colon or splenic flexure [14].

Thus, colon resections regardless of the region are segmental resections. This principle was introduced and accomplished with the sigmoid colon segment by Jean-Francois Reybard in 1833. Later this type of resection extended to the transverse colon, becoming a transversectomy. Also related to the name of this surgeon, Reybard is also linked with the first right hemicolectomy, performed in 1832.

3. Lymphatic drainage

Colic frame lymph nodes are present according to the Japanese Society for Cancer of the Colon and Rectum (JSCCR) in four areas:

- D1 or N1 lymphatic centers – epicolic/paracolic
- D2 or N2 lymphatic centers – intermediates
- D3 or N3 lymphatic centers – central
- D4 or N4 lymphatic centers – located on the anterior face of the large retroperitoneal vessels [18].

Thus, segmental, limited, or extensive resections for transverse colon cancers follow Hohenberger's recommendations for mesocolon excision and central vascular ligation [19, 20].

There are several comparative studies between D2 or D3 lymphadenectomy recommendations for locally advanced cancers, that often present themselves in the emergency department. They do not show a clear advantage of D3 over D2 but recommend performing D3 lymphadenectomy to obtain a radial resection margin and a larger number of lymph nodes necessary for accurate staging [21–23]. The minimum number of lymph nodes required for an accurate staging is 12 [2, 24, 25].

Transverse colon cancer frequently metastasizes to the lymph nodes of the infrapyloric lymph nodes, pancreatic cephalic nodules, and gastro-colic ligaments [26].

Another aspect used in surgical resections of transverse colon cancers is resection of the hepatic or splenic flexures. It is, therefore, necessary to define this flexure, anatomically. There is no general surgical concept but the most common limit is represented by a portion of 10 cm belonging to the ascending or descending colon, respectively 1/3 corresponding to the transverse colon. The splenic flexure is always located higher, and more angled, often creating an additional obstacle [14].

4. Therapeutic principles

4.1 Large bowel obstruction

Large bowel obstruction – is the most common complication of colorectal/rectal colon and transverse colon, representing about 77% of the entire volume of complications [27, 28]. The most common symptom is the lack of bowel movement in a patient with intestinal transit disorders. Due to the relatively large diameter of the proximal colon, ascending and transverse, the tumors become palpable, giant even, a long time before producing mechanical occlusion [29].

In this situation, the technical principle is segmental resection (**Figure 1**) represented by the right hemicolectomy, detailed by Kohler and Mikulicz or extended to the right, towards the left of the middle colic vessels followed by an ileocolic anastomosis or the segmental resection (transversectomy) followed by end-to-end anastomosis. There are divergent views and, in this regard, many articles and studies show that limited resections, such as transversectomy are more effective [24, 30].

If the location of the tumor is at the level of the hepatic flexure, then the common surgical procedure is a standard right hemicolectomy, with right omentectomy and

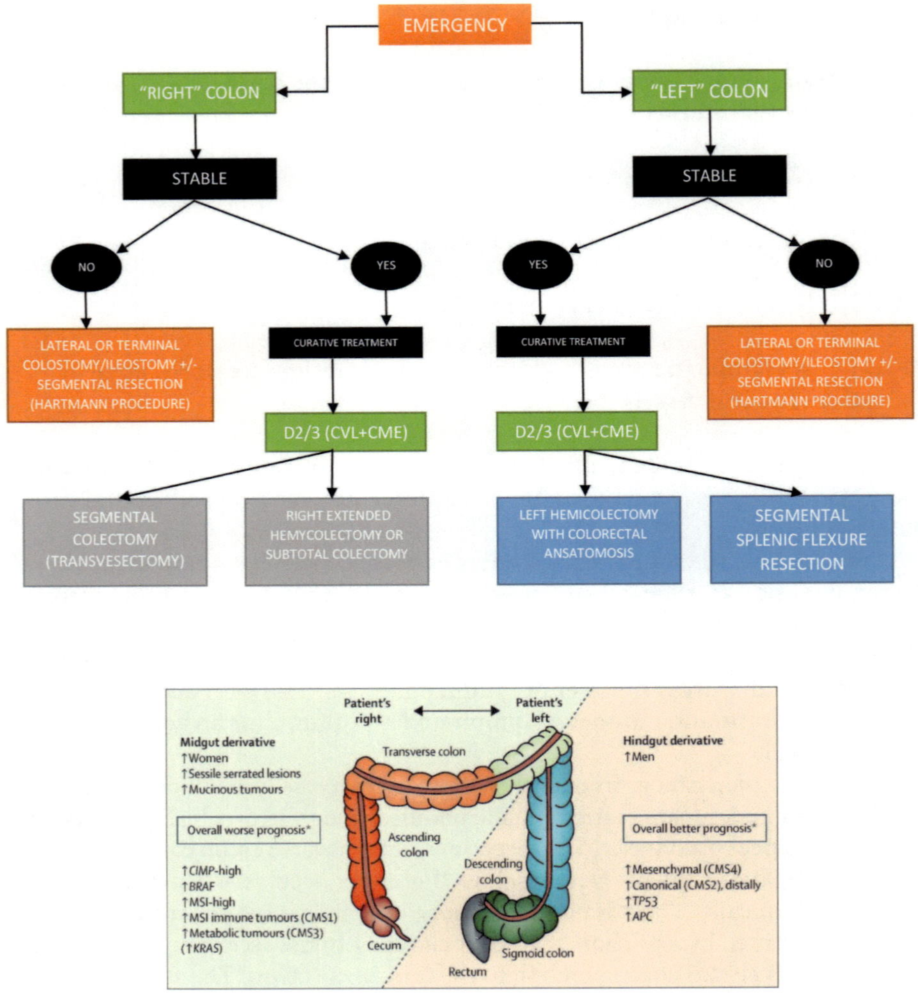

Figure 1.
Surgical approach of the colon.

ligation at the origin of the ileocolic vessels, right colic, and of the right branch of the middle colic vessels, followed by an ileo-colic end to end anastomosis (**Figure 2**).

If the obstructive tumor is located at the middle of the transverse colon, then you can opt for a transversectomy with omentectomy and resection of the mesocolon (**Figure 3**), and high ligation at the origin of the middle colic vessels. If the local anatomy is favorable, namely after an adequate mobilization of both the hepatic and the splenic flexure if we can obtain a resection margin of about 10 cm, then we can opt for a tension-free anastomosis. If the local anatomy is not favorable, it is recommended to perform an extended right hemicolectomy with omentectomy and high ligation of the vascular pedicles followed by an ileocolic anastomosis. This type of anastomosis is classified with the lowest fistula rate [24, 30–32].

If the occlusive tumor is located at the left third of the transverse colon, then an extended right hemicolectomy is recommended as long as we obtain an adequate distance resection margin as well as an adequate radial resection margin – all by maintaining the integrity of the visceral peritoneum sheets.

Location of the tumor at the level of the splenic flexure may be followed by segmental resection of the splenic angle, left omentectomy, resection of the mesocolon

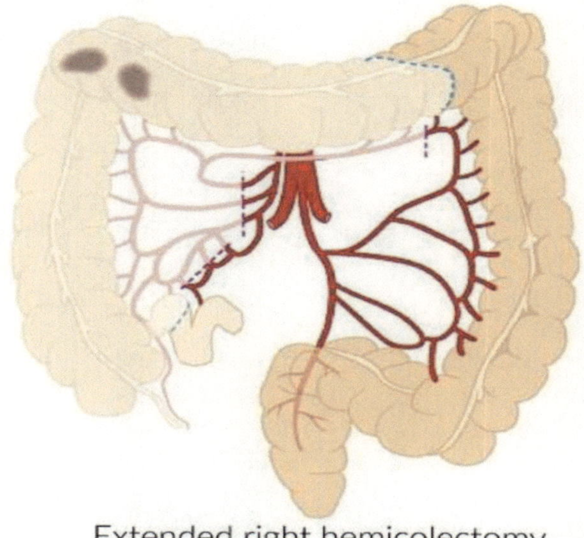

Figure 2.
D2/3 extended right hemicolectomy.

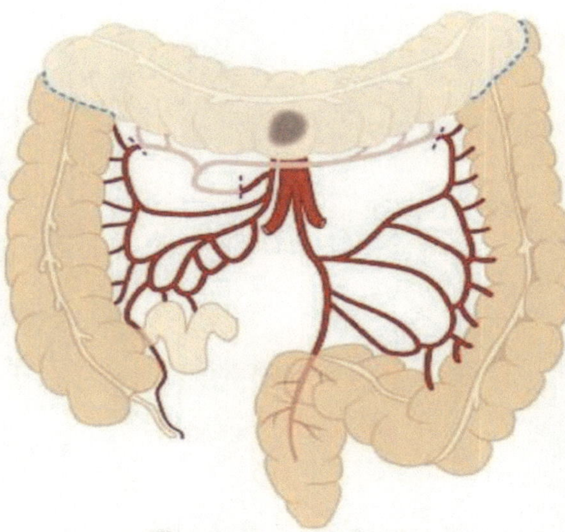

Figure 3.
D2/3 transverse colectomy.

and ascending branches of the left colic vessels, extended gastrocolic lymphadenectomy and colo colic anastomosis TT, or extended right hemicolectomy with omentectomy, mesocolon excision and extended gastro-colic lymphadenectomy, prepancreatic lymphadenectomy followed by an ileocolic end to end anastomosis (**Figure 4**) [28, 29].

The principle of diversion or the protection of an anastomosis using an ileostomy [28] has lost ground lately, being today only an exceptional indication [33].

In certain particular situations, like in an emergency, it is useful to practice a subtotal colectomy (**Figure 5**), as radical as possible with ileo sigmoid anastomosis.

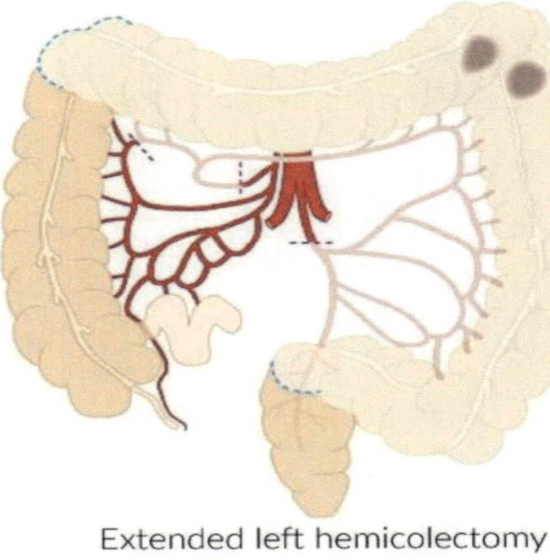

Figure 4.
D2/3 extended left hemicolectomy.

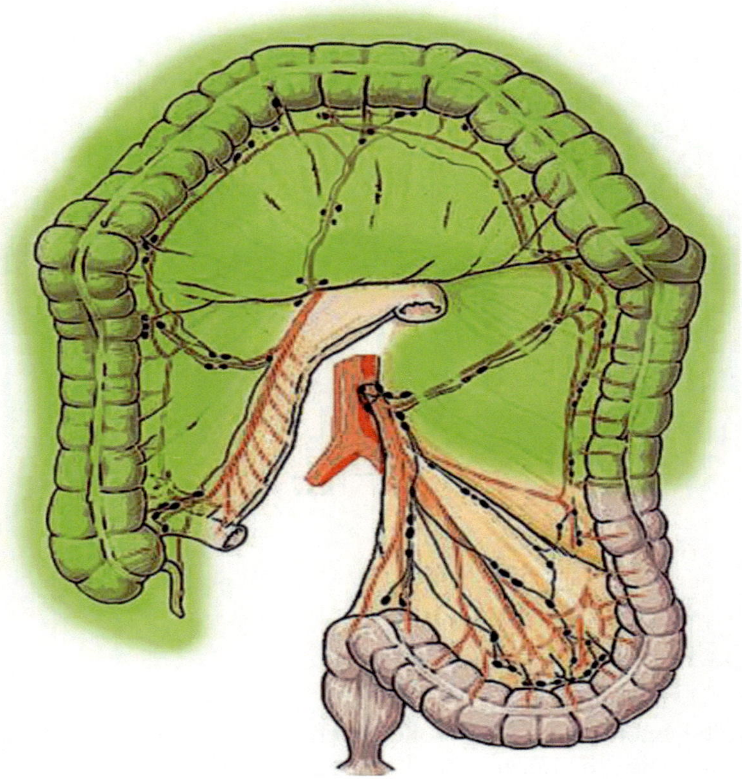

Figure 5.
D2/3 subtotal hemicolectomy.

The second indication for subtotal colectomy is the cecal diastatic perforation with the occlusive tumor in the transverse colon and the third indication for subtotal colectomy is synchronous tumors.

Extended right hemicolectomy is performed, in an emergency in about 73.7% of cases while left hemicolectomy is performed in 20% [2].

4.2 Tumor perforation with the peritoneal syndrome

Perforation followed by localized or generalized peritonitis is the second most common cause of complications in transverse colon cancer [3, 28].

Due to generalized peritonitis, septic shock, and multiple organ failure (MSOF), the patient becomes hemodynamically and respiratory unstable, leading to post-operative management governed by other principles, namely hydro electrolytic rebalancing and stabilization, exploratory laparotomy, identification of exact perforation site, and rapid surgical gestures.

Perforations in this situation are frequently diastatic and the most frequent localization is in the cecum region. In this situation, subtotal colectomy is required, followed by ileosigmoid anastomosis. In some rare cases, there is the possibility of parietal perforation through tumor necrosis and localized peritonitis, which prolongs the patient's addressability to the doctor. This situation is more common with the transverse colon or splenic flexure. However as long as the general condition of the patient is stable, a limited resection such as transversectomy can be attempted, but with the establishment of a diversion colostomy or by emptying the colon on the operating table with a first intent digestive anastomosis being recommended especially by Asian authors [28].

The hemorrhagic syndrome represents the 3rd emergency form of transverse colon cancer, the rarest form being an uncompensated hypovolemic shock with hemodynamic instability [28].

The presence of hemorrhage in cancer pathology is common in about 50% of cases [28]. The general form of manifestation, however, is occult hemorrhage, with minimal blood loss that does not suddenly undermine the patient. Thus, exsanguinating shock is rare [3].

If the endoscopic intervention cannot stop the hemorrhage or if embolization is not successful, then resection surgery is required when more than 6 units of blood [31] are transfused, followed by either a double colostomy or an anastomosis depending on the patient's hemodynamic stability [3, 28].

5. Discussions

The localization of the primary tumor in the transverse colon and the type of the emergency: occlusion, peritonitis with diastatic perforation or hemorrhage, as well as hemodynamic and respiratory stability of the patient, severity of hydroelectrolytic imbalance, require as emergency surgical treatment the following surgical therapeutic options (on cases that may benefit from surgical treatment):

- In the case of the unstable patient, performing a lateral (loop) or terminal colostomy or ileostomy, possibly associated with a segmental resection for an area of perforation or hemorrhage and the second surgery for curative resection with associated D2/3 lymphadenectomy and anastomosis.

- In the case of the stable patient, the intention will be curative surgical treatment and here an intervention with D2/3 lymphadenectomy and mesocolon resection is required according to the rule – CME and CVL imposed by Hohenberger. Depending on the location of the tumor hepatic flexure, standard transverse colon or splenic flexure, the presence of another synchronous tumor formation, vascular abnormalities or anatomical features of the transverse colon, high localization of the splenic flexure, the technical variants that can be achieved are represented by: segmental colectomy of the transverse colon or transversectomy, extended right colectomy, subtotal colectomy with CME and CVL Hohenberger and per-primal anastomosis TT, LL or LT, depending on local factors, technical possibilities – manual or mechanical and experience or preference of the surgeon.

Author details

Nicolescu Cosmin[1], Andrei Suciu Bogdan[1*], Adrian Tudor[1], Cristian Russu[2], Mircea Gherghinescu[2], Vlad Olimpiu Butiurca[2], Marian Botoncea[2], Catalin-Dumitru Cosma[2] and Călin Molnar[2]

1 Department of Anatomy and Embryology, George Emil Palade University of Medicine, Pharmacy, Science, and Technology of Targu Mures, Romania

2 Department of General Surgery, George Emil Palade University of Medicine, Pharmacy, Science, and Technology of Targu Mures, Romania

*Address all correspondence to: suciubogdanandrei@yahoo.com

References

[1] Cho MS, Baek SJ, Hur H, et al. Modified complete mesocolic excision with central vascular ligation for the treatment of right-sided colon cancer: Long-term outcomes and prognostic factors. Ann Surg 2015;261:708-715.

[2] Aleix Martínez-Pérez, Elisa Reitano, Paschalis Gavriilidis, et al. What is the best surgical option for the resection of transverse colon cancer? Ann Laparosc Endosc Surg 2019;4:69

[3] Xue-Fei Yang, Kai Pan-Dia. Diagnosis and management of acute complications in patients with colon cancer: Bleeding, obstruction, and perforation. Chin J Cancer Res 2014;26(3):331-340

[4] Sadler TW, ed. Langman's medical embryology. 13th edn. Wolters Kluwer/Lippincott Williams & Wilkins, 2015; 239e49.

[5] Takashi Ueki, Shuntato Nagai, Tatsuya Manabe et al. Vascular anatomy of the transverse mesocolon and bidirectional laparoscopic D3 lymph node dissection for patients with advanced transverse colon cancer. Surgical Endoscopy 2019;33:2257-2266

[6] Stelzner S, Hohenberger W, Weber K, et al. Anatomy of the transverse colon revisited with respect to complete mesocolic excision and possible pathways of aberrant lymphatic tumor spread. Int J Colorectal Dis. 2015;31:377-384.

[7] Langman J. Mesenteries and abdominal cavity. In: Medical Embryology. Vol 4. Baltimore, USA: The Williams & Wilkins Company; 1981. p. 149-155.

[8] Bertelsen CA, Kirkegaard-Klitbo A, Nielsen M, et al. Pattern of colon cancer lymph node metastases in patients undergoing central mesocolic lymph node excision: A systematic review. Dis *Colon rectum*. 2016;59(12):1209-1221.

[9] Mohamed E. Salem, Benjamin A. Weinberg, et al. Comparative molecular analyses of left-sided colon, right-sided colon, and rectal cancers. Oncotarget. 2017 Oct 17; 8(49): 86356-86368.

[10] Tejpar S, Stintzing S, Ciardiello F. Prognostic and predictive relevance of primary tumor location in patients with RAS wild-type metastatic colorectal cancer: Retrospective analyses of the CRYSTAL and FIRE-3 trials. JAMA Oncol. 2017;3(2):194-201.

[11] N. P. M. Brouwer, N. Hugen, and I. D. Nagtegaal. More extensive lymphadenectomy in colon cancer; how far are we willing to go for a biomarker? Tech Coloproctol. 2020; 24(7): 761-764.

[12] Hohenberger W, Weber K, Matzel K, Papadopoulos T, Merkel S. Standardized surgery for colonic cancer: Complete mesocolic excision and central ligation—Technical notes and outcome. Colorectal Dis. 2009;11(4):354-364.

[13] Heald RJ. The 'Holy Plane' of rectal surgery. J R Soc Med. 1988;81(9):503-508.

[14] Ellis H, Mahadevan V, eds Clinical anatomy. 13th edn, vols. 86e88. Wiley Blackwell, 2013; 94e8.

[15] M A Meyers. Griffiths' point: Critical anastomosis at the splenic flexure. Significance in ischemia of the colon AJR Am J Roentgenol 1976 Jan;126(1):77-94.

[16] Rossini F.P. (1975) The normal colon. In: Atlas of Coloscopy. Springer, New York, NY. https://doi.org/10.1007/978-1-4615-9650-9_12

[17] Moore KL, Dalley AF, Agur AMR, eds. Clinically oriented anatomy. 7th edn. Wolters Kluwer/Lippincott Williams & Wilkins, 2014; 246e53.

[18] Japanese Society for Cancer of the Colon and Rectum (JSCCR) guidelines 2019 for the treatment of colorectal cancer. International Journal of Clinical Oncology (2020) 25:1-42.

[19] Mori S, Kita Y, Baba K, et al. Laparoscopic complete mesocolic excision via combined medial and cranial approaches for transverse colon cancer. Surg Today 2017;47:643-649.

[20] Kotake K, Mizuguchi T, Moritani K, et al. Impact of D3 lymph node dissection on survival for patients with T3 and T4 colon cancer. Int J Colorectal Dis 2014;29:847-852.

[21] Resch A, Langner C. Lymph node staging in colorectal cancer: Old controversies and recent advances. World J Gastroenterol. 2013;19 (46):8515-8526.

[22] Hye Jin Kim, Gyu-Seog Choi. Clinical implications of lymph node metastasis in colorectal Cancer: Current status and future perspectives. Annals of Coloproctology 2019;35(3):109-117.

[23] Vilson Leite Batista, Antonio Carlos Ribeiro Garrido Iglesias, Fernando Athayde Veloso Madureira, et al. Adequate lymphadenectomy for colorectal cancer: a comparative analysis between open and laparoscopic surgery. Arq Bras Cir Dig. 2015 Apr-Jun; 28(2): 105-108.

[24] Matsuda T, Sumi Y, Yamashita K, Hasegawa H, Yamamoto M, Matsuda Y, et al. Optimal surgery for mid-transverse colon cancer: Laparoscopic extended right hemicolectomy versus laparoscopic transverse colectomy. World J Surg. 2018;42(10):3398-3404.

[25] Park IJ, Choi GS, Kang BM, Lim KH, Jun SH. Lymph node metastasis patterns in right-sided colon cancers: Is segmental resection of these tumors oncologically safe? Ann Surg Oncol. 2009;16(6):1501-1506.

[26] Bertelsen CA, Bols B, Ingeholm P, Jansen JE, Jepsen LV, Kristensen B, Neuenschwander AU, Gogenur I (2014) Lymph node metastases in the gastrocolic ligament in patients with colon cancer. Dis *Colon rectum* 57:839-845.

[27] Ferlay J, Shin HR, Bray F. GLOBOCAN 2008, Cancer incidence and mortality worldwide. 2012; 2012. Available at: http://globocan.iarc.fr

[28] Michele Pisano et al. 2017 WSES guidelines on colon and rectal cancer emergencies: obstruction and perforation, Pisano et al. World Journal of Emergency Surgery 2018; 13:36.

[29] Takeru Matsuda, Yasuo Sumi, Kimihiro Yamashita, et al. Optimal surgery for mid-transverse Colon Cancer: Laparoscopic extended right Hemicolectomy versus laparoscopic transverse colectomy. World J Surg 2018;42(10):3398-3404.

[30] Chong CS, Huh JW, Oh BY, Park YA, Cho YB, Yun SH, et al. Operative method for transverse colon carcinoma: Transverse colectomy versus extended colectomy. Dis *Colon rectum*. 2016;59(7):630-639.

[31] Carol A. Angel, Raul M. Bosio, The dilemmas of the transverse colon cancer: Segmental or extended right colectomy, laparoscopic hazards for the inexperienced surgeon. Ann Laparosc Endosc Surg 2019;4:4

[32] Milone M, Manigrasso M, Elmore U, Maione F, Gennarelli N, Rondelli F, et al. Short-and long-term outcomes after transverse versus extended colectomy for transverse colon cancer. A systematic review and meta-analysis. Int J Colorectal Dis. 2019;34(2):201-207.

[33] Ravo B, Reggio D, Frattaroli. Insertion of the coloshield through a colotomy after completion of a colonic anastomosis. Int J Color Dis 1991;6:46-48

Chapter 13

The Robotic Approach in Rectal Cancer

Ciprian Duta, Stelu Pantea, Dan Brebu, Amadeus Dobrescu, Caius Lazar, Kitty Botoca, Cristi Tarta and Fulger Lazar

Abstract

Since a robotic surgical system was developed in the early 1990s and the first robotic-assisted radical prostatectomy was reported in 2001, robotic surgery has spread in many surgical specialties, changing surgical management. Currently, compared to other colorectal procedures, robotic surgery appears to offer great benefits for total mesorectal excision for rectal cancer. Abdominal cavity other procedures such as right hemicolectomy and high anterior resection are relatively uncomplicated and can be performed easily by laparoscopic surgery. First reports have focused on the clinical benefits of robotic rectal cancer surgery compared with laparoscopic surgery. The indications for robotic and laparoscopic rectal cancer surgery are not different. The recently published results of the ROLARR trial, comparing robot-assisted TME to laparoscopic TME, show no advantages of robot assistance in terms of intraoperative complications, postoperative complications, plane of surgery, 30-day mortality, bladder dysfunction, and sexual dysfunction. A drawback of the study is the variability in experience of the participating surgeons in robotic surgery. After correction of this confounder, an advantage for robotic assistance was suggested in terms of risk of conversion to open surgery. For robotic rectal cancer surgery to become the preferred minimally invasive option, it must demonstrate that it does not have the technical difficulties and steep learning curve of laparoscopic surgery. Robotic surgery has several technical advantages over open and laparoscopic surgery. The system provides a stable operating platform, three-dimensional imaging, articulating instruments and a stable surgeon controlled camera which is mainly beneficial in areas where space and maneuverability is limited such as the pelvis.

Keywords: robotic treatment, rectal cancer, total mesorectal excision (TME), robotic surgery, laparoscopy

1. Introduction

Oncological surgery as it is known does not mean organ surgery, but it means the correct lymphadenectomy so that the oncological long-terms results are as expected. Rectal cancer surgery is a touchstone for any surgeon. The surgical technique has continuously progressed over the years and has been standardized with proven oncological results. After Richard Heald's contribution to the need to perform a complete excision of the mesorectum to have excellent control of locoregional spread of disease, surgeons quickly adopted the technique resulting in a significant improvement in local recurrence [1]. Then followed the revolution represented by the appearance of laparoscopy. Robotic surgery has brought a new lease of life to minimally invasive surgery due to its proven advantages. A shorter learning curve than laparoscopy, a lower conversion rate that has allowed an increasing number of patients to benefit from minimally invasive surgery [2, 3].

2. The minimally invasive approach to rectal cancer

Laparoscopy was a real revolution in surgery in the early 1990s. There are few examples in the history of surgery in which an innovative method has such a rapid and widespread spread throughout the world [4]. Of course, colorectal surgery has also faced the first attempts at laparoscopic surgery since the early 1990s, when the first published series of cases appeared [5–9].

The minimally invasive approach for colorectal neoplastic pathology had ups and downs. If initially laparoscopy began to be used especially for benign pathology, in the late 1990s it began to be approached more and more and neoplastic pathology. There have also been controversies related to this approach related to the quality of the specimens and the lymphadenectomy performed. There were also fears related to tumor dissemination at the level of the incision to extract the resection piece and the "chimney effect" with the possibility of metastases at the level of insertion of the trocars [10]. In the late 1990s, the first prospective studies appeared that showed the benefits of the laproscopic approach compared to the open approach, without repercussions related to the percentage of R0 resections or the increase in the number of parietal metastases [11–13].

Only in 2004 with the appearance of the COST study [14] and in 2005 of the CLASICC study [15] it was demonstrated that there are no differences between the laparoscopic and open approach in terms of 3-year recurrence rate, overall survival, number of excised lymph nodes and R0 resection percentage. But if we look to these studies carefully we can comment that most of the cases were related to the middle and upper locations and very few cases were related to low or ultra-low locations.

After that two other multicentric trials, aimed to specifically compare laparoscopic and open surgery in patients with rectal cancer, were the COLOR II trial [16] and the COREAN trial [17], enrolling respectively 1103 and 340 patients. In the COLOR II trial a complete or nearly complete TME was obtained in 92% of laparoscopic and 94% of open procedures; CRM positivity was 10% in both groups; distal margins were negative in 100% of both procedures. In the COREAN trial TME was complete/nearly complete in 92% (laparoscopic) and 88% (open) of patients; CRM was positive in 3% of laparoscopic and in 4% of open procedures; distal margins were negative in all patients in both procedures. In both COLOR and COREAN trials no significant differences were found regarding oncological outcomes, confirming the safety and feasibility of the laparoscopic approach for rectal cancer.

Even so, the global spread of the laparoscopic approach has been extremely slow. With a few exceptions, such as in the United Kingdom, South Korea, etc., the adoption rate has seen an upward but slow trend. In most countries, in centers with a high volume of colorectal interventions, the laparoscopic approach reaching in the period 2008–2015 a percentage that varied between 20 and 50%. If, however, we are talking about medium or low volume centers, the adoption rate was much lower. Another important element of increasing the number of cases was determined by the introduction in more and more centers of the ERAS program in colorectal surgery [18].

A study published on trends in the implementation of the minimally invasive approach in Canada and in the world in general showed that, except for South Korea and the United Kingdom where the percentage of minimally invasive approach in colorectal surgery exceeded 60%, otherwise the percentage varies between 20 and 40%. Finally, a series of strategies are issued to increase the use of the minimally invasive approach in colorectal surgery: increasing exposure to minimally invasive advanced surgery procedures, increasing the number of fellowship programs in minimally invasive surgery, intensive hands-on courses for young surgeons and programs of subsequent mentorship [19].

Despite the many benefits of the laparoscopic approach, there have been elements of slowing the spread on a large scale: the need for staff with expertise in both open surgery and laparoscopic surgery, relatively long learning curve, prolonged operation time, difficult positions for the surgeon maintained for a long time, the difficulty of performing an adequate dissection in case of a narrow pelvis, the need to change the operating device depending on the quadrant in which the operation is performed, etc.

The emergence of the AlaCaRT [20] and ACOSOGZ6051 [21] studies was a step backwards in terms of the ability of the laparoscopic approach to obtain oncological results at least comparable to the open approach. Even some of the lead authors of these studies have pointed out that the robotic approach may be an asset for minimally invasive rectal cancer surgery.

3. The robotic approach

Robotic surgery comes to replace the disadvantages of open surgery and many of those found in laparoscopy. It must be said from the beginning that we are not talking about a robotization of the surgical act, but about the fact that between the surgeon and the patient there is a high performance computer, which allows on the one hand a much finer surgery, with additional attention to detail. The disappearance of the tremor, with instruments that have 7 degrees of freedom, which make possible the access in the narrow spaces, and on the other hand allows the integration of an augmented reality by combining CT, MRI images, on the work screen. And we are talking about 3D images in which there is the possibility of using immunofluorescence with indocyanine green, so as to further visualize the vascularity or lymph node tissue that must be highlighted for a high quality oncological surgery. Fine tissues such as hypogastric nerve plexuses with a special role in maintaining potency are much better preserved when using robotic surgery in rectal cancer, and even more so in the case of large tumors or obese people with narrow pelvis.

This translates into a lower conversion rate, a reduced hospitalization, an easier learning curve and the ability to operate in confined spaces. Achieving a learning curve, which is half of that required for laparoscopy, requires the surgeon to master three unique concepts of robotic surgery, as outlined by Bokhari et al.: replacement of visual cues on tension and tissue manipulation instead of tactile feedback; aligning the robotic arms and trolley while operating remotely on the console, thus minimizing external collisions [22].

A recent retrospective study of 732 patients analyzing long-term oncologic outcomes using tilt score matching showed comparable survival between robotic and laparoscopic TME. In multivariate analysis, robotic surgery was a significant better prognostic factor for overall survival and cancer-specific survival [23]. The most recent and largest randomized clinical trial of laparoscopic or robotic approach for patients with rectal adenocarcinoma (ROLARR) demonstrated comparable oncological results [24].

With all the advantages that the robotic system has, there are also a number of disadvantages [25–27]. Of these, the absence of tactile sense is an important disadvantage. This is an important step in the learning curve so that you can get used to manipulating the tissues without over-pulling them and coordinating the pressure exerted by the instruments on the tissues only through the eye [28].

Another disadvantage was considered too long docking time, but this was shortened by the new generation of Da Vinci Xi robotic systems. After a learning curve of about 20 interventions, the docking time stabilized at a maximum of 15 minutes.

Another negative element that was attributed to the robotic system was also the fact that in the case of an intraoperative bleeding that would require conversion to the open approach, the time required to undo the robot may be too long. Today, however, with the improvements made to the robot, the undocking is done in a maximum of one minute [29].

Another difficulty in using robotic surgery rectal addressed is the possibility of collision between the robot arms.

The cost is a major disadvantage of the robotic approach in terms of rectal surgery. There are studies that show that robotic surgery is significantly more expensive than laparoscopic surgery. Baek et al. reported that hospital charges are 1.5 times higher for the robotic group compared to a laparoscopic group (USD 13,644 vs. USD 9,065, $P < 0.001$) [30]. On the other hand, Quijano et al. publishes a study on the cost-effectiveness comparison between the robotic and laparoscopic approach in rectal surgery. Even if the cost of hospitalization is really higher for the robotic approach, if we talk about quality adjusted life years then it seems that the robotic approach is superior to the laparoscopic one [31].

Disadvantages of robotic surgery include: increased operative time, lack of haptic feedback, remote location of the surgeon away from the operating table, inability to perform abdominal surgery in several quadrants and the cost of technology [25–27].

4. Indications of the robotic approach in rectal cancer

Patient selection is essential for surgeons at the beginning of the learning curve. The ideal candidate is the patient with a tumor located in the middle or upper rectum, in stage I or II, patient without previous abdominal interventions and with a normal BMI. With the gain of experience, the robotic approach proves its advantages exactly in cases where laparoscopy would have had relative contraindications. This includes obese, male patients with a narrow pelvis with tumors located in the lower rectum. In these cases the dissection can be performed successfully in small spaces, with articulated instruments, the quality of the total excision of the mesorectum to be superior even to the open approach. The three-dimensional view increased visibility allows a more precise visualization of the hypogastric nerve plexuses and their preservation as an extremely important objective in maintaining urinary and sexual functions.

5. Preoperative preparation

Preoperative preparation for colorectal robotic surgery is no different from laparoscopic surgery except in one significant way. Unlike laparoscopy, the surgeon is seated at the console, away from the operating table. That is why the role of a well-trained team is extremely important. The team ensures the correct handling of the robot's arms, in order to avoid the collision between the robot's arms during the intervention. The assistant surgeon will always be the one who will ensure the retraction of the structures to be dissected, will change the robot's instruments when necessary. There are also times during the operation when he will insert a stapler through which he will section the intestine, sometimes vascular sealing instruments or clips. Perhaps the most important role of the team is to be able, in case of need, to undock the robot in a very short time. That is why the permanent training of the team is very important.

Minimally invasive colorectal cancer surgery has also led to the widespread introduction of Enahenced Recovery After Surgery (ERAS) protocols. Within these protocols, an important role is represented by the preoperative preparation of the patients who are to have a colorectal intervention. The benefits are obvious in terms of reducing hospitalization, costs, postoperative infections, postoperative pain, facilitating faster resumption of intestinal transit and avoiding nausea or postoperative vomiting [18, 32].

As a preoperative preparation, an essential stage is represented by the patient's counseling, the discussion regarding the intervention, the postoperative evolution and the discharge criteria and the establishment of its compliance for the achievement of the criteria included in the protocol. The discussion is also important for the preparation of a possible stoma, either temporary protective or permanent, followed by marking the place of the future stoma. Avoiding a long period of fasting is important, the recommendation being to maintain a light fluid regime up to 2 hours before general anesthesia. The carbohydrate diet is encouraged in nondiabetic patients in an effort to reduce the increase in insulin resistance by starvation to which will be added the operating stress [33]. There is still controversy about intestinal preparation. The recommendation is for both mechanical and oral antibiotic preparation, which is associated with a decrease in the morbidity rate, including a decrease in the rate of infection in the incisions associated with the intervention [34]. Prophylaxis of deep vein thrombosis is achieved by preoperative administration of low molecular weight heparins. An important element is the multimodal analgesia that begins preoperatively by administering oral analgesics, along with antiemetics so that together with the measures taken intraoperatively to make an easy transition to the postoperative period and thus return the patient to normal much faster [35]. All will contribute to a reduced hospitalization with all the advantages that derive from it, including from the oncological point of view the faster initiation of the adjuvant treatments.

6. Operating setup

The first very important step is related to the positioning of the patient on the operating table. Given that the intervention can last a longer time in which the patient will sit in extreme positions. A Trendelenburg position sometimes accentuated at over 15 degrees for a long time requires effective cooperation with the anesthetic team, in terms of monitoring vital functions, cerebral edema, and last but not least the

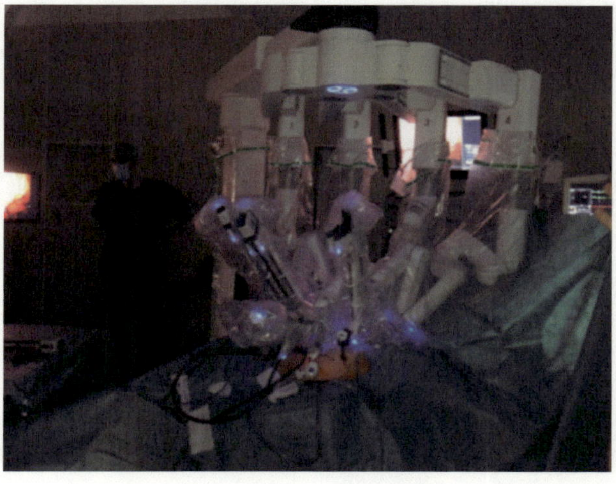

Figure 1.
Patient positioning.

existence of devices to prevent the patient from slipping by mounting shoulders, legs and arms, with protection of all pressure areas. The future positions of the robot's arms and the permanent possibility of the anesthetic team to have easy access to the airways must also be provided. The position of the table must be established from the beginning, because once the robot is fixed, the table cannot be changed (**Figure 1**). Recently the new table motion technology allowed robot and table movement in synchrony without having to undock the robot or reposition instruments.

The fourth generation of surgical robots, respectively da Vinci Xi, unlike the previous variants da Vinci S or Si, once fixed the position does not require its modification depending on the operating quadrant. After docking, the whole intervention can be done without the need for redocking, even if, for example, we perform splenic flexure mobilization first and after we go deep in the pelvis. The patient is placed in a modified lithotomy position, at least 15–20-degree Trendelenburg with the left side raised (**Figure 2**). The robot cart will be placed to the patient's

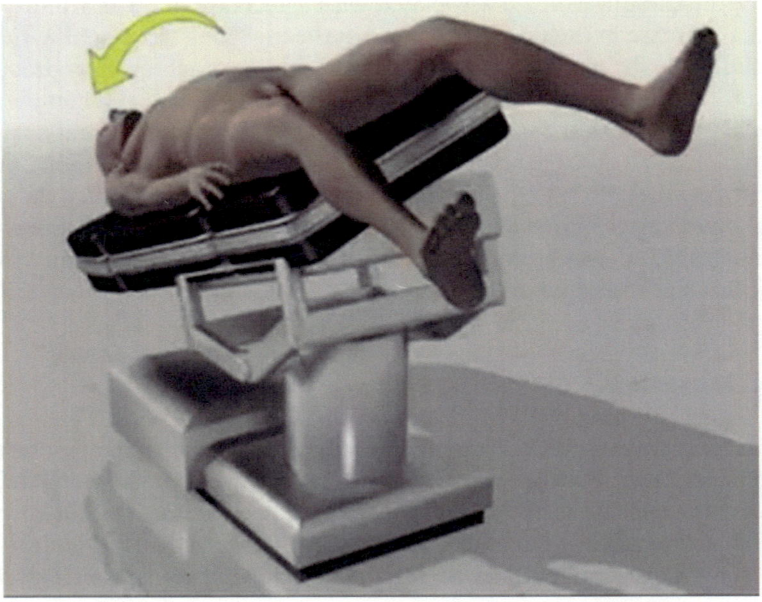

Figure 2.
Patient positioning 2015 Intuitive Surgical, Inc. with permission.

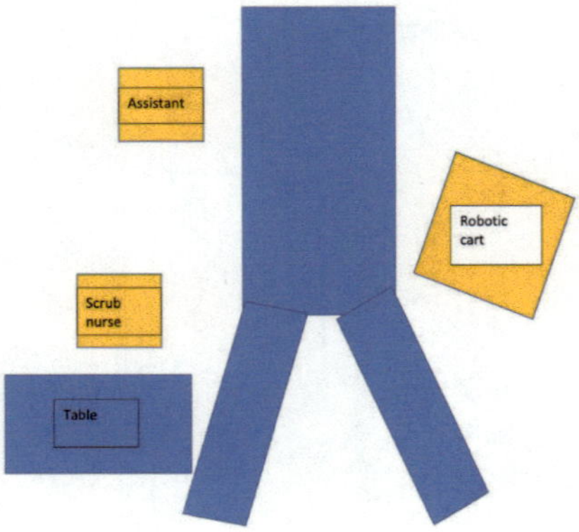

Figure 3.
Operative setup for robotic rectal surgery.

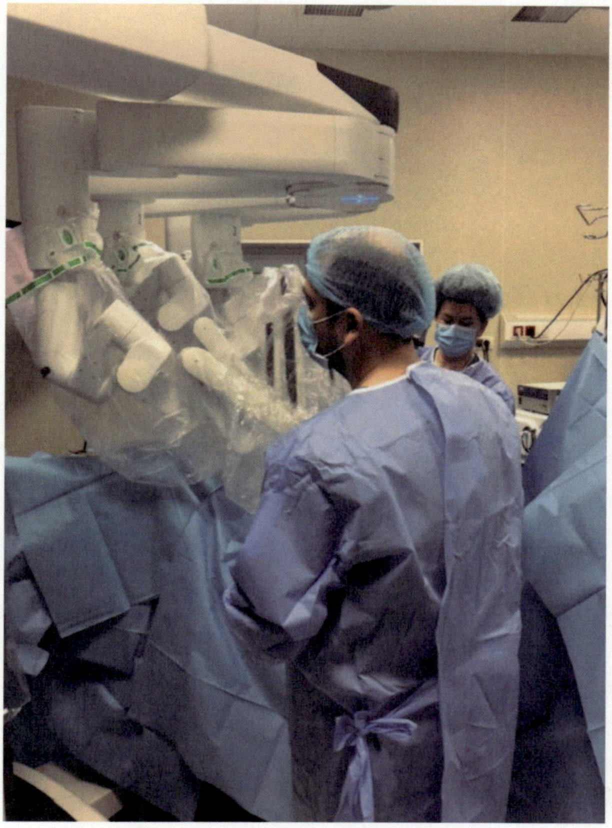

Figure 4.
Operative setup.

left. The assistant surgeon will be positioned to the patient's right. The scrub nurse will be set together with surgical instrument table at the patient's feet on the right (**Figures 3** and **4**).

7. Robotic low anterior resection of rectal cancer

After creating the pneumoperitoneum with the help of the Veres needle, the place of insertion of the future trocars for the 4 arms of the robot is marked. Unlike previous models for the Xi model, the 4 trocars of 8 mm must be placed in line. The distance between two trocars should be 6 to 8 cm. It starts with the trocar intended for the endoscope, which will be placed above the umbilical scar at about 3–4 cm on the right side (**Figure 5**). The insertion line of the following trocars should be slightly oblique between the right flank and the left hypochondrium. Thus, all stages of the intervention can be carried out without difficulty. In order for the possibility of losing pneumoperitoneum during the intervention and also for the immediate removal of the smoke resulting from electrocoagulation, the use of the AirSeal System Insufflation system is welcome. For this, the corresponding 12 mm trocar will be inserted in the right iliac fossa. Through this trocar, the assistant surgeon will introduce various tools: traction forceps, clip applicator, vessel sealing tools, linear staplers, etc. Sometimes, especially in obese patients, in order to maintain the intestinal loops in the right half of the abdomen, it is necessary to insert an additional trocar of 5 mm in the right hypochondrium (**Figure 6**).

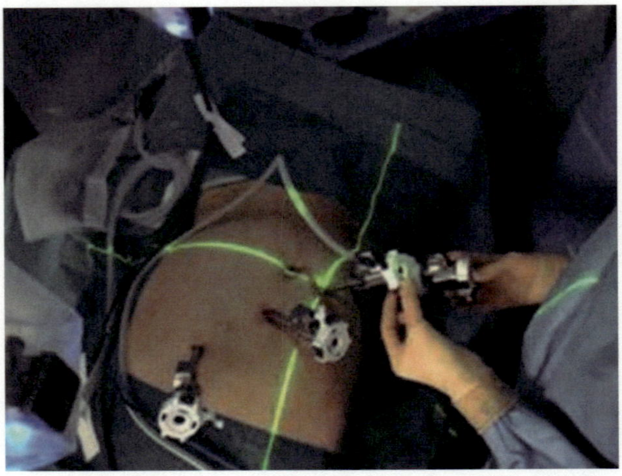

Figure 5.
Positioning of the cart.

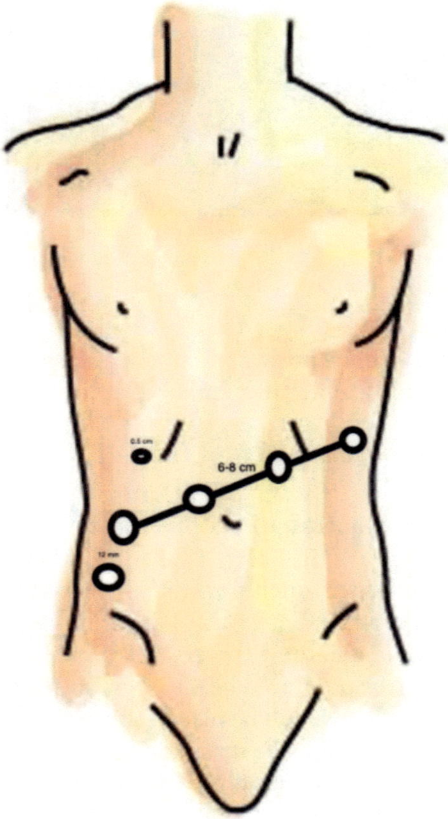

Figure 6.
Trocars positioning for robotic rectal surgery.

In the first stage of the operation, the large omentum is picked up and placed in the splenic fossa, after which the loops of small intestines are removed from the pelvis and kept in the right half of the abdomen, to have easy access from the duodenojejunal angle to the pelvis. In women, it is recommended that the uterus be raised to have enough working space in the pelvis. The uterus can be lifted either by using a uterine manipulator or by anchoring to the anterior abdominal wall with the help of a traction wire (**Figure 7**). The exploration of the peritoneal cavity begins by which the liver, colon and rectum are inspected with the identification of the area to be removed. At the same time, the anatomical landmarks are identified, and the length of the remaining colic partner is established, which will have to descend into the pelvis for the rectal anastomosis. In principle, there are two variants: a generous sigmoid loop sufficient for future anastomosis or a normal sigmoid loop and in this case, it will be necessary to perform a lowering of the splenic angle of the colon. In this situation it is good that the first stage of the intervention is this mobilization of the splenic flexion of the colon because it is a time-consuming step, which requires special attention to avoid damage to surrounding organs, spleen or tail of the pancreas. If done at the end of the procedure, when the surgeon is tired, the risks increase. The best approach of this part of procedure is to start the dissection from the medial to the lateral (**Figure 8**).

The vascular approach follows. The dissection must be performed in the vast majority of cases from the medial to the lateral. There are rare cases in which due

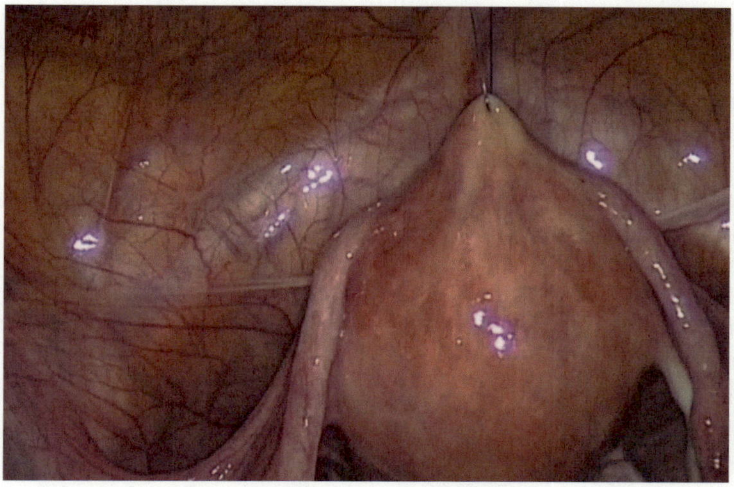

Figure 7.
Uterus mobilization.

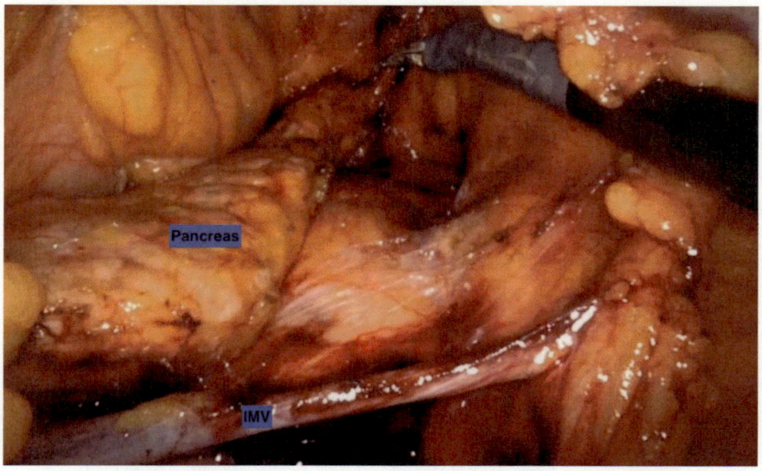

Figure 8.
Splenic flexure mobilization.

to local factors the dissection will take place starting from lateral. At this stage it is very important to correctly highlight the dissection space between the Toldt fascia and the Gerota fascia where we will identify the left ureteral and the genital vascular pedicle. The dissection at the level of the inferior mesenteric artery is performed meticulously for a correct and complete lymphadenectomy. For neoplastic pathology, high ligation of the inferior mesenteric artery is mandatory, followed by ligation of the inferior mesenteric vein (**Figure 9**).

After vascular time, the mesorectum can be completely dissected. Here the role of the robot becomes crucial for an accurate dissection, identification of hypogastric nerve plexuses and their preservation and maintenance in the avascular plane between the rectal fascia and the presacral fascia. At the level of the anterior wall, a complete dissection can also be performed at the level of the Denonvilliers fascia, with the highlighting of the seminal vesicles and the prostate lobes.

As a last stage, the lateral mobilization is performed, followed by the transection of the rectum with the help of linear staplers. They can be inserted through the AirSeal trocar or more recently through the staplers mounted on the robot's arms.

The specimen is currently extracted through a minimal Phanenstiel incision, protected by a system that covers the edges of the wound and thus avoids parietal dissemination. An alternative of extracting the specimen is the transanal extraction, in which the use of the robot proves once again its superiority over the laparoscopic approach [36]. The stapled rectal abutment is sectioned, and the colon is extracted transanal. After resection the specimen, the anvil is mounted either terminally or laterally and the colon is reintroduced into the peritoneal cavity. The stapler is inserted transanal and the rectal stump is circularly sutured around it, after which the anastomosis is created.

For a correct anastomosis, several principles must be observed: we need two healthy partners, well vascularized, with an adequate length and without tension in the future anastomosis. We must not forget that in most cases the tension does not exist at the level of the lateral portion, but at the level of the mesentery, which often appears as a rope at the level of the promontory.

The use of ICG in anastomosis perfusion testing has become a defining moment, especially since the robot is equipped as standard with the near-infrared firefly system (**Figure 10**) [37, 38].

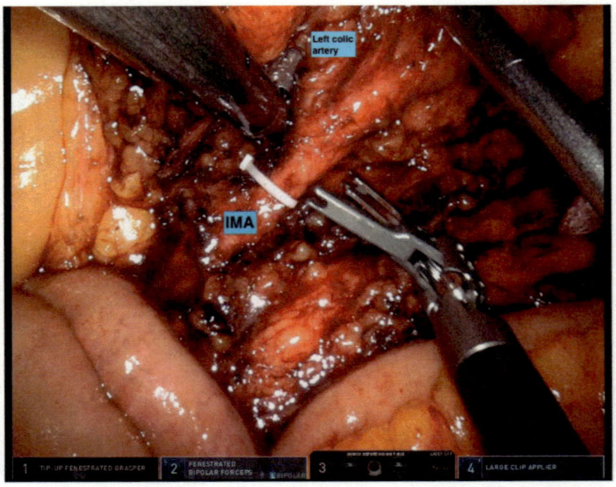

Figure 9.
Inferior mesenteric artery ligation.

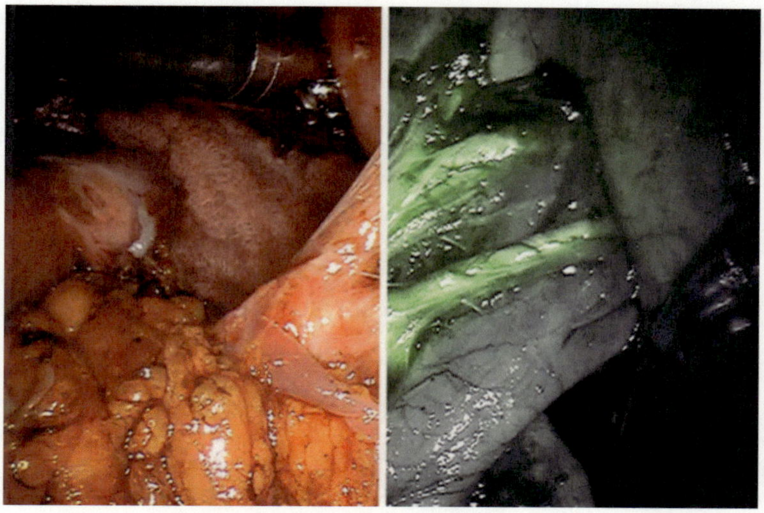

Figure 10.
Firefly fluorescence technology 2015 Intuitive Surgical, Inc. with permission.

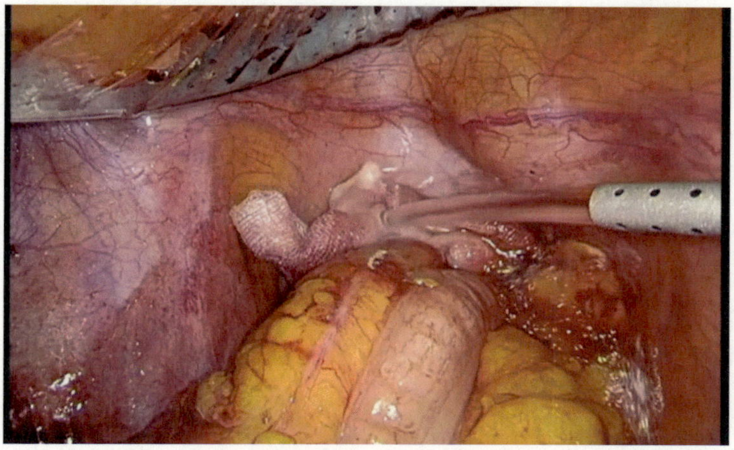

Figure 11.
Air test.

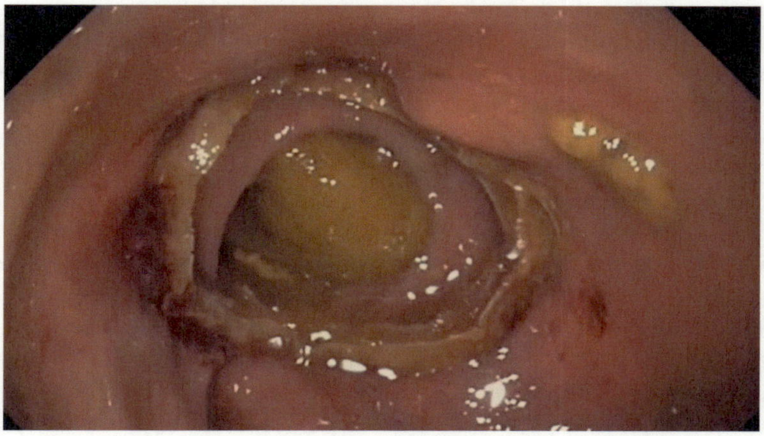

Figure 12.
Postoperative colonoscopy.

Finally, the colorectal anastomosis is checked by air test and colonoscopy. In this way we make sure that the anastomosis is sealed and there is no bleeding at the level of the stapling line (**Figures 11** and **12**).

8. Robotic abdominoperineal resection

The current indications for abdominoperineal resection are represented by:

- Rectal cancer that invades the levator ani muscle or the anal sphincter complex.
- Local recurrent rectal cancer.
- Rectal cancer in patients who cannot benefit of sphincter saving procedure due to poor functional status or comorbidities.
- Anal canal cancer: adenocarcinoma or squamous cell carcinoma.

There are no notable differences between the execution of the first steps. In general, the mobilization of the splenic flexure should not be performed, because the length of the sigmoid colon is sufficient to create a terminal colostomy. The differences occur in the dissection of the pelvic floor. For abdominoperineal resection, lateral dissection beyond the levator ani muscle is important for a lateral lymphadenectomy until the medial edge of the obturator fascia and down until the level of the ischiorectal fossa. If we compare the laparoscopic and the robotic approach, the superiority of the robot in performing the extra-levator resection is obvious. Robotic assisted sectioning of the levator ani muscle allows a precise dissection of the pelvic floor and shortens the perineal dissection time [39].

9. Robotic transanal total mesorectal excision (TaTME)

To improve the oncological and functional outcomes of the patients with rectal cancer new surgical techniques have been developed. It is known that the laparoscopic approach to rectal cancer with medium or lower location is a challenge due to the anatomy of a narrow pelvis and thus increases the risk of incomplete resection of the mesorectum with the possibility of an increased rate of local recurrences.

The introduction of single-port transanal surgery led to the development of the technique of complete excision of the transanal mesorectum [40, 41]. The first studies published by laparoscopic approach were published in 2010 [42]. The promoters of this approach claim that TaTME emphasize a number of benefits, namely a better quality of the specimen with a lower rate of circumferential resection involved, with a lower morbidity related to the extraction of the specimen and a much more sphincter saving procedures without compromising the oncological results.

The help of the robotic system is certain. Stable position, more ergonomic, the possibility of superior maneuverability in narrow spaces, with articulated instruments [43]. The first part of the intervention is performed normally with mesorectal dissection up to the level of the pelvic peritoneal fold. It then passes to the pelvic stage. Only three arms of the robot are used, and the use of AirSeal for smoke absorption is essential (**Figure 13**). It starts with a circular suture of the rectum about 1–2 cm below the tumor. The circular rectal wall is sectioned and after we reach the mesorectum plane, the complete dissection of the mesorectum

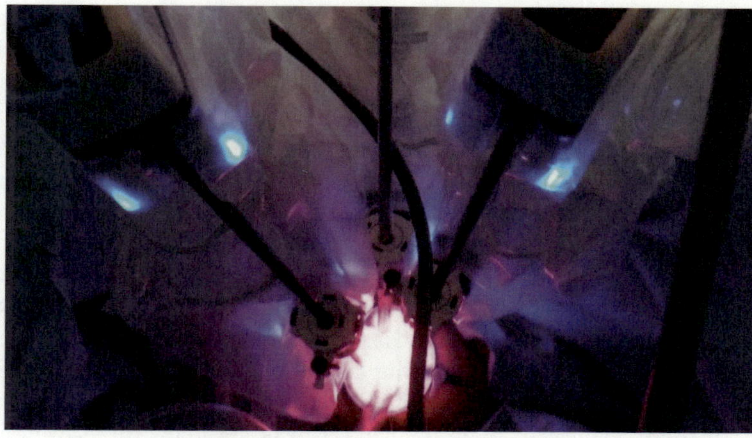

Figure 13.
Operative set-up for TaTME.

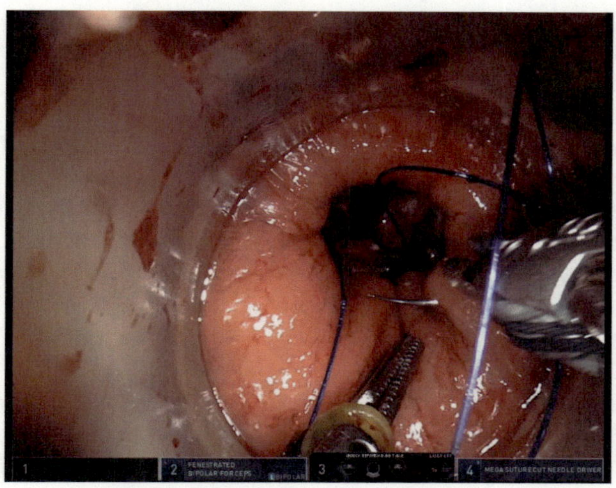

Figure 14.
Step 1 – transanal circular suture.

begins. The upper part will reach the peritoneal cavity, where the previously dissected mesorectal area will meet. The whole piece is extracted transanal and after the colorectal resection, the anvil of the stapler is mounted in the remaining colon, after which it is reintroduced in the peritoneal cavity. A circular bursa is performed at the level of the remaining anal canal and the stapler is inserted, performing a low or very low colorectal anastomosis (**Figure 14**).

10. Discussions

Colorectal laparoscopic surgery after the 1990s when viewed with considerable skepticism had a period of growth between 2000 and 2015 all over the world. According to studies published at that time, laparoscopy has a number of certain advantages over the open approach [11, 13]. However, it is obvious that it becomes extremely difficult to perform when there is relatively low visibility in a narrow pelvis or in different quadrants [14]. The learning curve for colorectal surgery is not small, on average a minimum of 90 interventions are required to overcome this learning curve. Miskovic et al. published in 2012 a meta-analysis related to the learning curve in laparoscopic surgery and shows that if we refer to the time of operation or blood loss more than 90 interventions are needed, but if we refer to the complication rate or conversion rate more than 150 procedures are needed [44].

After the publication of the ALaCaRT and ACOSOGZ6051 studies, the controversies resurfaced [20, 21]. There has been some delimitation between colon surgery and rectal surgery. For colon surgery, the laparoscopic approach is very good, with a clear distinction in terms of difficulty between right hemicolectomy and left colectomy. For rectal surgery, however, there have been controversies about the honesty of the laparoscopic approach compared to the open approach. Here rectal robotic surgery comes to replace all the disadvantages of laparoscopic surgery. The advantages of robotic surgery are obvious in terms of standard three-dimensional visibility, the ability to perform fine dissections in small spaces, difficult to access with tools with 7 degrees of freedom [45–48].

Although the first robotic operation for rectal cancer was performed in 2002 [49], published studies have been quite poor in comparing this approach to the laparoscopic or classical approach. Y. Cui et al. publishes in 2017 a meta-analysis which compares the robotic approach compared to the laparoscopic approach and which discusses only 9 studies that meet the eligibility conditions [50]. The following conclusions can be drawn from this meta-analysis. The robotic approach is superior to the laparoscopic approach in terms of intraoperative blood loss, length of hospital stays and postoperative morbidity rate. Only the time of the intervention was in favor of the laparoscopic approach. Another published meta-analysis which takes into account 5 eligible studies comparing 334 robotic interventions with 337 laparoscopic ones and which demonstrates the superiority of the robotic approach only in the lower conversion rate, but with a higher intervention time [51].

The findings of another study related to the robotic approach in rectal cancer published by Z. Azman highlight the benefits of this approach compared to the laparoscopic or open approach. Superior visualization, shorter learning curve, ergonomic position of the surgeon, lower conversion rate, lower blood loss, shorter hospitalization, lower morbidity rate and better preservation of sexual and urinary function are these robotic advantages [52].

The first randomized clinical trial (ROLARR Study) does not show statistically significant differences between the robotic and laparoscopic approach in any of the 8 end points studied [24]. Subsequent studies have shown a number of advantages of the robotic approach. Fleming et al. performs a meta-analysis comparing the robotic approach with the laparoscopic approach in terms of preserving urogenital function in men and concluding that urinary and erectile function is better in men undergoing the robot compared to conventional laparoscopic surgery for rectal cancer. The results in women did not identify a consistently more favorable result in any of the groups [53]. Another advantage of the robotic approach is found in obese patients, in whom hospitalization is lower and a re-admission to 30 days is rarer, with a faster recovery and a lower rate of postoperative complications, but with a longer duration of operation than the laparoscopic approach [54].

With the advent of novelties in robot instruments, vascular sealing instruments or robotic staplers bring obvious advantages in the easier and more precise development of interventions. In the future, with the advent of other robotic platforms with reusable tools, they will reduce costs and then this disadvantage of robotic surgery will disappear [55].

11. Conclusions

During the last two decades, advances in the surgical treatment of rectal cancer have drastically evolved into a more minimally invasive approach. The patients' need for a good or at least acceptable quality of life is one of the leading appearances of current rectal cancer surgery. Modern technologies, new surgical procedures, together with a deep knowledge of pelvic anatomy and oncological principles, may help the contemporary colorectal surgeon pursue the proper cancer treatment. The key could be tailored surgery, where the best technique is chosen on a case-by-case basis and the experience of the surgeon.

The field of minimally invasive medicine is going to evolve beyond our imagination. The abundance of techniques and technology should not defer the primary goal – patient's safety.

Author details

Ciprian Duta*, Stelu Pantea, Dan Brebu, Amadeus Dobrescu, Caius Lazar, Kitty Botoca, Cristi Tarta and Fulger Lazar
Department of Surgery, University of Medicine and Pharmacy, Timisoara, Romania

*Address all correspondence to: ciprian_duta@yahoo.com

References

[1] Heald RJ, Husband EM, Ryall RD. The mesorectum in rectal cancer surgery--the clue to pelvic recurrence? Br J Surg. 1982 Oct;69(10):613-616.

[2] Pigazzi A, Ellenhorn JD, Ballantyne GH, Paz IB. Robotic-assisted laparoscopic low anterior resection with total mesorectal excision for rectal cancer. Surg Endosc. 2006;20(10):1521-1525.

[3] Baik SH, Kang CM, Lee WJ, Kim NK, Sohn SK, Chi HS, et al. Robotic total mesorectal excision for the treatment of rectal cancer. J Robot Surg. 2007;1(1):99-102.

[4] Cuschieri A. Minimal access surgery: the birth of a new era. J R Coll Surg Edinb. 1990 Dec;35(6):345-347.

[5] Buess G, Manncke K, Merhan J, Lirici M. State of the art of laparoscopic colorectal surgery. Endosc Surg Allied Technol. 1993 Feb;1(1):3-12.

[6] Guillou PJ, Darzi A, Monson JR. Experience with laparoscopic colorectal surgery for malignant disease. Surg Oncol. 1993;2 Suppl 1:43-49.

[7] Wexner SD, Cohen SM, Johansen OB, Nogueras JJ, Jagelman DG. Laparoscopic colorectal surgery: a prospective assessment and current perspective. Br J Surg. 1993 Dec;80(12):1602-1605.

[8] Cohen SM, Wexner SD. Laparoscopic colorectal resection for cancer: the Cleveland Clinic Florida experience. Surg Oncol. 1993;2 Suppl 1:35-42.

[9] Darzi A, Super P, Guillou PJ, Monson JR. Laparoscopic sigmoid colectomy: total laparoscopic approach. Dis *Colon Rectum*. 1994 Mar;37(3):268-271.

[10] Akle CA. Early parietal recurrence of adenocarcinoma of the colon after laparoscopic colectomy. Port site metastasis after laparascopic colorectal surgery for cure of malignancy. Br J Surg. 1996 Mar;83(3):427.

[11] Milsom JW, Kim SH. Laparoscopic versus open surgery for colorectal cancer. World J Surg. 1997 Sep;21(7):702-705.

[12] Köckerling F, Rose J, Schneider C, Scheidbach H, Scheuerlein H, Reymond MA, Reck T, Konradt J, Bruch HP, Zornig C, Bärlehner E, Kuthe A, Szinicz G, Richter HA, Hohenberger W. Laparoscopic colorectal anastomosis: risk of postoperative leakage. Results of a multicenter study. Laparoscopic Colorectal Surgery Study Group (LCSSG). Surg Endosc. 1999 Jul;13(7):639-644.

[13] Khalili TM, Fleshner PR, Hiatt JR, Sokol TP, Manookian C, Tsushima G, Phillips EH. Colorectal cancer: comparison of laparoscopic with open approaches. Dis *Colon Rectum*. 1998 Jul;41(7):832-838.

[14] Kitano S, Inomata M, Sato A, Yoshimura K, Moriya Y; Japan Clinical Oncology Group Study. Randomized controlled trial to evaluate laparoscopic surgery for colorectal cancer: Japan Clinical Oncology Group Study JCOG 0404. Jpn J Clin Oncol. 2005 Aug;35(8):475-477.

[15] Guillou P, Quirke P, Thorpe H. Short-term endpoints of conventional versus laparoscopic-assisted surgery in patients with colorectal cancer (MRC CLASSIC trial): multicentre, randomised con- trolled trial. Lancet. 2005;365:1-9.

[16] van der Pas MH, Haglind E, Cuesta MA, Fu¨ rst A, Lacy AM, Hop WC et al. Laparoscopic versus open surgery for rectal cancer (COLOR II): Short-term outcomes of a randomised,

phase 3 trial. Lancet Oncol. 2013; 14(3):210-218.

[17] Kang SB, Park JW, Jeong SY, Nam BH, Choi HS, Kim DW et al. Open versus laparoscopic surgery for mid or low rectal cancer after neoadjuvant chemoradiotherapy (COREAN trial): Short-term outcomes of an open-label randomised controlled trial. Lancet Oncol. 2010; 11(7):637-645.

[18] Gustafsson UO, Scott MJ, Hubner M, Nygren J, Demartines N, Francis N, Rockall TA, Young-Fadok TM, Hill AG, Soop M, de Boer HD, Urman RD, Chang GJ, Fichera A, Kessler H, Grass F, Whang EE, Fawcett WJ, Carli F, Lobo DN, Rollins KE, Balfour A, Baldini G, Riedel B, Ljungqvist O. Guidelines for Perioperative Care in Elective Colorectal Surgery: Enhanced Recovery After Surgery (ERAS®) Society Recommendations: 2018. World J Surg. 2019 Mar;43(3):659-695.

[19] Hoogerboord M, Ellsmere J, Caycedo-Marulanda A, Brown C, Jayaraman S, Urbach D, Cleary S. Laparoscopic colectomy: trends in implementation in Canada and globally. Can J Surg. 2019 Apr 1;62(2):139-141.

[20] Stevenson AR, Solomon MJ, Lumley JW, Hewett P, Clouston AD, Gebski VJ, Davies L, Wilson K, Hague W, Simes J; ALaCaRT Investigators. Effect of Laparoscopic-Assisted Resection vs Open Resection on Pathological Outcomes in Rectal Cancer: The ALaCaRT Randomized Clinical Trial. JAMA. 2015 Oct 6;314(13):1356-1363.

[21] Fleshman J, Branda M, Sargent DJ, Boller AM, George V, Abbas M et al. Effect of Laparoscopic-Assisted Resection vs Open Resection of Stage II or III Rectal Cancer on Pathologic Outcomes: The ACOSOG Z6051 Randomized Clinical Trial. JAMA. 2015; 314(13):1346-1355.

[22] Bokhari MB, Patel CB, Ramos-Valadez DI, Ragupathi M, Haas EM. Learning curve for robotic-assisted laparoscopic colorectal surgery. Surg Endosc. 2011 Mar;25(3):855-860.

[23] Yamamoto S. Comparison of the perioperative outcomes of laparoscopic surgery, robotic surgery, open surgery, and transanal total mesorectal excision for rectal cancer: An overview of systematic reviews. Ann Gastroenterol Surg. 2020 Aug 29;4(6):628-634.

[24] Jayne D, Pigazzi A, Marshall H, Croft J, Corrigan N, Copeland J, Quirke P, West N, Rautio T, Thomassen N, Tilney H, Gudgeon M, Bianchi PP, Edlin R, Hulme C, Brown J. Effect of Robotic-Assisted vs Conventional Laparoscopic Surgery on Risk of Conversion to Open Laparotomy Among Patients Undergoing Resection for Rectal Cancer: The ROLARR Randomized Clinical Trial. JAMA. 2017 Oct 24;318(16):1569-1580.

[25] Hellan M, Stein H, Pigazzi A. Totally robotic low anterior resection with total mesorectal excision and splenic flexure mobilization. Surg Endosc. 2009;23(2):447-451.

[26] Kim YW, Lee HM, Kim NK, Min BS, Lee KY. The learning curve for robot-assisted total mesorectal excision for rectal cancer. Surg Laparosc Endosc Percutan Tech. 2012;22(5):400-405.

[27] Jimenez-Rodriguez RM, Diaz-Pavon JM, de la Portilla de Juan F, Prendes-Sillero E, Dussort HC, Padillo J. Learning curve for robotic-assisted laparoscopic rectal cancer surgery. Int J Color Dis. 2013;28(6):815-821.

[28] Park EJ, Baik SH. Robotic Surgery for Colon and Rectal Cancer. Curr Oncol Rep. 2016;18(1):5.

[29] Park S, Kim NK. The Role of Robotic Surgery for Rectal Cancer: Overcoming Technical Challenges in Laparoscopic

Surgery by Advanced Techniques. J Korean Med Sci. 2015;30(7):837-846.

[30] Baek SJ, Kim CH, Cho MS, Bae SU, Hur H, Min BS, Baik SH, Lee KY, Kim NK. Robotic surgery for rectal cancer can overcome difficulties associated with pelvic anatomy. Surg Endosc. 2015 Jun;29(6):1419-1424.

[31] Quijano Y, Nuñez-Alfonsel J, Ielpo B, Ferri V, Caruso R, Durán H, Díaz E, Malavé L, Fabra I, Pinna E, Isernia R, Hidalgo Á, Vicente E. Robotic versus laparoscopic surgery for rectal cancer: a comparative cost-effectiveness study. Tech Coloproctol. 2020 Mar;24(3):247-254.

[32] Cavallaro P, Bordeianou L. Implementation of an ERAS Pathway in Colorectal Surgery. Clin Colon Rectal Surg. 2019 Mar;32(2):102-108.

[33] Moya P, Soriano-Irigaray L, Ramirez JM, Garcea A, Blasco O, Blanco FJ, Brugiotti C, Miranda E, Arroyo A. Perioperative Standard Oral Nutrition Supplements Versus Immunonutrition in Patients Undergoing Colorectal Resection in an Enhanced Recovery (ERAS) Protocol: A Multicenter Randomized Clinical Trial (SONVI Study). Medicine (Baltimore). 2016 May;95(21):e3704.

[34] Rollins KE, Javanmard-Emamghissi H, Lobo DN. Impact of mechanical bowel preparation in elective colorectal surgery: A meta-analysis. World J Gastroenterol. 2018 Jan 28;24(4):519-536.

[35] Simpson JC, Bao X, Agarwala A. Pain Management in Enhanced Recovery after Surgery (ERAS) Protocols. Clin Colon Rectal Surg. 2019 Mar;32(2):121-128.

[36] Choi GS, Park IJ, Kang BM, Lim KH and Jun SH: A novel approach of robotic-assisted anterior resection with transanal or transvaginal retrieval of the specimen for colorectal cancer. Surg Endosc *23*: 2831-2835, 2005.

[37] Blanco-Colino R, Espin-Basany E. Intraoperative use of ICG fluorescence imaging to reduce the risk of anastomotic leakage in colorectal surgery: a systematic review and meta-analysis. Tech Coloproctol. 2018 Jan;22(1):15-23.

[38] Son GM, Kwon MS, Kim Y, Kim J, Kim SH, Lee JW. Quantitative analysis of colon perfusion pattern using indocyanine green (ICG) angiography in laparoscopic colorectal surgery. Surg Endosc. 2019 May;33(5):1640-1649.

[39] Douissard J, Obias V, Johnson CS, Hagen ME, Keller D, Ouellette JR, Hellan M. Totally robotic vs hybrid abdominoperineal resection: A retrospective multicenter analysis. Int J Med Robot. 2020 Apr;16(2):e2073.

[40] Marks JH, Marchionni C, Marks GJ. Transanal endoscopic micro- surgery in the treatment of select rectal cancers or tumors suspicious for cancer. Surg Endosc 2003;17(07):1114-1117

[41] Atallah S, Albert M, Larach S. Transanal minimally invasive surgery: a giant leap forward. Surg Endosc 2010;24(09): 2200-2205

[42] Sylla P, Rattner DW, Delgado S, Lacy AM. NOTES transanal rectal cancer resection using transanal endoscopic microsurgery and laparoscopic assistance. Surg Endosc 2010;24(05):1205– 1210

[43] Samalavicius NE, Janusonis V, Smolskas E, Dulskas A. Transanal and robotic total mesorectal excision (robotic-assisted TaTME) using the Senhance® robotic system - a video vignette. Colorectal Dis. 2020 Jan;22(1):114-115.

[44] Miskovic D, Ni M, Wyles SM, Tekkis P, Hanna GB. Learning curve and case selection in laparoscopic colorectal

surgery: systematic review and international multicenter analysis of 4852 cases. Dis *Colon Rectum*. 2012 Dec;55(12):1300-1310.

[45] D'Annibale A, Morpurgo E, Fiscon V, Trevisan P, Sovernigo G, Orsini C, et al. Robotic and laparoscopic surgery for treatment of colorectal diseases. Dis *Colon Rectum*. 2004;47(12):2162-2168.

[46] Spinoglio G, Summa M, Priora F, Quarati R, Testa S. Robotic colorectal surgery: first 50 cases experience. Dis *Colon Rectum*. 2008;51(11):1627-1632.

[47] Park JS, Choi GS, Lim KH, Jang YS, Jun SH. Robotic-assisted versus laparoscopic surgery for low rectal cancer: case-matched analysis of short-term outcomes. Ann Surg Oncol. 2010;17(12):3195-3202.

[48] Baik SH, Kwon HY, Kim JS, Hur H, Sohn SK, Cho CH, et al. Robotic versus laparoscopic low anterior resection of rectal cancer: short-term outcome of a prospective comparative study. Ann Surg Oncol. 2009;16(6):1480-1487.

[49] Hildebrandt U, Plusczyk T, Kessler K, Menger MD. Single-surgeon surgery in laparoscopic colonic resection. Dis *Colon Rectum*. 2003 Dec;46(12):1640-1645.

[50] Cui Y, Li C, Xu Z, Wang Y, Sun Y, Xu H, Li Z, Sun Y. Robot-assisted versus conventional laparoscopic operation in anus-preserving rectal cancer: a meta-analysis. Ther Clin Risk Manag. 2017 Sep 22;13:1247-1257.

[51] Prete FP, Pezzolla A, Prete F, Testini M, Marzaioli R, Patriti A, Jimenez-Rodriguez RM, Gurrado A, Strippoli GFM. Robotic Versus Laparoscopic Minimally Invasive Surgery for Rectal Cancer: A Systematic Review and Meta-analysis of Randomized Controlled Trials. Ann Surg. 2018 Jun;267(6):1034-1046.

[52] Mohd Azman ZA, Kim SH. A review on robotic surgery in rectal cancer. Transl Gastroenterol Hepatol. 2016 Mar 16;1:5.

[53] Fleming CA, Cullinane C, Lynch N, Killeen S, Coffey JC, Peirce CB. Urogenital function following robotic and laparoscopic rectal cancer surgery: meta-analysis. Br J Surg. 2021 Mar 12;108(2):128-137.

[54] Panteleimonitis S, Pickering O, Abbas H, Harper M, Kandala N, Figueiredo N, Qureshi T, Parvaiz A. Robotic rectal cancer surgery in obese patients may lead to better short-term outcomes when compared to laparoscopy: a comparative propensity scored match study. Int J Colorectal Dis. 2018 Aug;33(8):1079-1086.

[55] Tejedor P, Sagias F, Nock D, Flashman K, Naqvi S, Kandala NL, Khan JS. Advantages of using a robotic stapler in rectal cancer surgery. J Robot Surg. 2020 Apr;14(2):365-370.

Chapter 14

The Problem of the Colorectal Anastomosis

Sinziana Ionescu

Abstract

Colorectal anastomosis is defined as a surgical procedure in which the colon is attached to the remainder of the rectum after most or some part of it was removed during an intervention. A straight colorectal anastomosis implies a direct attachment, while a J-pouch colorectal anastomosis implies a previous creation of a reservoir, or "pouch" out of bowel material. The problem of colorectal anastomosis safety and outcome is among the most important and persistent issues in colorectal surgery, mainly due to the anastomotic leakage, a threatening and dangerous complication, with an incidence of up to 20% or even more in case of surgical oncology. Various prediction models and anastomosis testing techniques have been described in order to prevent or identify early any possible imperfection of the anastomosis, each with pros and cons. The measures generally used to increase the safety and reliability of the colorectal anastomosis are to evaluate the blood supply of the tissues anastomosed with indocyanine green, or to test the mechanical integrity of the anastomosis for leakage by employing air, methylene blue, or tension.

Keywords: colonic fistula, anastomotic leakage, colorectal anastomosis, colorectal surgery complications, total mesorectal excision (TME)

1. Introduction

An anastomosis is a surgical connection between two structures. It usually means a connection that is created between tubular structures, such as blood vessels or loops of the intestine. Surgeons can choose to join together the two parts of the intestine by using either sewing (sutures) or staples. Sewing by hand has been used successfully for over 100 years. However, stapling takes less time to perform. As with any intervention, anastomosis carries some risks. These include blood clots, bleeding, scarring, blockage, stricture, or abnormal narrowing, damage to the surrounding structures, and infections, all of which can lead to anastomotic leakage, sepsis, septic shock, or even death (**Figures 1** and **2**).

2. General aspects of bowel anastomoses and modern variations that impacted the outcome

Barbed sutures are available in a variety of both absorbable and nonabsorbable monofilament materials. Specifically, currently available bidirectional and unidirectional barbed suture materials include PDO, polyglyconate, poliglecaprone 25, glycomer 631, nylon, and polypropylene. A study performed by Wiggins [1]

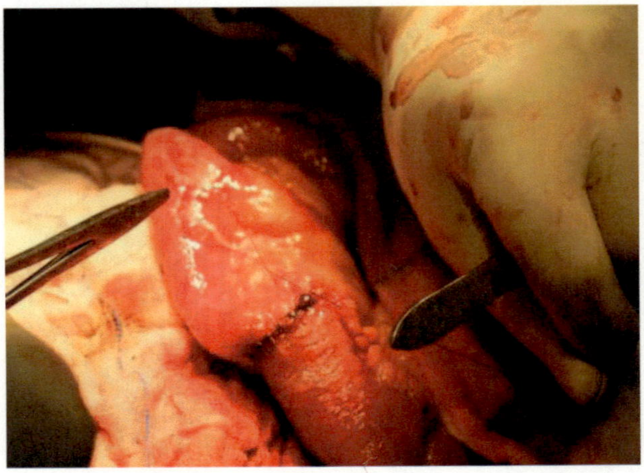

Figure 1.
Intraoperative aspect of an anastomosis performed manually at the level of the small bowel.

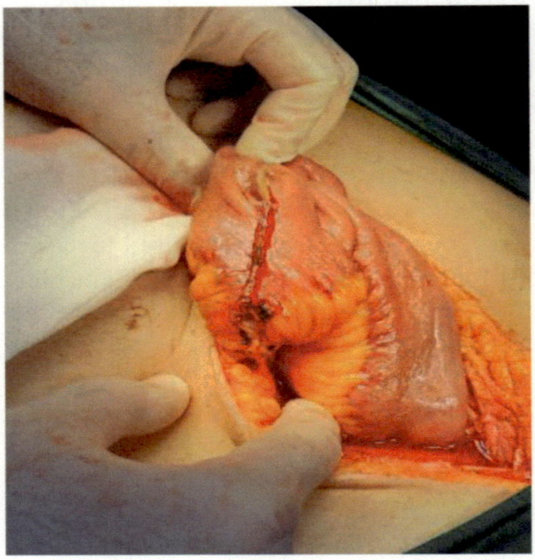

Figure 2.
Intraoperative aspect of an anastomosis performed mechanically at the level of the small bowel.

searched through a systematic review and meta-analysis for the benefits of barbed suture utilization in gastrointestinal anastomosis. The conclusion was that the use of barbed sutures for gastrointestinal anastomosis appears to be associated with shorter overall operative times. There was no difference in rates of complications (including anastomotic leak, bleeding, or stricture) compared with standard suture materials.

The study included consecutive CD patients with ileal/ileocolonic strictures who had SWE shear wave elastography within one week of surgical resection.

The SWE of the stenotic bowel wall was compared to the biofragmentable anastomosis ring used for gastrointestinal anastomoses in a literature review conducted by Bobkiewicz and coauthors [2].

The theoretical idea was that a biofragmentable anastomosis ring (BAR) could be used instead of manual and stapled anastomoses in the upper and lower GI tracts.

The aim of this study was to see how effective BAR was for bowel anastomoses using our own content. Methodologies: Between 2004 and 2014, a retrospective study was conducted on a total of 203 patients who underwent bowel surgery with

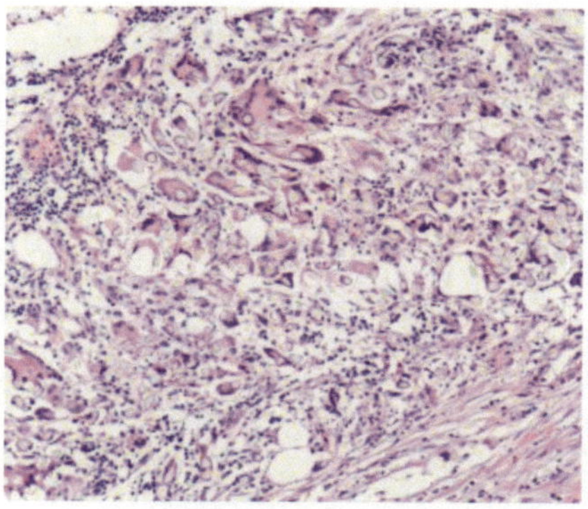

Figure 3.
Foreign body reaction at the level of the tissues containing suture material.

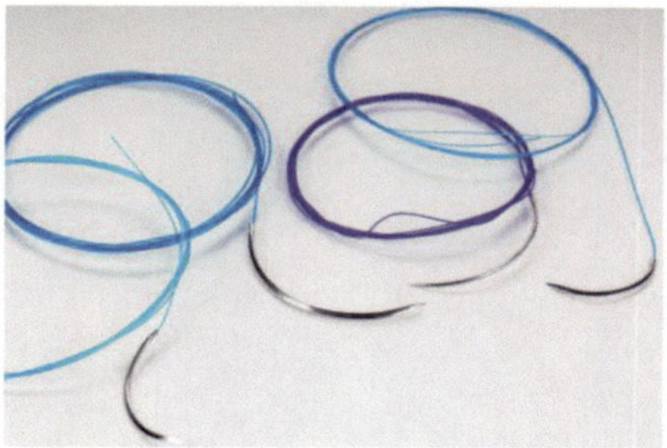

Figure 4.
Colorful surgical nylon monofilament suture with a curved needle.

BAR anastomosis in the upper and lower gastrointestinal tract. The study concluded that using BAR for GI tract anastomoses is an easy and quick procedure with a low rate of perioperative mortality (0.5%) and complication rates (**Figures 3** and **4**).

3. Colorectal anastomosis: General facts and variations of the techniques used

3.1 Manual versus mechanic

The ideal stapling device should be capable of rapid creation of an anastomosis with serosal apposition without the persistence of a foreign body or a foreign body reaction, which potentially contributes to early anastomotic dehiscence or late anastomotic stricture (**Figures 5** and **6**).

3.2 Debating issues of the mechanical colorectal anastomosis

While 2-row stapling has become normal in low anterior resections (LARs), it has no effect on morbidity or the incidence of AL.

Conducted by Nekliudov [3] is the first prospective, randomized clinical trial that compares the success rate of modern 3-row circular staplers to that of traditional 2-row staplers.

According to the hypothesis, the frequency of AL in the 3-row stapler group is not significantly higher than in the 2-row stapler group.

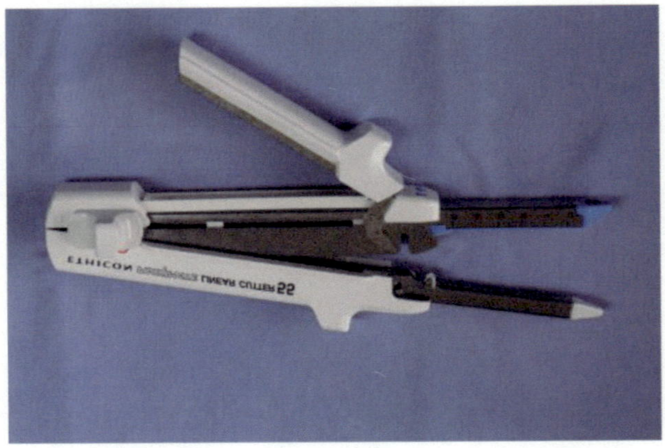

Figure 5.
Linear surgical stapler.

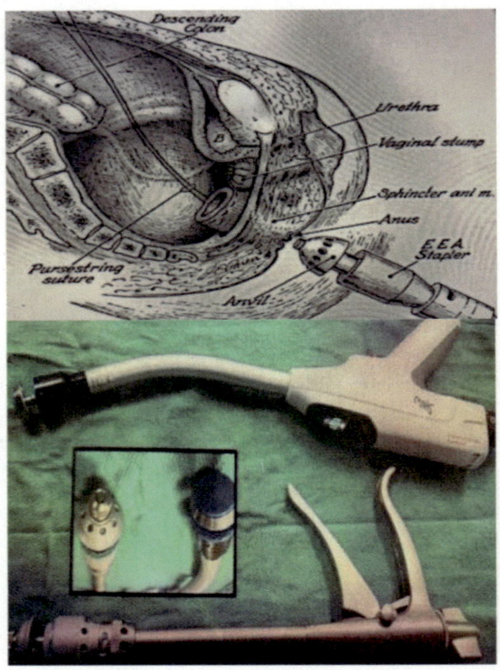

Figure 6.
(a and b) circular stapling device and its mode of appliance.

The rate of AL, as determined by imaging studies and measured using the Pearson chi-squared test and Fisher exact test, is the primary endpoint.

Secondary outcomes include AL severity (A, B, or C), anastomotic bleeding, postoperative complication rate (graded using the Clavien-Dindo classification), reintervention rate, stapler dysfunction rate, complications of nonfunctioning stoma, overall and cancer-specific quality of life (measured using short-form (36) questionnaire and quality-of-life (30) questionnaire core, respectively), fecal incontinence, and overall and cancer-specific quality of life.

Following the LAR, both patients will be tracked for a period of 12 months.

This is the first prospective randomized trial to look at the efficacy of 3-row staplers for colorectal anastomosis following rectal cancer surgery.

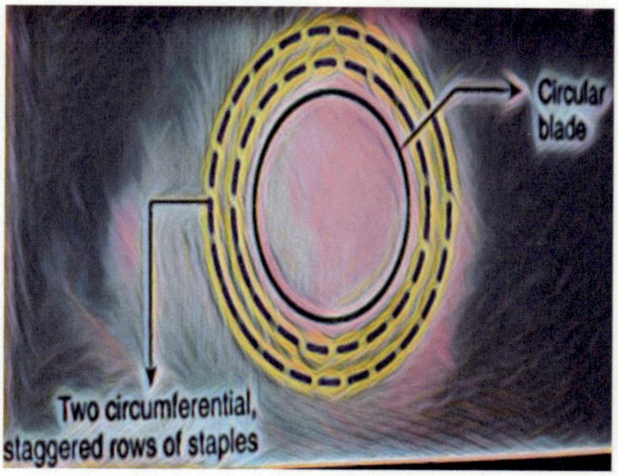

Figure 7.
2-row staple lines.

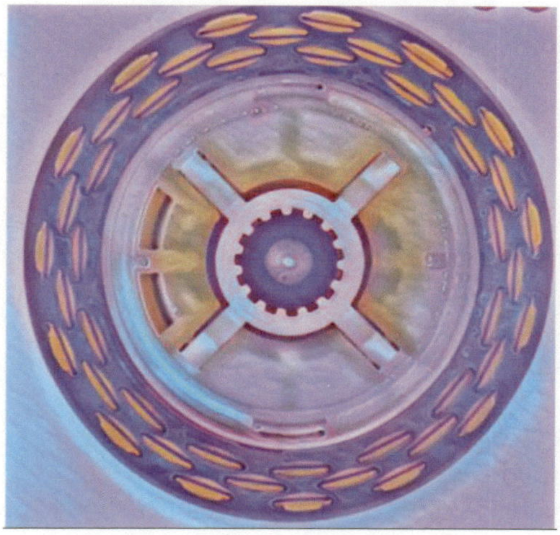

Figure 8.
3-row staple lines.

It could show that 3-row circular staplers are feasible in LAR in terms of short- and long-term patient outcomes (**Figures 7** and **8**).

3.3 MIS and colorectal anastomosis

A study performed by Jeong and coauthors [4] was assembled to report an institution's experiences with transanal total mesorectal excision (TME) of rectal cancer using single-port equipment and to discuss the feasibility and safety of the technique. In the institution mentioned, 10 patients (6:4) treated with transanal TME with colorectal anastomosis were examined (**Figure 9**).

In six of 10 patients, TME was done without the use of a laparoscope.

The average time spent on the operating table was 303.5 minutes.

The distal margin was 2.1 (0.2–4.2) cm on average.

The average number of lymph nodes harvested is 17.5.

Except for one patient who had an anastomotic leak, the majority of patients began dietary intake on POD 3 and were discharged on POD 7.

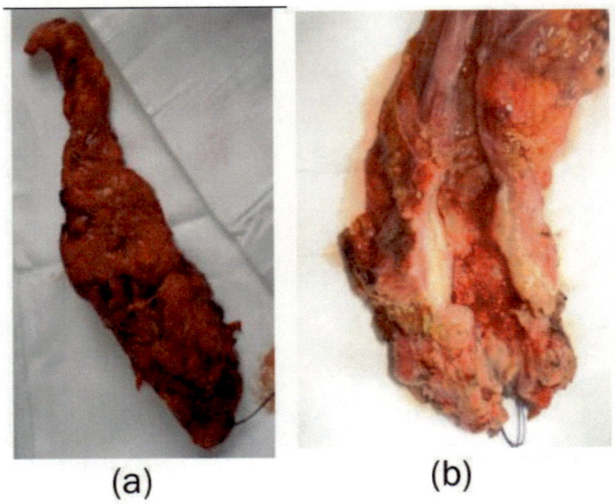

Figure 9.
Complete TME specimen (a) and sectioned (b) after abdomino-perineal resection with intact mesorectum.

The only postoperative complication was an anastomotic leak.

Conclusions: In selected cases of rectal cancer, pure natural orifice transluminal endoscopic surgery (NOTES) TME with coloanal anastomosis was found to be healthy and feasible.

4. Postoperative complications of colorectal anastomoses and their prevention

4.1 Anastomotic leakage

Anastomotic leak (AL) is a common problem in colorectal surgery, and its prevalence has remained steady in recent years.

The use of an intra-abdominal drain or mechanical bowel preparation to prevent AL has been shown to be ineffective and should be avoided.

The function of oral antibiotic preparation regimens should be explained and compared to other routes of administration, such as intravenous or enema, according to a study conducted by Meyer and coauthors [5].

Parallel to this, preoperative antibiotherapy should target pathogens that induce collagenase, as defined by the microbiome study.

Fluorescence angiography may minimize AL even further, resulting in major intraoperative improvements in surgical strategies.

Fluorescence angiography can be used more often.

There have been studies, such as the one by Gained and coauthors [6], that looked at the literature's connection between colorectal cancer recurrence, microbiome, and anastomotic leakage, and among the findings, one can find the aspect according to which the numerous mechanisms by which environmental factors act on the microbiome to alter its composition and function, with the net effect of adversely affecting oncological outcomes following surgery, are well documented and increasing.

Diet, antibiotic use, the procedures used to prepare the colon for surgery, and the physiological discomfort of the procedure are all examples of environmental causes.

Furthermore, using next-generation sequencing technologies to investigate the intestinal microbiome has the ability to affect cancer outcomes following colon resection. In a systematic review that targeted the endoscopic management of early postoperative complications, a literature search was performed by Clifford and coauthors [7] for published full text articles using the PubMed, Cochrane, and Scopus databases using the search criteria string "colorectal anastomotic ("leak" or "bleed")," "endoscopy," and "endoscopic management." Endoscopic therapy in the management of stable patients with colorectal anastomotic leaks appears safe and is associated with the high rates of technical performance in selected patients, according to a review of 89 papers.

The most suitable method, patient selection, and considering the practical and long-term consequences of this approach remain challenging.

To fully assess the function of these novel strategies, further data from large prospective cohort studies are needed.

Shalaby and coauthors [8] conducted another systematic review on endoluminal vacuum-assisted therapy as a salvage treatment for rectal anastomotic leakage and found the following findings among 476 articles identified, 17 studies reporting on 276 patients:

The weighted mean success rate was 853% (95% confidence interval [CI]: 801–905), with a median time from the start of EVT to full healing of 47 (range 40–105) days.

The weighted mean rate of stoma reversal was 759% (646–872%) across the studies.

After EVT, twenty-five patients (91%) needed additional interventions.

Thirty-eight patients (138%) experienced complications as a result of the procedure.

The weighted mean complication rate was 111% (60–162%) across all tests.

Preoperative radiotherapy, the absence of a diverting stoma, complications, and male sex were all found to be significantly associated with failure.

According to the findings of the study, EVT is linked to a high rate of full healing of anastomotic leakage and stoma reversal.

In appropriately selected patients with anastomotic leakage, it is a viable choice.

Colorectal cancer surgery is thought to involve "high tie" and "low tie" of the inferior mesenteric artery (IMA).

However, the blood supply of the anastomosis is closely linked to the ligation stage, which can increase the leakage rate, and it is unclear which technique confers a lower anastomotic leakage rate (AL) and survival advantage.

The aim of the literature review, as stated by Yang and coauthors [9], was to compare the efficacy and impact of IMA high ligation versus IMA low ligation on anastomotic leakage, lymph node yield rates, and 5-year survival.

Finally, after reviewing studies from 1990 to 2017, researchers came to the conclusion that neither the high-tie nor the low-tie approach has any data in terms of anastomotic leakage, harvested lymph nodes, or 5-year survival rates.

More RCT is needed.

A study conducted by Simianu and coauthors [10] looked at the recency effect, which means that people place disproportionate emphasis on events that occurred recently when making decisions, but the magnitude of this influence on surgeons' decisions is uncertain.

The use of preventative leak testing before and after colorectal operations with anastomotic leaks is examined in this study to see whether there is a recency effect in surgeons.

A prospective cohort of adult patients (aged 18 years) undergoing elective colorectal surgery at Washington State hospitals participating in the Surgical Care and Outcomes Assessment Program was used to develop the materials and methods (2006–2013).

The key outcome measure was the difference in leak monitoring between 6 months before and 6 months after an anastomotic leak.

A leak rate of 2.6% (n = 124) was found in 4854 elective colorectal operations performed by 282 surgeons at 44 hospitals.

The anastomosis was not checked in 40 leaks (32%), which were spread through 25 surgeons.

While the small sample size restricted the ability to detect an overall difference in leak testing use, 9 (36%) of the 25 surgeons increased their leak testing by 5% or more after leaks in cases where the anastomosis was not checked.

The above facts led to the conclusion that only one-third of qualified surgeons demonstrated the recency effect.

Understanding the degree to which the recency effect influences clinical decisions may be useful in developing quality management strategies that involve clinician's behavior change.

Wang and colleagues [11] contrasted many aspects of robot-assisted versus laparoscopic surgery for rectal cancer by reviewing 20 studies with a total of 5496 patients, divided into a robot-assisted surgery group (n = 2168, 39.4%) and a laparoscopic surgery group (n = 3328, 60.6%).

Longer operating period (OR: 0.48, 95% CI: 0.14, 0.82), lower conversion to open surgery rate (OR: 0.55, 95% CI: 0.44, 0.69), shorter LOS (Length Of Stay) (OR: −0.15, 95% CI: −0.30, 0.00), faster bowel function recovery (OR: −0.38, 95%

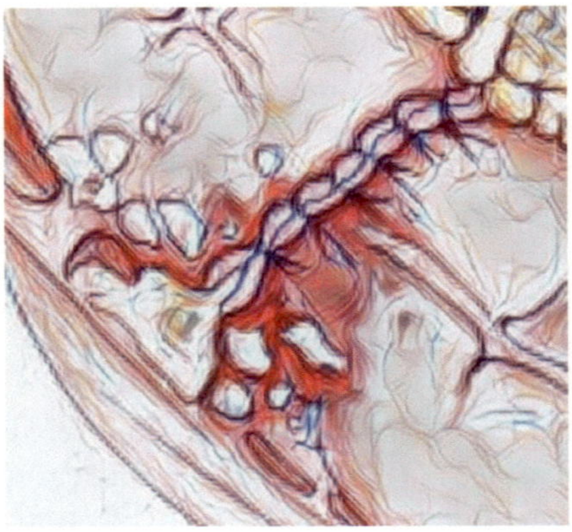

Figure 10.
Dehiscence at the level of the anastomosis.

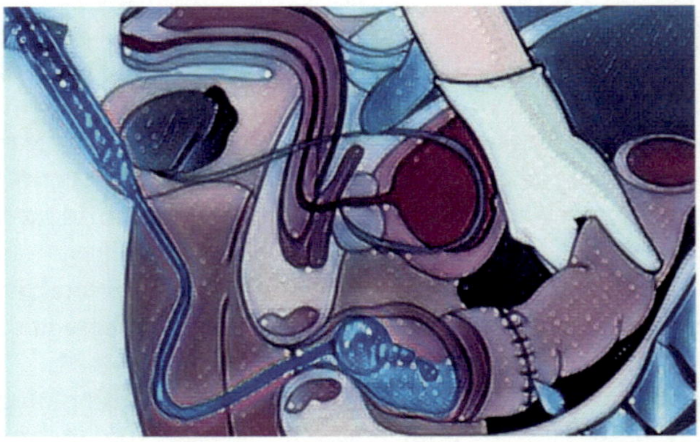

Figure 11.
Methylene blue test.

CI: −0.74, −0.02), and lower postoperative complications were all correlated with the robot-assisted surgery community (OR: 0.79, 95% CI: 0.65, 0.97).

There were no substantial differences between groups in EBL, anastomosis leak rate, or oncological outcomes such as the number of lymph nodes removed, the DRM, or the PCRM (**Figures 10** and **11**).

4.2 Postoperative ileus

Postoperative ileus generates a high impact on morbidity, hospital stay, and costs. Vergara Fernandez and coauthors [12] conducted a randomized controlled trial of 64 patients who had elective colorectal surgery with primary anastomosis in a tertiary referral center. Patients were divided into two groups: (i) those who chewed their gums (n = 32) and (ii) those who had a typical postoperative recovery (n = 32). Chewing gum after colorectal surgery was found to be associated with less postoperative ileus and vomiting, as well as improved flatus passage within the first 48 hours after surgery (**Figure 12**).

4.3 Anastomotic stenosis

It can sometimes be treated endoscopically, when surgery is contraindicated, by performing, as was found in a case report by Deng and team [13] with minimally invasive endoscopic approach was adopted to repair the obstruction. A needle knife was used to puncture the linear white scar, and contrast agent was injected under endoscopy and fluoroscopic guidance. Fluoroscopically, the proximal bowel was identified and a dual knife-mediated membrane puncture was performed. A guide-wire was then passed through the incision into the proximal bowel and progressive pneumatic dilatation was performed successively with a controlled radial expansion balloon dilator until a 1.8-cm-diameter dilation was achieved. After conventional balloon dilatation, the endoscope easily passed through the anastomosis without any patient discomfort. There were no postoperative signs of immediate or delayed complications (**Figure 13**).

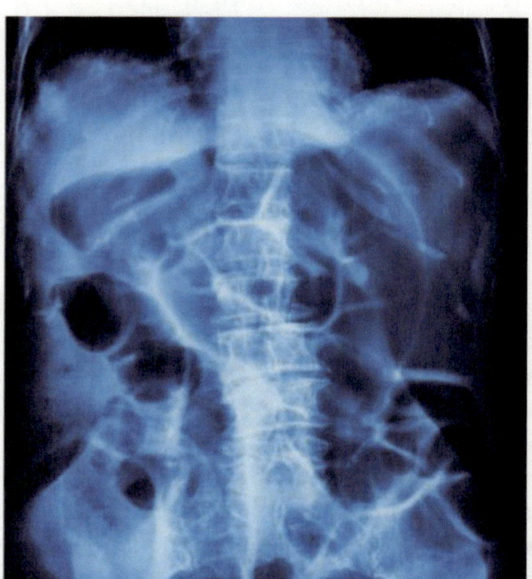

Figure 12.
Illustration of a simple abdominal X-ray exam in a patient with bowel obstruction.

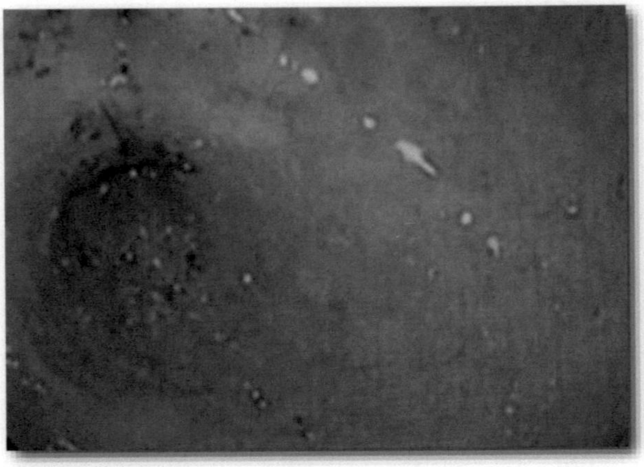

Figure 13.
Colonoscopic aspect of a anastomotic stenosis.

4.4 Anterior resection syndrome

Following TME, postoperative defecation dysfunctions known as "anterior resection syndrome" might appear.

Straight colorectal anastomosis (SCA), colon J-pouch (CJP), and side-to-end anastomosis are all common reconstruction techniques (SEA) (**Figures 14** and **15**).

There are no prospective, randomized, multi-center trials that compare their functional results, including long-term evaluations.

As a result, the primary endpoint of a study designed by Marti and collab [14] that included 336 patients from 15 hospitals who were randomized had a comparison of composite evacuation scores 12 months after TME as a primary endpoint.

Secondary endpoints included a comparison of composite evacuation and incontinence ratings at 6, 18, and 24 months after surgery, as well as morbidity and overall survival.

The study looked at the "per protocol" (PP) population, which complied with all-trial criteria, as well as the "intention-to-treat" (ITT) population.

At any time point, there were no statistically significant variations in the composite evacuation ratings of the PP and ITT populations.

Similarly, at any time point, there was no statistically significant difference in composite incontinence scores for the PP and ITT populations among the three trial weapons.

Conclusions: Within the scope of the investigation, surgeons in charge can continue to conduct intestinal continuity reconstruction following TME at their discretion.

In addition to the studies previously reported, Hou and collab [15] investigated whether the use of side-to-end anastomosis (SEA) in sphincter-preserving resection (SPR) is problematic and conducted a meta-analysis to compare the safety and efficacy of SEA with colonic J-pouch (CJP) anastomosis, which has been shown to improve postoperative bowel function.

The meta-analysis included a total of 864 patients from 10 RCTs.

At 12 months after SPR, patients who underwent SEA had a higher defecation frequency and a lower incidence of incomplete defecation than those who underwent CJP anastomosis with low heterogeneity and a lower incidence of incomplete defecation at 3 months after surgery.

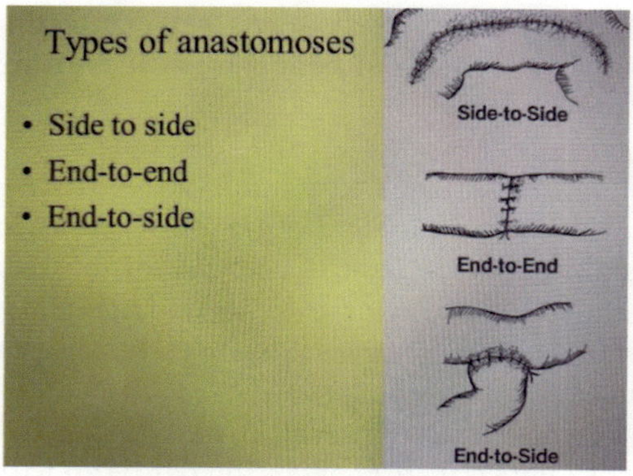

Figure 14.
Types of anastomoses illustrated.

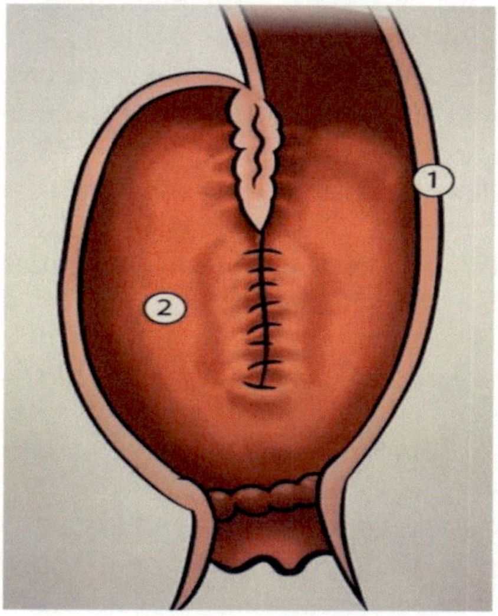

Figure 15.
Aspect of the J-pouch.

The SEA group also had a shorter operating period with no substantial heterogeneity.

The SEA group had a higher anorectal resting strain, but there was a lot of heterogeneity.

There were no significant differences between the groups in terms of efficacy outcomes such as defecation frequency, urgency, incomplete defecation, use of pads, enema, medications, anorectal squeeze pressure, and maximum rectal volume, or safety outcomes such as operating time, blood loss, use of protective stoma, postoperative complications, clinical outcomes, and complication rates.

In comparison with CJP anastomosis, the current evidence indicates that SEA is a successful anastomotic technique for achieving comparable postoperative bowel function without raising the risk of complications.

Shorter operating times, a lower occurrence of incomplete defecation three months after surgery, and improved sphincter function are all advantages of SEA.

However, after SPR, long-term defecation frequency should be closely monitored.

5. Intraoperative factors that interfere with the outcome of the anastomosis: testing methods of blood flow and patency at the level of the colorectal anastomosis

Assessing intraoperative perfusion with indocyanine green (ICG) and near-infrared (NIR) visualization can aid in selecting the degree of intestinal transection and subsequent anastomotic vascular sufficiency, according to the theory.

In a prospective study of nonselected patients undergoing any elective colorectal surgery with anastomosis in three tertiary hospitals over a 3-year span, NIR-ICG was used to look at anastomosis perfusion.

In addition to standard operator visual evaluation alone, a standard procedure was followed to evaluate NIR-ICG perfusion before and after anastomosis construction.

The researchers looked at 540 patients (median age 64 years, 279 men) who had surgery for neoplastic (330) and benign (174) pathology.

A total of 425 operations (853%) were initiated laparoscopically, with a 59% conversion rate.

In total, 220 patients (437%) had high anterior resection or reversal of Hartmann's procedure, and 90 patients (179%) had low anterior resection.

ICG angiography was effective in every patient, with leak rates of 24% (12 of 504) overall, 26% for colorectal anastomoses, and 3% for low anterior resection.

The anastomotic leak rates were lower when NIR-ICG imaging was used than in the participating centers from over 1000 related operations conducted with the same technique but without NIR-ICG technology. As a result, the study's findings were as follows:

Patients undergoing elective colorectal surgery should have their NIR-ICG levels checked on a regular basis.

The use of NIR-ICG can alter intraoperative decisions, potentially lowering anastomotic leak rates.

Kryzauskas conducted a systematic review and meta-analysis of publications, which included a total of 23 studies, with a total of 7115 patients, that were conducted to see whether intraoperative testing of the mechanical integrity and perfusion of the colorectal anastomosis could minimize the risk of AL. Intraoperative checks for the integrity (OR: 0.52, 95% CI: 0.34–0.82, P.001) and perfusion (OR: 0.40, 95% CI: 0.22–0.752, P.001) of the lower gastrointestinal tract anastomoses are linked to a substantially lower AL rate, according to a pooled study. The researchers came to the conclusion that intraoperative monitoring for anastomosis integrity or perfusion both reduced the AL dose. Studies combining these two anastomosis testing methods, especially intraoperative endoscopy and indocyanine green fluorescence angiography, could be very promising for further AL reduction. Since diabetes is a well-established independent factor that results in higher anastomotic leakage rates, the effects of biological sealants on colorectal anastomosis and their potential impact in patients with severe diabetes were studied in depth.

Fibrin sealants have been used to avoid anastomotic dehiscence in both laboratory and clinical trials.

We looked for existing evidence in the field by searching Medline (1966–2016) and Scopus (2004–2016). There is no evidence to support the use of fibrin sealants as a supplement in diabetic patients undergoing colorectal surgery at this time.

Experimental animal models with severe diabetes may be very useful in this area, and more research is required before fibrin sealants are used in a clinical environment.

In a systematic study and meta-analysis, Wu and team [16] analyzed the air leak test conducted intraoperatively.

The intraoperative air leak test (ALT) is a standard intraoperative test used to detect anastomosis that is mechanically inadequate.

The aim of this meta-analysis is to see whether ALT can help reduce postoperative colorectal anastomotic leakage (CAL).

The report included 22 experiments, with the following being the most notable.

According to the data, conducting an ALT using the recorded technique does not substantially reduce the clinical CAL rate, but it is still important due to the increased risk of CAL in ALT(+) cases.

Additional repairs, unfortunately, may not be successful in reducing this risk using current methods.

The findings of this study call for the standardization of ALT methodology and the creation of successful methods for repairing ALT(+) anastomoses.

A meta-analysis of randomized controlled trials on the use of suction drains following rectal surgery was conducted by Guerra and coauthors [17], and after looking at 760 patients from four RCTs that were eligible (RCT comparing drained with undrained anastomoses following rectal surgery), the use of drains showed little benefit in terms of anastomotic leak, pelvic complications, or reintervention.

On the other hand, the drained party had a slightly higher rate of postoperative bowel obstruction.

The researchers concluded that using pelvic drains routinely does not provide a major benefit in preventing postoperative complications following rectal surgery with extraperitoneal anastomosis.

Furthermore, a higher risk of bowel obstruction following surgery should be considered.

Non-surgery-based intraoperative risk factors for anastomotic healing also influence surgical outcome.

After analyzing 117 papers, a review by van Rooijen and team [18] provided an overview of potential modifiable risk factors that could play a role during the operation, and the results (the main outcome measure was the risk of anastomotic leakage and other postoperative complications during colorectal surgery) revealed that diabetes mellitus, hyperglycemia and a high HbA1c, anemia, and data on blood pressure, inotropes/vasopressors, oxygen supplementation, form of analgesia, and goal-directed fluid therapy are all unequivocal.

There was no research that looked into the effect of body core temperature or mean arterial pressure on CAL.

Subjective considerations including the surgeon's own evaluation of local perfusion and the visibility of the operating field have not been studied for incidence in CAL patients.

The findings revealed that in order to enhance colorectal treatment, both surgery-related and non-surgery-related risk factors that can be changed must be established.

In their ongoing attempt to minimize the number of CAL, surgeons and anesthesiologists can collaborate on these issues.

In the Netherlands, a multicenter cohort study is currently being conducted to determine individual intraoperative risk factors for CAL.

6. The anastomosis in an "emergency" setting, scared of a (potential) higher risk or do we still do the same?

In perforated diverticulitis, for example, there has been no consensus in the management, which is why the Shaban and coauthors [19] felt compelled to perform a systematic review and meta-analysis, particularly because many surgeons choose the Hartmann's procedure to avoid the risk of an anastomotic leak.

As a result, we proposed that in certain patients, resection with primary anastomosis is a healthy option.

The study found 1933 abstracts, of which 14 trials (2 RCTs, 4 prospective non-randomized, and 8 retrospective non-randomized) with 765 patients met the inclusion criteria, with 482 in the Hartmann's group and 283 in the primary anastomosis group.

Primary anastomosis had a slightly lower mortality rate (10.6%) than Hartmann's (20.7%) (p = 0.0003).

The rate of morbidity was also lower (41.8 vs. 51.2%) (p = 0.0483).

Primary anastomosis had a risk ratio of 0.92 in favor of mortality (p = 0.0019).

The average rate of anastomotic leak was 5.9%.

Resection and primary anastomosis should be considered as a feasible and secure operative technique in selected patients with perforated diverticulitis, according to the findings of the study.

However, there is a scarcity of high-level data, and further research is needed.

Resection with primary anastomosis (PRA) with or without diverting ileostomy (DI), Hartmann's procedure (HP), laparoscopic lavage (LL), and damage control surgery were among the aspects reviewed in another and more complicated approach to damage control strategy in perforated diverticulitis with generalized peritonitis performed by Sohn and team [20] (DCS).

DCS is divided into two levels.

Limited resection of the diseased colon, oral and aboral closure, lavage, and vacuum-assisted abdominal closure are all options for emergency surgery.

After proper resuscitation, a second look operation is performed: definitive reconstruction with colorectal anastomosis (±DI) or HP.

The inclusion criteria were fulfilled by eight observational studies involving 256 patients.

There was no randomized study available.

Purulent peritonitis affected 67% of the patients, while feculent peritonitis affected 30%. Hinchey stage II diverticulitis was observed in 3% of the patients. The Mannheim peritonitis index (MPI) was greater than 26 in 49% of the cases. In 73% of cases, a colorectal anastomosis was developed during the second surgery. DI was used in 15% of the above group. HP was given to the remaining 27%. The postoperative mortality rate was 9%, and the morbidity rate was 31%. The rate of anastomotic leak was 13%. Without a stoma, 55% of patients were discharged.

Conclusions: DCS is a safe treatment for acute perforated diverticulitis with generalized peritonitis, with a high incidence of colorectal anastomosis and stoma-free hospital discharge in more than half of patients.

7. Long-term surveillance of the anastomosis

Pickhardt [21] compared the accuracy of CT colonography versus optical colonoscopy for neoplastic involvement at the surgical anastomosis 1 year after curative-intent colorectal cancer resection for neoplastic involvement at the surgical anastomosis.

As part of a prospective, multicenter study, 201 patients (mean age 58.6 years; 117 men, 84 women) underwent same-day contrast-enhanced CT colonography and colonoscopy approximately 1 year (mean, 12.1 months; median, 11.9 months) after colorectal cancer resection.

Many of the patients enrolled had no clinical signs of illness and were found to have a low risk of recurrence (stage I–III).

Relevant intraluminal anastomotic pathology tends to be very rare 1 year after colorectal cancer resection in lower-risk cohorts, according to the findings.

Diagnostic contrast-enhanced CT colonography, unlike colonoscopy, successfully measures both the intraluminal and extraluminal dimensions of the anastomosis.

Yang and collab [22] investigated the use of stents as a bridge to surgery in the treatment of acute left-sided obstructive colorectal cancer.

In a meta-analysis of randomized controlled trials, the factor according to which the trials were conducted was taken into account.

The use of self-expanding metallic stents (SEMS) as a bridge to surgery in the treatment of acute left-sided obstructive colorectal cancer has remained contentious.

The following were the outcomes:

We chose 8 RCTs papers with a total of 497 instances.

The stent group had significantly lower directly stoma rates, significantly higher active primary anastomosis rates, and significantly lower post-procedural complication rates.

The stent party, on the other hand, had substantially higher tumor recurrence rates, leading to the following conclusions:

This meta-analysis confirms that SEMS placement can lower the rate of direct stomas and increase the rate of active primary anastomosis; however, it is linked to a higher rate of tumor recurrence.

8. Conclusions

Laparoscopic anterior resection (LAR) is nowadays routine practice in specialized high-volume centers, with equivalent oncological outcomes to open surgery. Anastomotic leakage (AL) remains one of the most threatening complications in colorectal surgery with the incidence of up to 20%. Therefore, recognition of the risk factors of postoperative complications is essential in order to be prevented. Moreover, one must underline the importance of some risk factors such as age, nutrition status of the patient, experience of the surgeon, and many other factors that influence outcome of colorectal surgery. Some risk factors can be modified before the intervention to prevent postoperative complications. Contrary to that, long-term postoperative complications may promote tumor recurrence and decrease survival.

Conflict of interest

The author declares no conflict of interest.

Author details

Sinziana Ionescu[1,2]

1 Bucharest Oncology Institute, Bucharest, Romania

2 Carol Davila University of Medicine and Pharmacy, Bucharest, Romania

*Address all correspondence to: sinzianaionescu30@gmail.com

References

[1] Wiggins T, Majid MS, Markar SR, Loy J, Agrawal S, Koak Y. Benefits of barbed suture utilisation in gastrointestinal anastomosis: A systematic review and meta-analysis. Annals of the Royal College of Surgeons of England. 2020;**102**(2):153-159. DOI: 10.1308/rcsann.2019.0106

[2] Bobkiewicz A, Studniarek A, Krokowicz L, Szmyt K, Borejsza-Wysocki M, Szmeja J, et al. Gastrointestinal tract anastomoses with the biofragmentable anastomosis ring: Is it still a valid technique for bowel anastomosis? Analysis of 203 cases and review of the literature. International Journal of Colorectal Disease. 2017;**32**(1):107-111. DOI: 10.1007/s00384-016-2661-z

[3] Nekliudov NA, Tsarkov PV, Tulina IA. Uni-center, patient-blinded, randomized, 12-month, parallel group, noninferiority study to compare outcomes of 3-row vs 2-row circular staplers for colorectal anastomosis formation after low anterior resection for rectal cancer. Medicine. 2019;**98**(24):e15978. DOI: 10.1097/MD.0000000000015978

[4] Jeong WJ, Choi BJ, Lee SC. Pure natural orifice transluminal endoscopic surgery for rectal cancer: Ta-TME and CME without abdominal assistance. Asian Journal of Surgery. 2019;**42**(2):450-457. DOI: 10.1016/j.asjsur.2018.08.010

[5] Meyer J, Naiken S, Christou N, Liot E, Toso C, Buchs NC, et al. Reducing anastomotic leak in colorectal surgery: The old dogmas and the new challenges. World Journal of Gastroenterology. 2019;**25**(34):5017-5025. DOI: 10.3748/wjg.v25.i34.5017

[6] Gaines S, Shao C, Hyman N, Alverdy JC. Gut microbiome influences on anastomotic leak and recurrence rates following colorectal cancer surgery. The British Journal of Surgery. 2018;**105**(2):e131-e141. DOI: 10.1002/bjs.10760

[7] Clifford RE, Fowler H, Govindarajah N, Vimalachandran D, Sutton PA. Early anastomotic complications in colorectal surgery: A systematic review of techniques for endoscopic salvage. Surgical Endoscopy. 2019;**33**(4):1049-1065. DOI: 10.1007/s00464-019-06670-9

[8] Shalaby M, Emile S, Elfeki H, Sakr A, Wexner SD, Sileri P. Systematic review of endoluminal vacuum-assisted therapy as salvage treatment for rectal anastomotic leakage. BJS Open. 2018;**3**(2):153-160. DOI: 10.1002/bjs5.50124

[9] Yang Y, Wang G, He J, Zhang J, Xi J, Wang F. High tie versus low tie of the inferior mesenteric artery in colorectal cancer: A meta-analysis. International Journal of Surgery. 2018;**52**:20-24. DOI: 10.1016/j.ijsu.2017.12.030

[10] Simianu VV, Basu A, Alfonso-Cristancho R, Thirlby RC, Flaxman AD, Flum DR. Assessing surgeon behavior change after anastomotic leak in colorectal surgery. The Journal of Surgical Research. 2016;**205**(2):378-383. DOI: 10.1016/j.jss.2016.06.075

[11] Wang X, Cao G, Mao W, Lao W, He C. Robot-assisted versus laparoscopic surgery for rectal cancer: A systematic review and meta-analysis. Journal of Cancer Research and Therapeutics. 2020;**16**(5):979-989. DOI: 10.4103/jcrt.JCRT_533_18

[12] Vergara-Fernandez O, Gonzalez-Vargas AP, Castellanos-Juarez JC, Salgado-Nesme N, Sanchez-Garcia RE. Usefulness of gum chewing to decrease postoperative ileus in colorectal surgery

with primary anastomosis: A randomized controlled trial. Revista de Investigación Clínica. 2016;**68**(6):314-318

[13] Deng S, Cao Y, Gu J, Wu K, Li J, Tao K, et al. Endoscopic diagnosis and treatment of complete anastomosis stenosis after colorectal resection without protective ileostomy: Report of two cases and literature review. The Journal of International Medical Research. 2020;**48**(4):300060520914833. DOI: 10.1177/0300060520914833

[14] Marti WR, Curti G, Wehrli H, Grieder F, Graf M, Gloor B, et al. Clinical outcome after rectal replacement with side-to-end, colon-J-pouch, or straight colorectal anastomosis following total mesorectal excision: A Swiss prospective, randomized, multicenter trial (SAKK 40/04). Annals of Surgery. 2019;**269**(5):827-835. DOI: 10.1097/SLA.0000000000003057

[15] Hou S, Wang Q, Zhao S, Liu F, Guo P, Ye Y. Safety and efficacy of side-to-end anastomosis versus colonic J-pouch anastomosis in sphincter-preserving resections: An updated meta-analysis of randomized controlled trials. World Journal of Surgical Oncology. 2021;**19**(1):130. DOI: 10.1186/s12957-021-02243-0

[16] Wu Z, van de Haar RC, Sparreboom CL, Boersema GS, Li Z, Ji J, et al. Is the intraoperative air leak test effective in the prevention of colorectal anastomotic leakage? A systematic review and meta-analysis. International Journal of Colorectal Disease. 2016;**31**(8):1409-1417. DOI: 10.1007/s00384-016-2616-4

[17] Guerra F, Giuliani G, Coletta D, Boni M, Rondelli F, Bianchi PP, et al. A meta-analysis of randomized controlled trials on the use of suction drains following rectal surgery. Digestive Surgery. 2018;**35**(6):482-490. DOI: 10.1159/000485139

[18] van Rooijen SJ, Huisman D, Stuijvenberg M, Stens J, Roumen RMH, Daams F, et al. Intraoperative modifiable risk factors of colorectal anastomotic leakage: Why surgeons and anesthesiologists should act together. International Journal of Surgery. 2016;**36**(Pt A):183-200. DOI: 10.1016/j.ijsu.2016.09.098

[19] Shaban F, Carney K, McGarry K, Holtham S. Perforated diverticulitis: To anastomose or not to anastomose? A systematic review and meta-analysis. International Journal of Surgery. 2018;**58**:11-21. DOI: 10.1016/j.ijsu.2018.08.009

[20] Sohn M, Agha A, Iesalnieks I, Gundling F, Presl J, Hochrein A, et al. Damage control strategy in perforated diverticulitis with generalized peritonitis. BMC Surgery. 2021;**21**(1):135. DOI: 10.1186/s12893-021-01130-5

[21] Pickhardt PJ, Edwards K, Bruining DH, Gollub M, Kupfer S, Lubner SJ, et al. Prospective trial evaluating the surgical anastomosis at one-year colorectal cancer surveillance: CT colonography versus optical colonoscopy and implications for patient care. Diseases of the Colon and Rectum. 2017;**60**(11):1162-1167. DOI: 10.1097/DCR.0000000000000845

[22] Yang P, Lin XF, Lin K, Li W. The role of stents as bridge to surgery for acute left-sided obstructive colorectal cancer: Meta-analysis of randomized controlled trials. Revista de Investigación Clínica. 2018;**70**(6):269-278. DOI: 10.24875/RIC.18002516

Chapter 15

Surgery for Colorectal Cancer in Older People

Alexia Farrugia and John Camilleri-Brennan

Abstract

Life expectancy has been increasing, and an increasing number of older patients are presenting with colorectal cancer. Surgical management of colorectal cancer in these patients poses a unique challenge, requiring a multidisciplinary team approach, as they have more comorbidities and lower functional reserves. An accurate diagnosis, a thorough patient assessment and individualized treatment is crucial in order to achieve the best possible outcome. While the overall postoperative mortality rates were significantly higher in the over 75 age group, it seems that age itself is not a risk factor for surgery. Older patients presented with more locally advanced disease, a factor that increased the overall postoperative mortality. Comorbid conditions increase the risk of postoperative mortality in these patients. When comparing different age groups with similar American Society of Anesthesiologists (ASA) scores, no significant difference was found in postoperative mortality. Laparoscopic surgery was shown to be beneficial for the elderly, with low morbidity and mortality and a shortened hospital stay. Patients with rectal cancer benefit from transanal endoscopic surgery as a primary procedure or as part of a 'watch and wait' strategy following neoadjuvant chemoradiotherapy. Early elective surgery and the avoidance of emergency major surgery whenever possible, by for example the use of stents followed by elective resection in cases of colonic obstruction, will help improve outcomes.

Keywords: surgery, colorectal cancer, rectal cancer, older patients, laparoscopic surgery, endorectal surgery

1. Introduction

Colorectal cancer (CRC) is the third most common cancer worldwide, and the second leading cause of cancer-related deaths. Approximately 1.8 million new cases of CRC and 900,000 colorectal cancer-related deaths were recorded in 2018. The incidence of CRC is increasing worldwide. About 60% of CRC patients are over the age of 70 years at diagnosis, and about 40% are aged over 75 years [1].

The global population is aging. In fact, according to the World Health Organization, 11% of the world's population was over 60 years old in 2006, with an expected rise to 22% by 2050. A majority of these elderly patients are frail and have a number of comorbid illnesses and lower functional reserves, as well as potential psychological and social care issues [2].

Surgical resection is the standard treatment for CRC. The surgical management of these patients is challenging, requiring a multidisciplinary team approach. An accurate diagnosis, a thorough patient assessment and individualized treatment is crucial in order to achieve the best possible outcome.

2. Surgical assessment of the older patient

The number of older people undergoing surgery, both open and laparoscopic, has been increasing over the years. This increase is mainly attributed to improvements in living conditions, longer life expectancy, advances in surgical, and anesthetic techniques, as well as changes in the expectations of both the patient and the clinician. Despite all this, older surgical patients remain at increased risk of developing adverse postoperative outcomes when compared to younger patients.

A thorough assessment of an older patient with colorectal cancer is, therefore, important in order to aid therapeutic decisions [3–8]. Functional levels vary widely. At one end of the spectrum are patients who are robust and able to tolerate surgical and oncological treatment well, while at the other end are patients who are frail and unable to tolerate even minor procedures without the risk of life-threatening complications.

Treatment decisions are clear at either end of this spectrum, but less clear otherwise. Formal assessments are, therefore, necessary to identify those at risk of functional decline and to determine the degree of frailty of these older patients. The results of these assessments may, thus, help in tailoring the treatment to the individual patient. When choosing between various treatment options, the quality of life is at least as important for these patients as the cancer-specific or surgical outcome [9].

A number of factors are taken into account during the assessment of the older patient with colorectal cancer. These include:

1. Estimating life expectancy based on functional evaluation and comorbidities.

2. Estimating the risk of cancer-related morbidity. This is achieved by accurately staging of the tumor, and by assessment of tumor aggressiveness, the risk of recurrence and tumor progression.

3. Evaluation, using the comprehensive geriatric assessment (CGA), of the conditions that could interfere in the treatment of the patient's cancer. The CGA is defined by the British Geriatrics Society as a 'multidimensional interdisciplinary diagnostic process focused on determining a frail older person's medical, psychological and functional capability in order to develop a coordinated and integrated plan for treatment and long-term follow-up.'

4. Assessment of the patient's goals and expectations of treatment. An important aspect of this assessment is quality of life. Quality of life is a multidimensional construct, representing an individual's subjective perception of physical, social, and psychological well-being, as well as satisfaction with the balance between disease control and adverse effects of treatment. There are generic and disease-specific instruments that can be used to measure quality of life. These instruments include SF-36, QLQ-C30, and QLQ-CR38 [9].

Elements of the CGA, especially comorbidity, functional status, frailty, and cognitive dysfunction, are consistently associated with adverse treatment outcomes such as toxicity and mortality.

It is beneficial for all older patients with cancer to receive a complete geriatric assessment. In fact, a meta-analysis by Ellis et al. in 2011 [3] has shown that patients who received a formal CGA in secondary care were more likely to be alive and in their own homes at 12 months follow-up. However, a complete CGA is time-consuming. Studies show that frailty screening methods are useful in the selection of those patients who will benefit from a complete CGA or further assessment. These frailty screening methods include:

1. Timed up and go. This test assesses mobility, balance, walking ability, and risk of falls in older adults. Patients, who require more than 10 seconds to perform the exercise, those who need to use their arms to get up, or those who perform an erroneous trajectory, will need a full CGA [8];

2. Seven-item physical performance. This test 'assesses multiple domains of physical function using observed performance of tasks that simulate activities of daily living of various degrees of difficulty.' This test takes 10 min to perform. If the total result is less than 20, a CGA would be beneficial. It has been demonstrated to be more sensitive than the Karnofsky performance status in recognizing patients with a higher risk of functional decline;

3. Vulnerable elders survey 13 (VES-13) [10]. This is a 'simple function-based tool for screening community-dwelling populations to identify older persons at risk for health deterioration.' Scores that are equal or above three indicate a higher risk of functional deterioration and a four-fold increased probability of death within the next 2 years. A complete CGA is then indicated [11–14]. If the score is less than three, the patient can receive the standard treatment recommended for adult patients according to the tumor stage.

The concept of 'frailty' continues to develop and expand. Criteria used by Fried et al. [15] include an assessment of weight loss, physical exhaustion, physical activity level, grip strength, and speed of walking. Any degree of frailty measured by the Hopkins Frailty Score [16] has been linked to a worse postoperative outcome after surgery for colorectal cancer. Core features of frailty include impairments in multiple and interrelated systems, resulting in a reduced ability to tolerate stressful events. This is associated with an increase in vulnerability to severe complications with cancer treatment, which may then lead to an increase in overall mortality [17, 18].

Wieland and Hirth recommend that the CGA should include the following [19, 20]:

1. Functional status: Evaluation of dependency in daily activities using scales such as Barthel and Lawron, the TITAN scale, and the Karnofsky index. Functional decline in an elderly patient is a predictor of short- and medium-term mortality, independent of the disease process [21];

2. Comorbidity: The Charlson comorbidity index predicts 1-year mortality in patients with coexisting illnesses. Sarcopenia (skeletal muscle depletion) in older patients is related to infection, requirements for rehabilitation following surgery, and length of hospital stay;

3. Socio-economic evaluation: The elderly population is at a greater risk of social deprivation. The social situation of the older patient should, therefore, always be evaluated, and any cases of social isolation identified and dealt with through the social services;

4. Nutritional status: A useful tool is the mini nutritional assessment. Patients who are identified as being undernourished, with a recent loss of more than

5% weight or a body mass index less than 19, should be assessed and managed appropriately in conjunction with the dieticians;

5. Cognitive status: The mini-mental state examination is useful in this regard. The impact of depression and dementia on the treatment of colorectal cancer is not well known, but it has been identified as one of the determinant factors in receiving inadequate treatment;

6. Geriatric syndromes: The presence of geriatric syndromes, such as urinary and fecal incontinence and risk of falls, is an indicator of frailty [22]. A full assessment of the cognitive and emotional state is particularly important in older cancer patients. Polypharmacy, with the risk of drug interactions, is common in these patients;

7. Surgical risk: The American Society of Anesthesiologists (ASA) classification continues to be one of the most reliable predictors of postoperative morbidity and mortality. Multiple studies have shown that the presence of comorbidities increases the risk of postoperative complications, and this is more evident in patients over 70 years of age;

8. An evaluation of the patient's views and expectations on the aims of treatment. The ideal treatment of the older adult patient with cancer starts with a careful delineation of goals through conversation. Studies show that older patients want to be informed about the diagnosis and prognosis of their disease [23, 24].

Multidisciplinary team working involves specialties such as oncologists, surgeons, gastroenterologists, radiotherapists, anesthetists, radiologists, and pathologists. This has become essential in the management of elderly patients with cancer. It is recommended that older patients with colorectal cancer should be treated in hospitals, where the expertise is available to provide the most favorable surgical and oncologic treatment outcomes.

Balducci [25] studied the role of CGA in the selection of treatment for cancer. Patients were placed into three groups depending on the severity of frailty symptoms and signs:

1. Functionally independent patients without any important comorbidities. These patients may be suitable to receive standard cancer-specific treatment such as surgery;

2. Functionally dependent patients with two or less comorbidities. These patients could benefit from a modified cancer-specific treatment such as a less extensive surgical resection, as for example a transanal resection of a rectal cancer instead of an anterior resection;

3. Partially dependent patients with three or more comorbidities or the presence of a geriatric syndrome. Palliative or best supportive care is usually recommended for these patients.

3. Outcome of elective surgery in the older patient

There is no consensus about the optimal surgical management of older people with colorectal cancer, whose fitness varies from very fit to very frail individuals.

This population is undertreated compared with younger patients, with a comparatively lower percentage of patients being operated on. Older cancer patients are recruited less often to clinical trials than younger patients and are therefore under-represented in publications about cancer treatment [26].

Surgical risk stratification remains one of the most important aspects in the management of older patients [27]. Age is associated with an increased mortality following elective colorectal resection, with a mortality of up to 15.6% in patients who are older than 80 years of age. Patients with higher levels of comorbidities are expected to have significantly higher rates of complications, longer hospital stays, and mortality [28].

The American Society of Anaesthetists (ASA) score is the most commonly used parameter to compare comorbidities in younger and older patients. Whereas Vironen et al. [29] and Li et al., [30] concluded that there were multiple interobserver errors in computing the ASA scores, and therefore ASA scores were considered to be of limited in use for surgical patients, other studies concluded otherwise. Significant differences in the ASA scores between the younger and older groups were shown by Symeonidis et al. [31], Khan et al., [32], Marusch et al. [33], and Gurevitch et al. [34].

Symeonidis et al. showed that there was a significant difference in mortality rate for those having an ASA score of two or more when compared to those with a lower ASA score [31]. This paper also correlated an increased postoperative mortality rate to a higher TNM score. On the other hand, Vironen et al. [29] demonstrated that when comparing two groups over and under 75 years of age, but with similar ASA scores, there was no significant difference in postoperative mortality. In this case, the postoperative mortality rate was shown to be low throughout, no matter the ASA score. It seems that there was considerable interobserver inconsistency of classification, making the ASA score too imprecise to use with regards to making a treatment decision.

Schwandner et al. [35] included 298 patients who had undergone laparoscopic or laparoscopic-assisted procedures for colorectal surgery. The morbidity in patients above 70 years of age and that in patients below 70 years of age showed no statistically significant difference. Also, two patients above 70 years of age died versus one patient below that age. They concluded 'if preoperative assessment of comorbid conditions and perioperative care was ensured, laparoscopic procedures were shown to be safe options in the elderly. The outcome of laparoscopic colorectal surgery in patients older than 70 years is similar to that noted in younger patients. Advanced age is no contraindication for laparoscopic colorectal surgery.' Tan et al. [36] studied 727 patients with an age of 70 years and over who underwent laparoscopic and open colorectal cancer surgery. The 30-day mortality was significantly lower in the laparoscopic arm compared to open colectomy (1.3 vs. 4.6%). Laparoscopic colectomy was deemed safe in older patients and not associated with a higher morbidity.

Ong et al. [37] included 90 patients who were 80 years of age or older and who had undergone colorectal cancer surgery. A morbidity of 21% and a 30-day mortality of 1.1% were reported. Basili et al. [38] reported their experience with 248 patients who had undergone colorectal cancer surgery. Patients were divided into four age groups: less than 65 years, 66 to 74 years, 75 to 84 years, and more than 85 years of age. The 30-day mortalities were 0% for under 75 years of age, and 6% and 7%, respectively, for patients with ages from 75 to 84 years and those older than 85 years. However, none of these results was significant.

In a large multicenter prospective observational study in Germany on 16,142 patients who were younger than 80 years of age and 2932 who were 80 years of age or older, Marusch et al. [33] reported an overall morbidity of 35.4% with a significant difference ($p < 0.001$) between patients less than 80 years of age (33.9%) and those more than 80 years of age (43.5%). Significant differences were also found between the morbidity for emergency surgery ($p < 0.001$) and that for elective surgery ($p < 0.001$). The 30-day postoperative mortality rate also differed significantly ($p < 0.001$), 2.1% and 7.2% for those less than 80 years of age and those more than 80 years of age, respectively. Despite these significant results, they concluded that age alone should not be a limitation for surgery.

In a recent retrospective study by Shalaby et al. [39], the outcome of colorectal cancer surgery between two groups of patients was compared. The mean ages were 85 years in group A (range, 80 to 104 years) and 55.3 years in group B (range, 13 to 79 years). Both groups were manually matched for body mass index, ASA score, Charlson Comorbidity Index, and procedure performed. The overall 30-day postoperative mortality rate was 1% of total 200 patients, both of these two patients were in group A. However, this observation had no statistical significance. No intraoperative complications were encountered in either group. The 30-day postoperative morbidity rates in groups A and B were 28 and 26%, respectively. However, these differences between the groups were not statistically significant.

Marusch et al. [33] demonstrated a significant difference ($p < 0.001$) in the postoperative mortality rate between the groups (in this case, cohort 1 was under 65, cohort 2 was 65–79 and cohort 3 was over 80 years old). The differences were significant in both emergency ($p = 0.004$) and elective surgery ($p < 0.001$). The tumor stage differed significantly between the cohorts, which may be a reason for the increased mortality in the older age groups.

Andereggen et al. [40] demonstrated a postoperative mortality rate of 5% and a 67% 5-year survival, with 57% of deaths occurring in this period being unrelated to cancer. This was similar to the 60% 5-year survival shown by Vironen et al. [29]. Hermans et al. [41] demonstrated a mortality rate of 16% in those over 75 years and 5% in those under 75 years ($p < 0.01$), and between the two groups, there were no significant differences in comorbidities except for cardiovascular problems, which were more prevalent in the elderly group ($p < 0.01$, with 49% of all patients in the elderly group and 25% of all patients in the younger group having cardiovascular problems).

Gurevitch et al. [34] also found a significant difference in postoperative mortality between the younger and older groups ($p < 0.01$), though the cutoff age, in this case, was 80. In this study, emergency surgery was also considered, and there was a higher risk of postoperative mortality in the emergency setting ($p < 0.001$). Poor functional status, as well as the ASA score, was assessed in this case and there was a significant difference ($p < 0.05$) of 8% in the under 80 cohort and 32% in the over 80 cohort. Symeonidis et al. [31] showed that more elderly patients presented for emergency surgery when compared to younger patients (29.7 vs. 15.7%), $p < 0.001$). Hermans et al. [41] demonstrated a 22% emergency presentation in the over 75 age group and a 9% emergency presentation in the younger age group ($p < 0.05$) thus concurring with the conclusion of Symeonidis et al.. On the other hand, Khan et al. [32] noted that although 17.9% of the elderly group presented as an emergency when compared to 12.1% of the younger group, the difference was not significant ($p = 0.25$).

Leong et al. [42, 43] demonstrated increased morbidity and mortality rates following emergency surgery in the older colorectal cancer patients. The crude mortality rate was 27.5%. The most common cause of death was pneumonia, causing 38% of deaths. Other causes included sepsis and acute myocardial infarction, each causing 19% of deaths. A high ASA score was associated with a higher mortality ($p = 0.04$), and in this study, 52.5% of patients had an ASA score of III or IV. With regards to postoperative morbidity, 81% of total patients presented with postoperative complications. Pneumonia was once again the commonest complication (38%), followed by wound infection (16% of complications). Renal impairment, prolonged ileus, and fluid overload each caused 14% of total complications. In this study, it was also shown that Duke's staging had no impact on the mortality ($p = 0.48$) or morbidity ($p = 0.51$).

Li et al. [30], using the Score of the Association of Coloproctology of Great Britain and Ireland (ACPGBI), showed that ACPGBI scores showed a higher concordance between predicted probability of postoperative mortality and the actual postoperative outcome than ASA scores. Roscio et al. used the Charlson comorbidity index (CCI) where a score of more than three was associated with twice the mortality rate of those scoring less than three. Mamidanna et al. [44] found that there was a significant difference in the mortality rate between patients younger and older than 75 ($p < 0.01$), and the rate was related to the presence of comorbidities.

With regards to the incidence of local postoperative complications, such as surgical site infections, in the older patient, the overall incidence was similar to a younger age group. In fact, Khan et al. [32] showed that when comparing the incidence of local postoperative complications in elective surgery, there was no difference ($p = 0.39$). However, systemic complications were higher in the older age group ($p < 0.05$), and higher ASA scores, as well as the tumor site, had a predictive effect on postoperative complications. In fact, those with an ASA score of two or higher were 2.9 times more likely to have systemic complications (CI 1.30–6.25). Older patients have the same rate of postoperative complications as younger patients with similar clinical status. Symeonidis et al. [31] demonstrated that while elderly patients demonstrated an increased morbidity ($p = 0.002$), this was dependent on their previous health status as shown by the ASA score and tumor stage.

Vironen et al. [29] studied patients with ASA scores one or two and compared them with patients of ASA score three or four. The overall complication rate was not significantly different between these two groups ($p = 0.07$). They also found no significant difference in the complication rates between those under 75 and those older than 75 ($p = 0.31$) with similar ASA scores. On the other hand, Marusch et al. [33] found significant differences in risk factors between the cohorts (cohort 1 was under 65, cohort 2 was 65–79, and cohort 3 was over 80 years old) ($p < 0.001$) when it came to preoperative risk factors such as cardiovascular or pulmonary conditions, or diabetes mellitus. Intraoperative complication rates did not differ significantly between the cohorts, but they differed in the case of systemic complications. General complications following emergency surgery also differed between age groups ($p = 0.002$). Local postoperative complications, such as anastomotic leaks, wound infection, and postoperative ileus, were significantly different for both emergency ($p = 0.006$) and elective surgery ($p < 0.001$) between the age groups. Gurevitch et al. [34] also found that when considering general postoperative complications there were no significant differences between the age groups, though there were significant differences in the presence of comorbidities and ASA scores between the cohorts (both $p = 0.0001$). However, certain general complications, such as pulmonary, cardiovascular, and urinary tract infections, were more common in the elderly. This was also demonstrated by Hermans et al. [41], who recorded significantly higher rates of wound infections, cases of pneumonia, urinary tract infections, and electrolyte disturbances in the over 75 age group ($p < 0.05$). However, unlike the study conclusions of Gurevitch et al., Hermans et al. demonstrated a significant difference in complications between younger (32%) and older (50%) age groups ($p < 0.01$).

Law et al. [45] found that the complication rate following elective surgery did not differ significantly in older and younger patients (36.8 vs. 30.1%, $p = 0.141$), but the ASA score was related to the morbidity of patients ($p = 0.042$). The concomitant medical diseases were also highly related to the morbidity ($p = 0.033$). Jin et al. [46] also demonstrated a significant differences in ASA scores between patients over and under 75, with 42.7% of the younger age group with a score of 2 or more, and 77.8% of the older age group with an ASA score of 2 or more ($p = 0.01$). They also found a significant difference in the BMI, with younger patients having a higher BMI than older patients $p = 0.035$.

Older patients who are deemed to be clinically and biochemically optimized for surgery may still have poor outcomes. As discussed earlier, the concept of frailty can be used to identify patients who require further investigation before surgery. Patients with a high frailty score had a higher risk of developing major complications. Decreased survival in older (more than 75 years) patients after surgery has mainly been attributed to differences in early mortality [47–49]. The rate of cardiovascular complications increases significantly with age. Pulmonary complications are also twice as common. Postoperative complications are more severe in older patients [50–53]. The occurrence of a complication was associated with a significantly increased risk of mortality at 6 months. Dekker et al. noted that the overall 6-month mortality was four times higher in older patients than in younger patients (14 *vs.* 3.3%; $P < 0.0001$) as was the 1-year mortality rate (20.1 *vs.* 5.1%) [54]. Older patients with colorectal cancer who survived the first postoperative year, however, had the same overall cancer-related survival as younger patients.

These results, therefore, confirm that the emphasis should be on survival and minimizing postoperative complications during the first postoperative year. These aims are achieved by the use of prehabilitation programs. These programs help correct malnutrition and optimize cardiovascular and pulmonary function [55].

4. Outcome of emergency surgery in the older patient

Emergency surgery should be avoided if possible. The presence of obstruction or perforation increases the perioperative mortality rate in older patients. Several studies show the correlation between advanced age, mortality, and emergent surgery. Kurian et al. [56] reported a postoperative 30-day mortality rate of 28% in emergency surgery compared to only 5% in elective surgery. Morse et al. [57] found similar outcomes in patients older than 80 years in open surgery for colonic cancer. Similarly, the results of the study by Louis et al. [58] found a close correlation between advanced age, high ASA grade, and emergency surgery. A study by Zerib et al. found that no patient with an ASA grade of three or more survived an emergency colectomy more than 6 months [59]. Modini et al. [60] reported a six-fold higher 30-day postoperative mortality in older patients more than 80 years of age when compared to younger patients. Basili et al. and McGillicuddy et al. noted that although morbidity and mortality rates in older patients could be similar to that of younger patients in elective surgery, these rates could be up to nine times higher in cases of emergency surgery [38, 61]. Patients over 70 years of age after emergency surgery have been shown to have a higher rate of postoperative myocardial infarction, and this complication is associated with a six-fold increase in postoperative mortality. Other common complications are pulmonary failure, acute renal failure, and sepsis; anastomotic leakage also occurred more frequently in older patients after emergency colorectal surgery and presented a significant association with postoperative mortality [62–64].

A feasible alternative management to emergency surgery for colonic obstruction could be the endoscopic placement of stents, especially in acute left-sided colonic obstruction. These self-expanding metallic stents alleviate obstruction and allow the clinician to optimize the patient's clinical condition. In some cases, subsequent elective surgery may take place. Stents are, however, associated with a risk of colonic perforation and bleeding [65].

5. Outcome after laparoscopic surgery in the older patient

Laparoscopic surgery has been shown to reduce postoperative pain, allowing a decreased use of opioid analgesia, reducing postoperative ileus, and a reduced hospital stay [66]. In addition, laparoscopic surgery is beneficial to the older patient since it is associated with a reduced risk of cardiovascular and pulmonary complications, reduced intraoperative blood loss, and a quicker recovery of gastrointestinal function. For example, Chaudhary et al. demonstrated that elective laparoscopic surgery for colorectal cancer was associated with lower rates of pneumonia and cardiopulmonary complications when compared to open surgery [67]. Pinto et al. compared postoperative complications between groups of older patients, with similar ASA and BMI scores, having open and laparoscopic surgery. The laparotomy group had higher overall complication rates compared to the laparoscopic group (49.1 *vs.* 22.6%, $p = 0.0007$). The main differences were in the postoperative medical complications, with 38.8% of the laparotomy group and 21% of the laparoscopy group having medical complications ($p = 0.01$). Other complications, such as wound infections, anastomotic leaks, and deep vein thrombosis, were not significantly different between the two groups [68]. Stocchi et al. [69] found that the preoperative functional status of older patients following laparoscopic surgery was more frequently maintained at the time of discharge. In a randomized trial including 553 patients, Frasson et al. [66] had similarly concluded that laparoscopy should be the first choice in elderly patients operated on for CRC because it increases the preservation of functional status, allowing a higher rate of independence during the postoperative period and discharge and a faster postoperative recovery. Compared to open surgery, laparoscopic surgery is also beneficial to the older patient due to a lower inflammatory response and lower surgical stress.

6. Enhanced recovery after surgery (ERAS) programs for the older patients

Various studies have confirmed that older patients benefit from enhanced recovery after surgery (ERAS) programs in the same way as younger patients [70]. ERAS programs advocate the avoidance of bowel preparation, the restriction of opiate use, and early mobilization. The advantages of participation in an ERAS program are significant, with benefits noted primarily in the length of stay, readmission rates, and reoperation rates. Although overall complications are higher, there does not seem to be an increased risk of aspiration pneumonia in the older patient following early commencement of oral feeding.

7. Delayed discharge home after surgery for colorectal cancer

Delays in the discharge of older patients from the acute hospital may be attributed to various factors. A study from our institution by Pizzuto et al. noted 'the reasons for delayed discharge of patients were due to social care issues, in particular, due to delays in transfer home because of the lack of a package of care or to a community hospital due to a lack of beds' [71], even when the postoperative recovery of the older patient was uneventful. Pizzuto et al. and others advocate the early involvement of the local geriatric services in order to minimize avoidable acute hospital stays, a situation referred to as 'bed blocking.' Care of the elderly physicians may help by optimizing the medical management and addressing the psychosocial needs of these patients. Well-organized and coordinated hospital and community geriatric services, are therefore necessary to help improve outcomes such as survival and ensure that the older cancer patients recovering from cancer surgery reside in their own homes [72, 73].

Despite the aforementioned risks, some older patients do very well after curative surgery for colorectal cancer, but unfortunately, others will not [74, 75]. It is quite clear from the literature that the risks and benefits of surgery for CRC in the elderly have not been clearly reviewed [74]. There is, therefore, still no agreement on how actively the older patients should be treated and when not to offer them surgery, which could lead to physical disability and a worse quality of life. Over 74% of patients interviewed in a study by Ahmed et al. stated that they would refuse, or be reluctant, to receive treatment leading to severe functional impairment [75]. Therefore, the discussions with older patients and their significant others regarding treatment options should be made with careful consideration of life expectancy, morbidity and mortality, quality of life (physical, social, and psychological aspects), as well as the possibility of never returning home and needing permanent residential care.

8. Rectal cancer surgery in the older patients

The treatment of older patients with rectal cancer differs from that of colonic cancer, so it deserves a special mention. Surgery for rectal cancer takes longer to carry out than surgery for colonic cancer of a similar stage, thus increasing the risk of systemic complications. The risk of local complications after curative restorative surgery for rectal cancer, such as anastomotic leak, and pelvic abscess, is also higher than for colonic surgery. Therefore, in general, a more conservative approach in the treatment of rectal cancer in the older patient is preferred to more radical treatment in order to avoid high rates of postoperative morbidity [76].

The aim of rectal cancer surgery in older patients should be a reduction in local recurrence, as well as improvement in quality of life. Rather than age itself, the frailty of patients and preoperative sphincter function should determine the type of surgery for rectal cancer [77, 78]. Some older patients are keen to avoid a permanent stoma and may accept a higher risk of local recurrence to achieve this. However, sphincter preservation in older patients could result in poor functional results, especially in those with preexisting rectal and sphincter dysfunction. Studies have shown that older patients with the 'anterior resection syndrome' have a very poor quality of life. Patients with a risk of developing these functional bowel problems, following restorative rectal resection, should therefore be identified preoperatively and counseled appropriately on the construction of a stoma [79]. Although stomas are not without their problems, such as herniation and prolapse, a properly constructed stoma can lead to functional independence and enhanced quality of life.

Bhangu et al. [80] analyzed the results of local resection of rectal cancer in older patients, using techniques such as transanal resection of tumor (TART), transanal endoscopic microsurgery (TEMS), and transanal minimally invasive surgery (TAMIS). They showed that, in patients with pT1 tumors, local excision achieved the same results as radical surgery. However, in patients having local resection of pT2 cancers, the survival is less compared to radical surgery in the general population. The difference with the general population is most likely due to the prevalence of comorbidities in the older patient group, with the older patients not being fit for radical surgery or chemoradiotherapy. Transanal endoscopic surgery can, therefore, be considered as suitable palliative treatment option in such patients.

Chemoradiotherapy (CRT) or radiotherapy (RT) alone may be used instead of, or as an adjunct to, surgery for rectal cancer. Studies have shown that older patients with rectal cancer are treated less often with RT [81–83]. Fewer older patients are likely to receive preoperative RT with proportionately more receiving palliative RT instead [84]. Older patients with stage II or III rectal cancer who are fit enough for surgery are generally fit enough for preoperative neoadjuvant RT. Although the tolerability and response rates are similar to those seen in younger patients, Stockholm I and II trial results have shown the distinct side effects of neoadjuvant radiotherapy in older patients. Such side effects, which include deep vein thrombosis, femoral neck and pelvic ring fractures, small bowel obstruction, and fistulas, were significantly more prevalent after preoperative radiotherapy in the older age group [77, 81].

A number of patients who undergo neoadjuvant CRT have a complete pathological response. A complete pathological response means that there is no detectable residual rectal cancer on sigmoidoscopy or MRI. A strategy known as 'watch and wait' was proposed and pioneered by Habr-Gama et al. for these patients in order to spare them unnecessary resection [85]. They published a series of 'watch and wait' in 70 patients with tumor stages of pT2- and pN1-2 who were treated with CRT. Forty-seven patients had a complete clinical response, with 8 (17%) developing an early recurrence and four had a late recurrence. All had subsequent radical R0 surgery and were disease-free 56 months later. This could be an option for patients who are not considered fit for surgery. It does not have to be considered as a palliative treatment as such, but a possible standard treatment with a 50% probability of cure in frail elderly patients [80].

A study by Smith et al. [86] showed that older patients, because of their higher surgical risk, obtained the greatest benefit from the 'watch and wait' policy with an improved survival at 1 year after treatment. More recently, the results of a joint study between Glasgow University and Memorial Sloan Kettering in New York [87] concluded 'a watch and wait strategy for select rectal cancer patients who had a clinical complete response after neoadjuvant therapy resulted in excellent rectal preservation and pelvic tumor control; however, in the watch and wait group, worse survival was noted along with a higher incidence of distant progression in patients with local regrowth vs those without local regrowth.'

The groups of patients that present a significant regression of their rectal cancer with neoadjuvant CRT, and especially those with lymph node regression (ypN0), could be candidates for alternative treatments without needing radical surgery. Transanal endoscopic surgical techniques could be used in these patients [80]. Local excision following CRT is associated with a 15% risk of recurrence. In older patient with comorbidities, such a risk may be an acceptable alternative to radical surgery [87–91].

9. Conclusion

The aim of surgery for colorectal cancer in the older patient is not only to optimize survival but also the improvement of quality of life and keeping postoperative complications to a minimum. Though some significant differences are present in postoperative morbidity and mortality rates between the young and old, chronological age alone should not be the deciding factor for surgery. Physiological rather than chronological age should determine the management of cancer in each individual, with due regard to comorbid illnesses. Therefore, risk stratification based on comorbidities, and biochemical and physiological markers could help to decide whether to perform surgery, what type of surgery, and the timing of surgery. Careful preoperative clinical assessment and prehabilitation programs are required in order to optimize outcomes. Laparoscopic surgical techniques should be employed whenever possible. Patients with rectal cancer benefit from transanal endoscopic surgery as a primary procedure or as part of a 'watch and wait' strategy following neoadjuvant chemoradiotherapy. Early elective surgery and the avoidance of emergency major surgery whenever possible, by for example the use of stenting followed by elective resection in cases of colonic obstruction, will help improve outcomes.

Author note

This chapter has been originally presented with the title "Surgery for colorectal cancer in the elderly: Is it safe"? at the Tripartite Colorectal Meeting of the American Society of Colon & Rectal Surgeons (ASCRS), Association of Coloproctology of Great Britain & Ireland (ACPGBI) and the Colorectal Surgical Society of Australia and New Zealand, in association with the European Society of Coloproctology (ESCP), 30th June to 3rd July 2014, Birmingham, UK.

It was published in abstract form in Colorectal Disease 2014, Vol.16, issue S2.

Author details

Alexia Farrugia[1,2] and John Camilleri-Brennan[1,2*]

1 Sandwell General Hospital, Sandwell and West Birmingham Hospitals NHS Trust, England, UK

2 Forth Valley Royal Hospital, Stirlingshire, Scotland UK and the University of Glasgow, Glasgow, Scotland, UK

*Address all correspondence to: johncbrennan@doctors.org.uk

References

[1] Available from: http://www.ncin.org.uk/cancer_information_tools/ukcis

[2] Schmoll HJ, Van Cutsem E, Stein A, Valentini V, Glimelius B, Haustermans K, et al. ESMO consensus guidelines for management of patients with colon and rectal cancer. A personalized approach to clinical decision making. Annals of Oncology. 2012;**23**:2479-2516

[3] Ellis G, Whitehead MA, O'Neill D, Langhorne P, Robinson D. Comprehensive geriatric assessment for older adults admitted to hospital. Cochrane Database of Systematic Reviews. 6 Jul 2011;(7):CD006211

[4] Extermann M, Hurria A. Comprehensive geriatric assessment for older patients with cancer. Journal of Clinical Oncology. 2007;**25**:1824-1831

[5] Naeim A, Reuben D. Geriatric syndromes and assessment in older cancer patients. Oncology (Williston Park). 2001;**15**:1567-1577, 1580 discussion 1581, 1586, 1591

[6] Ingram SS, Seo PH, Martell RE, Clipp EC, Doyle ME, Montana GS, et al. Comprehensive assessment of the elderly cancer patient: The feasibility of self-report methodology. Journal of Clinical Oncology. 2002;**20**:770-775

[7] Hamaker ME, Jonker JM, de Rooij SE, Vos AG, Smorenburg CH, van Munster BC. Frailty screening methods for predicting outcome of a comprehensive geriatric assessment in elderly patients with cancer: A systematic review. The Lancet Oncology. 2012;**13**:e437-e444

[8] Gill TM, Baker DI, Gottschalk M, Peduzzi PN, Allore H, Byers A. A program to prevent functional decline in physically frail, elderly persons who live at home. The New England Journal of Medicine. 2002;**347**:1068-1074

[9] Camilleri-Brennan J, Steele RJC. Prospective analysis of quality of life and survival following mesorectal excision for rectal cancer. The British Journal of Surgery. 2001;**88**:1617-1622

[10] Rockwood K, Mitnitski A. Frailty defined by deficit accumulation and geriatric medicine defined by frailty. Clinics in Geriatric Medicine. 2011;**27**:17-26

[11] Monfardini S, Gridelli C, Pasetto LM, Soubeyran P, Droz JP, Basso U. Vulnerable and frail elderly: An approach to the management of the main tumour types. European Journal of Cancer. 2008;**44**:488-493

[12] Luciani A, Ascione G, Bertuzzi C, Marussi D, Codecà C, Di Maria G, et al. Detecting disabilities in older patients with cancer: Comparison between comprehensive geriatric assessment and vulnerable elders survey-13. Journal of Clinical Oncology. 2010;**28**:2046-2050

[13] Monfardini A, Basso U, Fiduccia P, Brunello A, Baretta Z, Soldà C. Can the short screening test vulnerable elders survey 13 (VES-13) substitute for the time-consuming comprehensive geriatric assessment (CGA) to identify vulnerable/frail elderly breast cancer patients? Journal of Clinical Oncology. 2010;**28**(suppl. 9114):15s

[14] Monfardini S, Giordano G, Sandri R, Gnocchi PL, Galetti G. Bringing geriatrics into oncology or also oncology into geriatrics? Annals of Oncology. 2012;**23**:801

[15] Fried LP, Tangen CM, Walston J, Newman AB, Hirsch C, Gottdiener J, et al. Frailty in older adults: Evidence for a phenotype. The Journals of Gerontology. Series A, Biological Sciences and Medical Sciences. 2001;**56**:M146-M156

[16] Revenig LM, Canter DJ, Taylor MD, Tai C, Sweeney JF, Sarmiento JM, et al. Too frail for surgery? Initial results of a large multidisciplinary prospective study examining preoperative variables predictive of poor surgical outcomes. Journal of the American College of Surgeons. 2013;**217**:665-670.e1

[17] Balducci L. New paradigms for treating elderly patients with cancer: The comprehensive geriatric assessment and guidelines for supportive care. The Journal of Supportive Oncology. 2003;**1**:30-37

[18] Basso U, Tonti S, Bassi C, Brunello A, Pasetto LM, Scaglione D, et al. Management of Frail and not-Frail elderly cancer patients in a hospital-based geriatric oncology program. Critical Reviews in Oncology/Hematology. 2008;**66**:163-170

[19] Wieland D, Hirth V. Comprehensive geriatric assessment. Cancer Control. 2003;**10**:454-462

[20] Millan M, Merino S, Caro A, Feliu F, Escuder J, Francesch T. Treatment of colorectal cancer in the elderly. World Journal of Gastrointestinal Oncology. 2015;**7**(10):204-220

[21] Monfardini S. What do we know on variables influencing clinical decision-making in elderly cancer patients? European Journal of Cancer. 1996;**32A**:12-14

[22] Darlene Gabea U, Ronnie A. Preoperative evaluation of the elderly surgical patient. In: Rosenthal RA, Zenilman ME, Katlic MR, editors. Principles and Practice of Geriatric Surgery. New York: Springer-Verlag; 2001. pp. 126-143

[23] Kemeny MM, Busch-Devereaux E, Merriam LT, O'Hea BJ. Cancer surgery in the elderly. Hematology/Oncology Clinics of North America. 2000;**14**:169-192

[24] Ajaj A, Singh MP, Abdulla AJ. Should elderly patients be told they have cancer? Questionnaire survey of older people. BMJ. 2001;**323**:1160

[25] Balducci L. Management of cancer in the elderly. Oncology. 2006;**20**:135-143

[26] Townsley CA, Selby R, Siu LL. Systematic review of barriers to the recruitment of older patients with cancer onto clinical trials. Journal of Clinical Oncology. 2005;**23**:3112-3124

[27] Tan KY, Kawamura YJ, Tokomitsu A, Tang T. Assessment for frailty is useful for predicting morbidity in elderly patients undergoing colorectal cancer resection whose comorbidities are already optimized. American Journal of Surgery. 2012;**204**:139-143

[28] Faiz O, Haji A, Bottle A, Clark SK, Darzi AW, Aylin P. Elective colonic surgery for cancer in the elderly: An investigation into postoperative mortality in English NHS hospitals between 1996 and 2007. Colorectal Disease. 2011;**13**:779-785

[29] Vironen JH, Sainio P, Husa AI, Kellokumpu IH. Complications and survival after surgery for rectal cancer in patients younger than and aged 75 years or older. Diseases of the Colon and Rectum. 2004;**47**:1225-1231

[30] Li WH, Lau T, Wong KK, Chan A, Cheung MT. Colorectal cancer surgery of octogenarians in Hong Kong: Who will survive? Hong Kong Medical Journal. 2011;**17**:358-364

[31] Symeonidis D, Christodoulidis G, Koukoulis G, Spryidakis M, Tepetes K. Colorectal cancer surgery in the elderly: Limitations and drawbacks. Techniques in Coloproctology. 2011;**15**(Suppl. 1):S47-S50

[32] Khan MR, Bari H, Zafar SN, Raza SA. Impact of age on outcome after

colorectal cancer surgery in the elderly – A developing country perspective. BMC Surgery. 2011;**11**:17

[33] Marusch F, Koch A, Schmidt U, Zippel R, Gastmeier J, Pross M, et al. Impact of age on the short-term postoperative outcome of patients undergoing surgery for colorectal carcinoma. International Journal of Colorectal Disease. 2002;**17**:177-184

[34] Gurevitch AJ, Davidovitsh B, Kashtan H. Outcome of right colectomy for cancer in octogenarians. Journal of Gastrointestinal Surgery. 2009;**13**: 100-104

[35] Schwandner O, Schiedeck THK, Bruch HP. Advanced age—Indication or contraindication for laparoscopic colorectal surgery? Diseases of the Colon and Rectum. 1999;**42**:356-362

[36] Tan WS, Chew MH, Lim IA, Ng KH, Tang CL, Eu KW. Evaluation of laparoscopic versus open colorectal surgery in elderly patients more than 70 years old: An evaluation of 727 patients. International Journal of Colorectal Disease. 2012;**27**:773-780

[37] Ong ES, Alassas M, Dunn KB, Rajput A. Colorectal cancer surgery in the elderly: Acceptable morbidity? American Journal of Surgery. 2008;**195**:344-348

[38] Basili G, Lorenzetti L, Biondi G, Preziuso E, Angrisano C, Carnesecchi P, et al. Colorectal cancer in the elderly. Is there a role for safe and curative surgery? ANZ Journal of Surgery. 2008;**78**:466-470

[39] Shalaby M, Di Lorenzo N, Franceschilli L, Perrone F, Angelucci GP, Quareisma S, et al. Outcome of colorectal surgery in elderly populations. Annals of Coloproctology. 2016;**32**:139-143

[40] Anderegenn E, Ris F, Gervaz P, Bucher P, Morel P. Outcome of surgery for rectal cancer in octogenarians. Swiss Medical Weekly. 2006;**136**:185-188

[41] Hermans E, van Shaik PM, Prins HA, Ernst MF, Dautzenberg PJL, Bosscha K. Outcome of colonic surgery in elderly patients with colon cancer. Journal of Oncology. 2010;**2010**:865908

[42] Leong QM, Aung MO, Ho CK, Sim R. Emergency colorectal resections in Asian octogenarians: Factors impacting surgical outcome. Surgery Today. 2009;**39**:575-579

[43] Roscio F, Bertoglio C, De Luca A, Frigerio A, Galli F, Scandroglio I. Outcomes of laparoscopic surgery for colorectal cancer in elderly patients. Journal of the Society of Laparoendoscopic Surgeons. 2011;**5**:315-321

[44] Mamidanna R, Eid-Arimoku L, Almoudarin AM, Burns EM, Bottle A, Aylin P, et al. Poor 1-year survival in elderly patients undergoing nonelective colorectal resection. Diseases of the Colon and Rectum. 2012;**55**:788-796

[45] Law WL, Choi HK, Ho JW, Lee YM, Seto CL. Outcomes of surgery for mid and distal rectal cancer in the elderly. World Journal of Surgery. 2006;**30**:598-604

[46] Jin L, Inoue N, Sato N, Matsumoto S, Kanno H, Hashimoto Y, et al. Comparison between surgical outcomes of colorectal cancer in younger and elderly patients. World Journal of Gastroenterology. 2011;**17**(12):1642-1648

[47] Mäkelä JT, Kiviniemi H, Laitinen S. Survival after operations for colorectal cancer in patients aged 75 years or over. The European Journal of Surgery. 2000;**166**:473-479

[48] Hill AL, Russell MM. The special needs of elderly patients. Seminars in Colon and Rectal Surgery. 2013;**24**: 200-208

[49] Bouassida M, Charrada H, Chtourou MF, Hamzaoui L, Mighri MM, Sassi S, Azzouz MM, Touinsi H. Surgery for colorectal cancer in elderly patients: How could we improve early outcomes? Journal of Clinical and Diagnostic Research. 2015;**9**:4-8

[50] Sanoff HK, Bleiberg H, Goldberg RM. Managing older patients with colorectal cancer. Journal of Clinical Oncology. 2007;**25**:1891-1897

[51] Doat S, Thiébaut A, Samson S, Ricordeau P, Guillemot D, Mitry E. Elderly patients with colorectal cancer: Treatment modalities and survival in France. National data from the ThInDiT cohort study. European Journal of Cancer. 2014;**50**:1276-1283

[52] Bergman H, Ferrucci L, Guralnik J, Hogan DB, Hummel S, Karunananthan S, et al. Frailty: An emerging research and clinical paradigm--issues and controversies. The Journals of Gerontology. Series A, Biological Sciences and Medical Sciences. 2007;**62**:731-737

[53] Scandrett KG, Zuckerbraun BS, Peitzman AB. Operative risk stratification in the older adult. The Surgical Clinics of North America. 2015;**95**:149-172

[54] Dekker JW, Gooiker GA, Bastiaannet E, van den Broek CB, van der Geest LG, van de Velde CJ, et al. Cause of death the first year after curative colorectal cancer surgery; a prolonged impact of the surgery in elderly colorectal cancer patients. European Journal of Surgical Oncology. 2014;**40**:1481-1487

[55] Ugolini G, Ghignone F, Zattoni D, Veronese G, Montroni I. Personalized surgical management of colorectal cancer in elderly population. World Journal of Gastroenterology. 2014;**20**:3762-3777

[56] Kurian A, Suryadevara S, Ramaraju D, Gallagher S, Hofmann M, Kim S, et al. In-hospital and 6-month mortality rates after open elective vs open emergent colectomy in patients older than 80 years. Diseases of the Colon and Rectum. 2011;**54**:467-471

[57] Morse BC, Cobb WS, Valentine JD, Cass AL, Roettger RH. Emergent and elective colon surgery in the extreme elderly: Do the results warrant the operation? The American Surgeon. 2008;**74**:614-618 discussion 618-619

[58] Louis DJ, Hsu A, Brand MI, Saclarides TJ. Morbidity and mortality in octogenarians and older undergoing major intestinal surgery. Diseases of the Colon and Rectum. 2009;**52**:59-63

[59] Zerbib P, Kulick JF, Lebuffe G, Khoury-Helou A, Plenier I, Chambon JP. Emergency major abdominal surgery in patients over 85 years of age. World Journal of Surgery. 2005;**29**:820-825

[60] Modini C, Romagnoli F, De Milito R, Romeo V, Petroni R, La Torre F, et al. Octogenarians: An increasing challenge for acute care and colorectal surgeons. An outcomes analysis of emergency colorectal surgery in the elderly. Colorectal Disease. 2012;**14**:e312-e318

[61] McGillicuddy EA, Schuster KM, Davis KA, Longo WE. Factors predicting morbidity and mortality in emergency colorectal procedures in elderly patients. Archives of Surgery. 2009;**144**:1157-1162

[62] Chiappa A, Zbar AP, Bertani E, Biella F, Audisio RA, Staudacher C. Surgical outcomes for colorectal cancer patients including the elderly. Hepato-Gastroenterology. 2001;**48**(38):440-444

[63] Moghadamyeghaneh Z, Mills SD, Carmichael JC, Pigazzi A, Stamos MJ. Risk factors of postoperative myocardial infarction after colorectal surgeries. The American Surgeon. 2015;**81**:358-364

[64] Bakker IS, Grossmann I, Henneman D, Havenga K, Wiggers T. Risk factors for anastomotic leakage and leak-related mortality after colonic cancer surgery in a nationwide audit. The British Journal of Surgery. 2014;**101**:424-432 discussion 432

[65] Guo MG, Feng Y, Zheng Q, Di JZ, Wang Y, Fan YB, et al. Comparison of self-expanding metal stents and urgent surgery for left-sided malignant colonic obstruction in elderly patients. Digestive Diseases and Sciences. 2011;**56**:2706-2710

[66] Frasson M, Braga M, Vignali A, Zuliani W, Di Carlo V. Benefits of laparoscopic colorectal resection are more pronounced in elderly patients. Diseases of the Colon and Rectum. 2008;**51**:296-300

[67] Chaudhary BN, Shabbir J, Griffith JP, Parvaiz A, Greenslade GL, Dixon AR. Short-term outcome following elective laparoscopic colorectal cancer resection in octogenarians and nonagenarians. Colorectal Disease. 2012;**14**(6):727-730

[68] Pinto RA, Ruiz D, Edden Y, Weiss EG, Nougeras JJ, Wexner SD. How reliable is laparoscopic colorectal surgery compared with laparotomy for octogenarians? Surgical Endoscopy. 2011;**25**:2692-2698

[69] Stocchi L, Nelson H, Young-Fadok TM, Larson DR, Ilstrup DM. Safety and advantages of laparoscopic vs. open colectomy in the elderly: Matched-control study. Diseases of the Colon and Rectum. 2000;**43**:326-332

[70] Bagnall NM, Malietzis G, Kennedy RH, Athanasiou T, Faiz O, Darzi A. A systematic review of enhanced recovery care after colorectal surgery in elderly patients. Colorectal Disease. 2014;**16**:947-956

[71] Pizzuto M, Buhagiar GJ, Camilleri-Brennan J. A prospective analysis of inappropriate delays to surgical patient discharge in a teaching general hospital. International Journal of Surgery. 2018;**55**:S72

[72] Dhesi J. Improving outcomes in older people undergoing elective surgery. The Journal of the Royal College of Physicians of Edinburgh. 2010;**40**:348-353

[73] Tan KY, Tan P, Tan L. A collaborative transdisciplinary "geriatric surgery service" ensures consistent successful outcomes in elderly colorectal surgery patients. World Journal of Surgery. 2011;**35**:1608-1614

[74] Neuman HB, O'Connor ES, Weiss J, Loconte NK, Greenblatt DY, Greenberg CC, et al. Surgical treatment of colon cancer in patients aged 80 years and older: Analysis of 31,574 patients in the SEER-Medicare database. Cancer. 2013;**119**:639-647

[75] Ahmed S, Howel D, Debrah S. The influence of age on the outcome of treatment of elderly patients with colorectal cancer. Journal of Geriatric Oncology. 2014;**5**:133-140

[76] Manceau G, Karoui M, Werner A, Mortensen NJ, Hannoun L. Comparative outcomes of rectal cancer surgery between elderly and non-elderly patients: A systematic review. The Lancet Oncology. 2012;**13**:e525-e536

[77] De Caluwé L, Van Nieuwenhove Y, Ceelen WP. Preoperative chemoradiation versus radiation alone for stage II and III resectable rectal cancer. Cochrane Database of Systematic Reviews. 2013;**2**:CD006041

[78] Serra-Rexach JA, Jimenez AB, García-Alhambra MA, Pla R, Vidán M, Rodríguez P, et al. Differences in the therapeutic approach to colorectal cancer in young and elderly patients. The Oncologist. 2012;**17**:1277-1285

[79] Camilleri-Brennan J, Steele RJC. Quality of life after treatment for rectal cancer. British Journal of Surgery. 1998;**85**(8):1036-1043

[80] Bhangu A, Kiran RP, Audisio R, Tekkis P. Survival outcome of operated and non-operated elderly patients with rectal cancer: A surveillance, epidemiology, and end results analysis. European Journal of Surgical Oncology. 2014;**40**:1510-1516

[81] Jung B, Pahlman L, Johannson R, Nilsson E. Rectal cancer treatment and outcome in the elderly: An audit based on the Swedish rectal cancer registry 1995-2004. BMC Cancer. 2009;**9**:68

[82] Ayanian JZ, Zaslavsky AM, Fuchs CS, Guadagnoli E. Use of adjuvant chemotherapy and radiation therapy for colorectal cancer in a population-based cohort. Journal of Clinical Oncology. 2003;**21**:1293-1300

[83] Chang GJ, Skibber JM, Feig BW. Are we undertreating rectal cancer in the elderly? An epidemiologic study. AnnSurg. 2007;**246**:215-221

[84] Martijn H, Vulto JC. Should radiotherapy be avoided or delivered differently in elderly patients with rectal cancer? European Journal of Cancer. 2007;**43**:2301-2306

[85] Habr-Gama A, Perez RO, Nadalin W, Sabbaga J, Ribeiro U, Silva e Sousa AH, et al. Operative versus nonoperative treatment for stage 0 distal rectal cancer following chemoradiation therapy: Long-term results. Annals of Surgery. 2004;**240**:711-717 discussion 717-718

[86] Smith FM, Rao C, Oliva Perez R, Bujko K, Athanasiou T, Habr-Gama A, et al. Avoiding radical surgery improves early survival in elderly patients with rectal cancer, demonstrating complete clinical response after neoadjuvant therapy: Results of a decision-analytic model. Diseases of the Colon and Rectum. 2015;**58**:159-171

[87] Smith JJ, Strombom P, Chow OS, Roxburgh C, et al. Assessment of a watch-and-wait strategy for rectal cancer in patients with a complete response after neoadjuvant therapy. JAMA Oncology. 2019;**5**(4):e185896

[88] Engelen SM, Beets-Tan RG, Lahaye MJ, Lammering G, Jansen RL, van Dam RM, et al. MRI after chemoradiotherapy of rectal cancer: A useful tool to select patients for local excision. Diseases of the Colon and Rectum. 2010;**53**:979-986

[89] Perez RO, Habr-Gama A, Lynn PB, São Julião GP, Bianchi R, Proscurshim I, et al. Transanal endoscopic microsurgery for residual rectal cancer (ypT0-2) following neoadjuvant chemoradiation therapy: Another word of caution. Diseases of the Colon and Rectum. 2013;**56**:6-13

[90] Kim CJ, Yeatman TJ, Coppola D, Trotti A, Williams B, Barthel JS, et al. Local excision of T2 and T3 rectal cancers after downstaging chemoradiation. Annals of Surgery. 2001;**234**:352-358 discussion 358-359

[91] Garcia-Aguilar J. Transanal endoscopic microsurgery following neoadjuvant chemoradiation therapy in rectal cancer: A word of caution about patient selection? Diseases of the Colon and Rectum. 2013;**56**:1-3